ABSITE SLAYER

Dan J. Becha

NOTICE

Medicine is an ever-changing science. As new research and clinical experience broaden our knowledge, changes in treatment and drug therapy are required. The authors and the publisher of this work have checked with sources believed to be reliable in their efforts to provide information that is complete and generally in accord with the standards accepted at the time of publication. However, in view of the possibility of human error or changes in medical sciences, neither the authors nor the publisher nor any other party who has been involved in the preparation or publication of this work warrants that the information contained herein is in every respect accurate or complete, and they disclaim all responsibility for any errors or omissions or for the results obtained from use of the information contained in this work. Readers are encouraged to confirm the information contained herein with other sources. For example and in particular, readers are advised to check the product information sheet included in the package of each drug they plan to administer to be certain that the information contained in this work is accurate and that changes have not been made in the recommended dose or in the contraindications for administration. This recommendation is of particular importance in connection with new or infrequently used drugs.

ABSITE SLAYER

EDITORS

Dale A. Dangleben, MD, FACS
Associate Program Director
Clerkship Director
Department of Surgery
Lehigh Valley Health Network
Allentown, Pennsylvania

James Lee, MD
PGY5
Department of Surgery
Lehigh Valley Health Network
Allentown, Pennsylvania

Firas Madbak, MD
PGY5
Department of Surgery
Lehigh Valley Health Network
Allentown, Pennsylvania

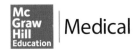

New York   Chicago   San Francisco   Lisbon   London   Madrid   Mexico City
Milan   New Delhi   San Juan   Seoul   Singapore   Sydney   Toronto

ABSITE Slayer

1 2 3 4 5 6 7 8 9 0 CTP/CTP 18 17 16 15 14 13

ISBN 978-0-07-180416-5
MHID 0-07-180416-1

This book was set in Minion Pro by Thomson Digital.
The editors were Brian Belval and Robert Pancotti.
The production supervisor was Sherri Souffrance.
Project management was provided by Asheesh Ratra, Thomson Digital.
The text designer was Alan Barnett; the cover designer was Anthony Landi.
China Translation & Printing Services, Ltd. was printer and binder.

Library of Congress Cataloging-in-Publication Data

ABSITE slayer / editors, Dale A. Dangleben, James Lee, Firas Madbak.
  p. ; cm.
  ISBN 978-0-07-180416-5 (book : alk. paper)
  ISBN 0-07-180416-1 (book : alk. paper)
  ISBN 978-0-07-180417-2 (ebook)
  ISBN 0-07-180417-X (ebook)
  I. Dangleben, Dale A. II. Lee, James, 1979- III. Madbak, Firas.
  [DNLM: 1. Surgical Procedures, Operative—Examination Questions. WO 18.2]
6170076—dc23
                                        2012045904

I would like to thank my wife and children
for their continued support and patience through this project.
I would also like to thank my residents for their role in completing the book.

Dale A. Dangleben, MD, FACS

CONTENTS

Contributors ix

Introduction: General Test-Taking Tips xiii
Dale A. Dangleben, James Lee,
Firas Madbak, and Courtney Edwards

1 Cell Biology 1
Peter Bechtel

2 Hematology 11
Christine Du

3 Transplant and Immunology 23
Arjumand Ali

4 Infection and Antibiotics 37
Dale A. Dangleben, James Lee, and
Firas Madbak

5 Pharmacology......................................47
Peter Bechtel

6 Anesthesia.......................................55
Patty T. Liu

7 Fluids/Electrolytes/Nutrition...........................63
Firas Madbak

8 Surgical Oncology 81
Ryan Lawless

9 Wound Healing...95
Ramon Garza III

10 Head and Neck.....................................103
Jonathan M. Lee and Margaret M. Moore

11 Breast 113
Christine Du and Daniel Barnas

12 Endocrine 131
Danielle Press and Patty T. Liu

13 Abdominal Wall and Hernias.......................155
Dale A. Dangleben and James Lee

14 Stomach 173
Rona Altaras and Dale A. Dangleben

15 Hepatobiliary......................................189
Firas Madbak

16 Pancreas 203
Firas Madbak

17 Spleen...215
Ryan Lawless

18 Esophagus 225
Timothy Misselbeck and James Lee

19 Small Intestine.................................245
James Lee and Dale A. Dangleben

20 Colorectal 265
Carlos Glanville, Anton Kelly,
and Dale A. Dangleben

21 Trauma...281
Dale A. Dangleben, Rovinder Sandhu,
and Firas Madbak

22 Critical Care 309
Dale A. Dangleben, Firas Madbak,
and Jayme Lieberman

23 Burns..325
Karin McConville

24 Vascular 335
Samuel N. Steerman and Jason Davis

25 Pediatrics 355
Doug Lehman, Jarom Gilstrap,
and Anthony Georges

26 Plastic and Reconstructive Surgery 379
Ramon Garza III

27 Thoracic Surgery 389
Timothy Misselbeck

28 Orthopedics.....................................409
Joshua Gish and Scott Sexton

29 Neurosurgery...................................421
Joshua Gish

30 Obstetrics and Gynecology 429
Leon Plowright and
Christine Chen

31 Statistics...441
Lung Ching Lee and
Dale A. Dangleben

32 Ethics and Professionalism 449
Robert D. Barraco and
Stephen E. Lammers

Index 455

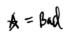

☆ = Bad

CONTRIBUTORS

Arjumand Ali, MD
General Surgeon
Department of Surgery
Lehigh Valley Health Network
Allentown, Pennsylvania
Chapter 3—Transplant and Immunology

Rona Altaras, MD, FACS
Trauma Critical Care Fellow
Department of Surgery
Lehigh Valley Health Network
Allentown, Pennsylvania
Chapter 14 — Stomach

Daniel Barnas, MD
Breast Surgeon
Department of Surgery
Lehigh Valley Health Network
Allentown, Pennsylvania
Chapter 11 — Breast

Robert D. Barraco, MD, MPH, FACS, FCCP
Chief, Sections of Geriatric Trauma
    and Trauma Outreach
Chair, Institutional Ethics Committee
Lehigh Valley Health Network
Department of Surgery
Lehigh Valley Health Network
Allentown, Pennsylvania
Chapter 32 — Ethics and Professionalism

Peter Bechtel, MD
PGY4
Department of Surgery
Lehigh Valley Health Network
Allentown, Pennsylvania
Chapter 1 — Cell Biology
Chapter 5 — Pharmacology

Christine Chen, MD
The Permanente Medical Group
Department of Obstetrics & Gynecology
Daly City, California
Chapter 30 — Obstetrics and Gynecology

Lung Ching Lee, MD
PGY2
Department of Surgery
Lehigh Valley Health Network
Allentown, Pennsylvania
Chapter 31 — Statistics

Dale A. Dangleben, MD, FACS
Associate Program Director
Clerkship Director
Department of Surgery
Lehigh Valley Health Network
Allentown, Pennsylvania
Chapter 4 — Infection and Antibiotics
Chapter 13 — Abdominal Wall and Hernias
Chapter 14 — Stomach
Chapter 19 — Small Intestine
Chapter 20 — Colorectal
Chapter 21 — Trauma
Chapter 22 — Critical Care
Chapter 31 — Statistics

Jason Davis, MD
PGY4
Department of Surgery
Lehigh Valley Health Network
Allentown, Pennsylvania
Chapter 24 — Vascular

Christine Du, MD
PGY4
Department of Surgery
Lehigh Valley Health Network
Allentown, Pennsylvania
Chapter 2 — Hematology
Chapter 11 — Breast

Courtney Edwards, MD
PGY3
Lehigh Valley Health Network
Allentown, Pennsylvania
Introduction: General Test-Taking Tips

Ramon Garza III, MD
PGY3, Plastic Surgery
Department of Surgery
Lehigh Valley Health Network
Allentown, Pennsylvania
Chapter 9 — Wound Healing
Chapter 26 — Plastic and Reconstructive Surgery

Anthony Georges, MD
Pediatric Surgeon
Department of Surgery
Lehigh Valley Health Network
Allentown, Pennsylvania
Chapter 25 — Pediatrics

Jarom Gilstrap, MD
PGY 2, Plastic Surgery
Department of Surgery
Lehigh Valley Health Network
Allentown, Pennsylvania
Chapter 25 — Pediatrics

Joshua Gish, MD
PGY3
Department of Surgery
Lehigh Valley Health Network
Allentown, Pennsylvania
Chapter 28 — Orthopedics
Chapter 29 — Neurosurgery

Carlos Glanville, MD
Colorectal Fellow
Orlando Health
Orlando, Florida
Chapter 20 — Colorectal

Anton Kelly, MD
PGY3
Department of Surgery
Easton Hospital
Easton, Pennsylvania
Chapter 20 — Colorectal

Stephen E. Lammers, PhD
Helen H.P. Manson Professor of the English Bible
    Emeritus, Lafayette College
Ethics Program Consultant
Lehigh Valley Health Network
Allentown, Pennsylvania
Chapter 32 — Ethics and Professionalism

Ryan Lawless, MD
PGY4
Department of Surgery
Lehigh Valley Health Network
Allentown, Pennsylvania
Chapter 8 — Surgical Oncology
Chapter 17 — Spleen

James Lee, MD
PGY5
Department of Surgery
Lehigh Valley Health Network
Allentown, Pennsylvania
Chapter 4 — Infection and Antibiotics
Chapter 13 — Abdominal Wall and Hernias
Chapter 18 — Esophagus
Chapter 19 — Small Intestine

Jonathan M. Lee, MD
PGY5, Otorhinolaryngology
University of Pennsylvania Health System
Philadelphia, Pennsylvania
Chapter 10 — Head and Neck

Doug Lehman, MD
PGY5
Department of Surgery
Lehigh Valley Health Network
Allentown, Pennsylvania
Chapter 25 — Pediatrics

Jayme Lieberman
Trauma/Critical Care
Department of Surgery
Lehigh Valley Health Network
Allentown, Pennsylvania
Chapter 22 — Critical Care

Patty T. Liu, MD
PGY4
Department of Surgery
Lehigh Valley Health Network
Allentown, Pennsylvania
Chapter 6 — Anesthesia
Chapter 12 — Endocrine

Firas Madbak, MD
PGY5
Department of Surgery
Lehigh Valley Health Network
Allentown, Pennsylvania
Chapter 4 — Infection and Antibiotics
Chapter 7 — Fluids/Electrolytes/Nutrition
Chapter 15 — Hepatobiliary
Chapter 16 — Pancreas
Chapter 21 — Trauma
Chapter 22 — Critical Care

Karin McConville, MD
PGY5
Department of Surgery
Lehigh Valley Health Network
Allentown, Pennsylvania
Chapter 23 — Burns

Timothy Misselbeck, MD
Cardiothoracic Surgeon
Department of Surgery
Lehigh Valley Health Network
Allentown, Pennsylvania
Chapter 18 — Esophagus
Chapter 27 — Thoracic Surgery

Margaret M. Moore, MD
PGY3
Department of Surgery
Lehigh Valley Health Network
Allentown, Pennsylvania
Chapter 10 — Head and Neck

Leon Plowright, MD
Urogynecology Fellow
Cleveland Clinic Florida
Weston, Florida
Chapter 30 — Obstetrics and Gynecology

Danielle Press, MD
PGY 5
Department of Surgery
Lehigh Valley Health Network
Allentown, Pennsylvania
Chapter 12 — Endocrine

Rovinder Sandhu, MD, FACS
Trauma/Critical Care
Department of Surgery
Lehigh Valley Health Network
Allentown, Pennsylvania
Chapter 21 — Trauma

Scott Sexton, MD
Assistant Chief
Division of Orthopaedics
Department of Surgery
Lehigh Valley Health Network
Allentown, Pennsylvania
Chapter 28 — Orthopedics

Samuel N. Steerman, MD
Vascular Surgery Fellow
Eastern Virginia Medical School
Norfolk, Virginia
Chapter 24 — Vascular

INTRODUCTION: GENERAL TEST-TAKING TIPS

1. The night before the test should not be devoted to an "all-nighter" or intense review. Read a few things to ease your conscience but spend time having a good meal and, more importantly, getting a good night's sleep.

2. Beware of the urge to change answers. Statistically, your first answer is correct more often than a changed answer.

3. If you know an answer is correct but can't remember why, the reason may not matter. For the sake of the test—so you don't get too hung up on one single question—just answer the question and move on.

4. Don't get bogged down by wordy or long questions. Often the last sentence or two tells the primary question being asked.

5. The best prep for the ABSITE is RESIDENCY and a small amount of daily formal study. Always do what you do in real life: stabilize patients before the OR, never send an unstable patient to the CT scanner, and always remember to differentiate sick patients from non-sick patients.

6. "Get to two": these exams are usually about narrowing the answers to two likely choices. Then go back to look for the clues to sort out these final options.

7. Study hard in order to treat your patients in the best way possible, not to take an exam.

8. As noted in tip #1, it is a bad idea to try to study the night before an ABSITE exam. This can lead to finding information that you have not totally mastered and may affect your confidence for the exam. If you are going to review a topic, choose a topic in which you are well versed to boost your confidence for the exam.

9. Layer your clothing for the exam. You never know what the room temperature will be like.

10. Eat breakfast but avoid eating heavy foods. Bring snacks to the test.

11. Questions are generally "fluff free." There is little fluff in the questions. If they wanted you to know more, they would have told you! The absence of clues toward a particular decision is a clue that you should NOT be moving in that direction.

12. It is unwise to devote excessive time and energy to a difficult question. Mark difficult questions and return to them after you have gone through the entire test.

13. Consider bringing Tylenol and Ibuprofen for muscle aches or headaches.

14. Remember to underline key words.

15. The test writers love the "thoughtless trap." For example, they will give you a patient with colon CA that needs an operation, but they will also mention the patient had an MI last week. You have to factor the MI into your decision. Read the questions carefully: there is usually more than enough time.

16. Remember, the ABSITE is an endurance test. Pace yourself wisely and take a short break if necessary to get back on track.

17. They want you to get it right! Only a handful of questions are designed to separate out the 99th percentile from the 98th percentile. Most of the questions on the senior exam are basic management decisions with most of the clues pointing you in one direction.

Dale A. Dangleben, MD, FACS
James Lee, MD
Firas Madbak, MD
Courtney Edwards, MD

CHAPTER 1
Cell Biology

Peter Bechtel

CELL WALL

Which cell wall component increases membrane fluidity?
Cholesterol

What are the 3 main lipid classes found in the cell membrane?
Phospholipids, cholesterol, and glycolipids

What percentages of protein, carbohydrate, and lipid compose the plasma membrane?
Protein: 60%, carbohydrate: 1% to 10%, and lipid: 40%

What are the most common phospholipids in the plasma membrane?
Phosphatidylethanolamine and phosphatidylcholine

Which portion of the cell wall provides capacitance (ability to store charge)?
Lipid portion of plasma membrane

Which portion provides ability to resist charge?
Protein portion

What is the difference between surface antigens in the ABO system versus HLA system?
ABO = glycolipids
HLA = glycoproteins

Name the adhesion molecules that anchor a cell to other cells *or* the extracellular matrix:
Desmosomes/hemidesmosomes

Cell-cell occluding junctions that form an impermeable barrier:
Tight junctions

Toxic portion of lipopolysaccharide complex:
Lipid A

CELL STRUCTURES

Name the thin filaments that interact with myosin:
Actin

Name the thick filaments that slide along actin utilizing ATP:
Myosin

Intermediate filament found in hair and nails:
Keratin

Intermediate filament found in muscle:
Desmin

Intermediate filament found in fibroblasts:
Vimentin

Form specialized cellular structures such as mitotic spindles, cilia, and neuronal axons; forms lattice inside the cell to aid in transport of organelles in cell:
Microtubules

Specialized microtubule that form spindle fibers during cell division:
Centriole

Structural component of cell that synthesizes exported proteins:
Rough endoplasmic reticulum

Structural component of cell that detoxifies drugs and is involved with lipid/steroid synthesis:
Smooth endoplasmic reticulum

Structural component of a cell that uses carbohydrates to modify proteins and targets proteins to lysosomes:
Golgi apparatus

Structure inside the cell that has a double membrane with an outer membrane that is continuous with the rough endoplasmic reticulum:
Nucleus

Structure inside the nucleus where ribosomes are made:
Nucleolus

Cell structure responsible for energy production:
Mitochondria

GENETICS

Consists of proteins, histones, and double-stranded helical DNA
Chromosomes

Adenine and guanine are examples of:
Purines

Cytosine, thymidine, and uracil are examples of:
Pyramidines

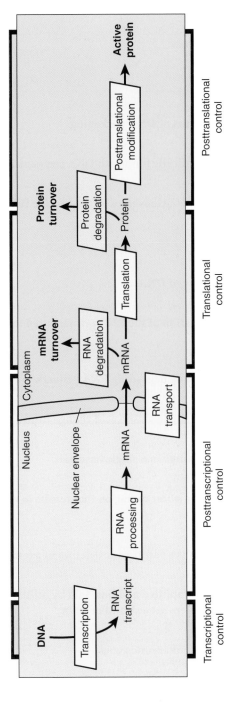

FIGURE 1-1. Four major steps in the control of eukaryotic gene expression. Transcriptional and posttranscriptional control determine the level of mRNA that is available to make a protein, whereas translational and posttranslational control determine the final outcome of functional proteins. Note that posttranscriptional and posttranslational controls consist of several steps. (*Reproduced from Brunicardi FC, Andersen DK, Billiar TR, et al. Schwartz's Principles of Surgery. 9th ed. http://www.accessmedicine.com. Copyright © The McGraw-Hill Companies, Inc. All rights reserved.*)

Process by which ribosomes use mRNA as a template for synthesis of proteins:
Translation

Process by which RNA polymerase uses a DNA strand for synthesis of mRNA:
Transcription

Place where transcription takes place:
Nucleus

Sequence of the start codon:
AUG

Coils of DNA that are the basic units of DNA packaging:
Nucleosomes

Small basic proteins that nonspecifically bind with DNA segments:
Histones

Formed by the coiling of 6 or more nucleosomes by the histone H1:
Solenoids

Proteins are synthesized from:
mRNA

Enzyme involved in the unwinding of DNA:
DNA helicase

Enzyme used to catalyze the formation of the RNA primers used to initiate DNA synthesis:
DNA primase

Enzyme that links DNA fragments by degrading RNA primers:
DNA ligase

Type of mutation that results in a single amino acid change from a point mutation:
Missense mutation

Type of mutation resulting in a change in a single base pair:
Point mutation

Type of mutation occurring from a point mutation that results in replacement of an amino acid with a stop codon:
Nonsense mutation

Type of mutation that occurs with the addition or deletion of a few base pairs:
Frameshift mutation

Technique by which DNA can be amplified a billion-fold by utilizing synthesized primers/oligonucleotides to complement a strand of DNA:
Polymerase chain reaction

Noncoding regions that interrupt eukaryotic genes:
Introns

Process by which introns are removed from an RNA transcript:
Splicing

RECEPTORS AND SIGNALS

Platelet-derived growth factor, epidermal growth factor, and transforming growth factor alpha belong to this receptor family:
Tyrosine kinase receptor

Activated by calcium and diacylglycerol:
Protein kinase C

Activated by cAMP:
Protein kinase A

Enzyme that converts membrane phosphoinositols into IP3 and DAG:
Phospholipase C

Mediates release of calcium from sarcoplasmic reticulum in muscle, endoplasmic reticulum, and mitochondria:
IP3

Works with calcium to activate protein kinase C:
DAG

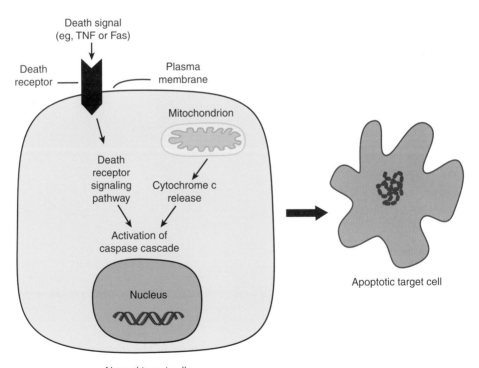

FIGURE 1-2. A simplified view of the apoptosis pathways. Extracellular death receptor pathways include the activation of Fas and tumor necrosis factor receptors, and consequent activation of the caspase pathway. Intracellular death pathway indicates the release of cytochrome c from mitochondria, which also triggers the activation of the caspase cascade. During apoptosis, cells undergo DNA fragmentation, nuclear and cell membrane breakdown, and are eventually digested by other cells. *(Reproduced from Brunicardi FC, Andersen DK, Billiar TR, et al. Schwartz's Principles of Surgery. 9th ed. http://www.accessmedicine.com. Copyright © The McGraw-Hill Companies, Inc. All rights reserved.)*

Enzyme that breaks down ATP to cAMP with release of pyrophosphate:
Adenylate cyclase

Most critical component in neovascularization in tumor metastases:
VEGF receptor

Cellular process under the precise control of different extra- and intracellular signals and follows a fixed sequence of events leading to cell death:
Apoptosis

Steroid hormones bind receptor in:
Cytoplasm

Thyroid hormone binds receptor in:
Nucleus

Examples of cAMP-dependent hormones:
TSH, ACTH

CELL TRANSPORT

Type of cell transport that uses concentration gradient as a driving force:
Diffusion (CO_2, O_2, and urea)

Type of diffusion that utilizes a carrier and is saturable:
Facilitated diffusion

Type of cell transport that requires ATP for energy:
Active transport

CELLULAR ENERGY

One glucose molecule generates:
Two ATP and 2 pyruvate molecules

Name of cycle where NADH and $FADH_2$ are created from the 2 pyruvate molecules produced from the breakdown of glucose.
Krebs cycle

Overall number of ATP generated from 1 molecule of glucose:
38 ATP: 36 from Krebs cycle + 2 ATP from glycolysis

Process by which amino acids and lactic acid via the Cori cycle are converted into glucose:
Gluconeogenesis

Name the breakdown product of fat metabolism that cannot be converted back into pyruvate:
Acetyl CoA

Lipases act on lipids to form:
Fatty acids and monoacylglycerols

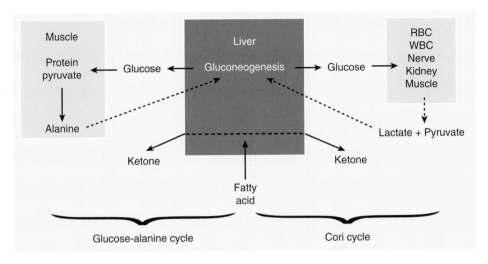

FIGURE 1-3. The recycling of peripheral lactate and pyruvate for hepatic gluconeogenesis is accomplished by the Cori cycle. Alanine within skeletal muscles can also be used as a precursor for hepatic gluconeogenesis. During starvation, such fatty acid provides fuel sources for basal hepatic enzymatic function. RBC, red blood cell; WBC, white blood cell. *(Reproduced from Brunicardi FC, Andersen DK, Billiar TR, et al. Schwartz's Principles of Surgery. 9th ed. http://www.accessmedicine.com. Copyright © The McGraw-Hill Companies, Inc. All rights reserved.)*

Fatty acid utilization:
Short chain = direct transport to liver
Long chain = packaged into micelles into lymph

CELL CYCLE

Most variable part of the cell cycle that determines cell cycle length:
G1

Part of cell cycle where protein synthesis and chromosomal duplication occur:
S

Growth factors affect the cell during this phase of the cell cycle:
G1

Phase between S phase and M phase:
G2

Part of cell cycle where nucleus divides:
M

Tumor cells are most sensitive to radiation during this stage of the cell cycle:
M

Phase of mitosis where chromosomes shorten, nucleolus and nuclear envelope disappear, and spindle apparatus forms:
Prophase

Phase of mitosis where centromeres align on the equatorial plate, spindle fibers attach to the centromeres, and centromeres duplicate:
Metaphase

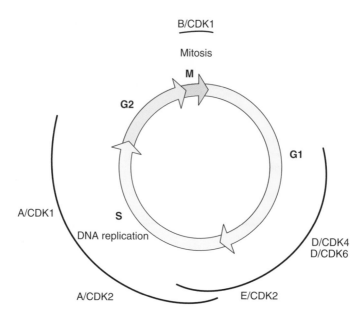

FIGURE 1-4. The cell cycle and its control system. M is the mitosis phase, when the nucleus and the cytoplasm divide; S is the phase when DNA is duplicated; G1 is the gap between M and S; G2 is the gap between S and M. A complex of cyclin and cyclin-dependent kinase (CDK) controls specific events of each phase. Without cyclin, CDK is inactive. Different cyclin/CDK complexes are shown around the cell cycle. A, B, D, and E stand for cyclin A, cyclin B, cyclin D, and cyclin E, respectively. *(Reproduced from Brunicardi FC, Andersen DK, Billiar TR, et al. Schwartz's Principles of Surgery. 9th ed. http://www.accessmedicine.com. Copyright © The McGraw-Hill Companies, Inc. All rights reserved.)*

Phase of mitosis where chromatids migrate to opposite poles:
Anaphase

Phase when nucleolar and nuclear envelope re-form and chromosomes decondense:
Telophase

MULTIPLE CHOICE QUESTIONS

1. **Erythrocytes use glycolysis primarily as a source of energy in the form of**
   A. ATP to power active membrane transport
   B. ATP to maintain cytoskeleton integrity
   C. NADH to power protein synthesis
   D. NADPH to initiate DNA replication
   E. NADH to reduce oxidized glutathione

2. **A defect in cholesterol metabolism or other sources of bile would cause difficulties in digestion because bile is needed for**
   A. Emulsification of dietary fat for easier access of stomach lipases
   B. Denaturation of dietary proteins for easier digestion by proteases
   C. Micelle incorporation of lipids for easier digestion by lipases
   D. Neutralization of stomach acid
   E. Stimulation of pancreatic secretions

3. **Cyclins are proteins that serve as signals to control progression of cells around the cell cycle. Cyclin signals are transmitted via**
   A. Histone acetylases
   B. Protein kinases
   C. DNA methylases
   D. Specific proteases
   E. Small, interfering RNAs (siRNA)

4. **Which of the following is a correct match?**
   A. G cell—pepsinogen
   B. Chief cell—Gastrin
   C. Parietal cell—HCl and intrinsic factor
   D. Mucous cells—Cholecystekinin

5. **Platelet activation, muscle contraction, pancreatic secretion, and glycogen degradation act via which intracellular signal mechanism?**
   A. cAMP second messenger signaling
   B. Calmodulin-induced calcium release
   C. Protein kinase A activation
   D. IP3 and DAG induced activation of protein kinase C

6. **Base deficit and serum lactate correlate with mortality in trauma by reflecting which of the following systemic changes from normal physiology?**
   A. Myoglobin induced ATN progressing to renal failure
   B. Hyoperfused end organs relying on energy generated via aneorobic metabolism
   C. Skeletal muscle sarcomere unregulated release of calcium and diacylglycerol
   D. Injured organ trauma induced apoptosis releasing corresponding intravascular waste cellular products

7. **Which of the following clinical scenarios regarding metabolism is false or implausible?**
   A. An elderly patient on indomethacin, oxazepam, aspirin, and acetaminophen becomes jaundiced after overwhelming UDP-glucuronic acid transferase enzymes.
   B. A 26-year-old female on oral contraceptives conceives after a course of antibiotics.
   C. A 56-year-old with atrial fibrillation on warfarin is admitted with spontaneous hematemesis after starting ciprofloxacin/metronidazole therapy for diverticulitis.
   D. A traumatically injured 38-year-old with no past medical history develops coma and cerebral infarction from profound hypoglycemia within 30 minutes of injury.

8. **Which mechanism explains ultraviolet light as a risk factor for skin cancers?**
   A. UV-B light is absorbed by DNA strands causing pyrimidine dimers
   B. Increased number of melanocytes after prolonged tanning leads to proliferation errors
   C. Vitamin D activation includes free radicals as a side product
   D. Sunlight induces collagen breakdown, leading to sheer stress injury

9. **Select the incorrect statement from below.**

A. Aerobic metabolism provides the most efficient, most proliferative process to convert glucose into ATP in humans.

B. Hepatocyte metabolism of toxins includes cytochrome P-450 enzymes, UDP-glucuronyl transferases, glutathione S-transferases, and sulfotransferases.

C. The entirety of chromosomal DNA is contained within the nucleus in formation with histone proteins.

D. Phase I reactions change endogenous substances solubility while Phase II reactions change their chemical structure.

ANSWERS

1. **Answer: A.** B would be correct if it listed NADPH instead of ATP. C is incorrect because the cell does not make its own proteins. D is incorrect because RBCs lack nuclei and therefore do not replicate any DNA. E would be correct if it listed NADPH instead of NADH.

2. **Answer: C.** The stomach does not produce lipases. Bile micelle incorporation is not related to protease activity. Bile does not affect acidic pH of stomach effluent. Pancreas secretions are stimulated by hormones, not bile.

3. **Answer: B.** Histone acetylases and DNA methylases play a role in DNA configuration, while proteases are not involved in cell messenging. siRNA is part of gene expression, not directly related to cell messenging.

4. **Answer: C.** G cell = gastrin, chief cell = pepsinogen, parietal cell = HCl and intrinsic factor, mucous cell = mucous/bicarbonate.

5. **Answer: D.** B is false because IP3 binding to endoplasmic reticulum releases calcium. A and C are false because they belong to the protein kinase A system.

6. **Answer: B.** Lactate production is associated with hypoperfusion in trauma. Myoglobin can cause ATN or renal failure in trauma but should not directly alter BD or lactate. Sarcomere release of calcium is implicated in malignant hyperthermia.

7. **Answer: D.** D is the false scenario. Glycogen stores can supply necessary glucose for anaerobic metabolism even in intense need for 20 to 90 minutes, after which depleted, anaerobic metabolism would attempt to meet the needs of the patient in scenario D.

8. **Answer: A.** B is incorrect because melanocyte number is constant as part of neural crest migration as an embryo. C is incorrect because free radicals are not involved. D is incorrect because collagen is unrelated to DNA sequence.

9. **Answer: D.** Phase I reactions change chemical structure while Phase II reactions change solubility.

CHAPTER 2
Hematology

Christine Du

Hematology requires lots of memorization. Important topics to look over include bleeding disorders and anticoagulants. These are basic questions you don't want to miss.

THE COAGULATION PATHWAY

Sequence of the intrinsic pathway of coagulation:
Prekallikrein + HMW kininogen + Factor XII + exposed collagen → activates Factor XI → activates Factor IX, combines with Factor VIII → activates Factor X, combines with Factor V → converts prothrombin (Factor II) into thrombin. Thrombin converts fibrinogen into fibrin.

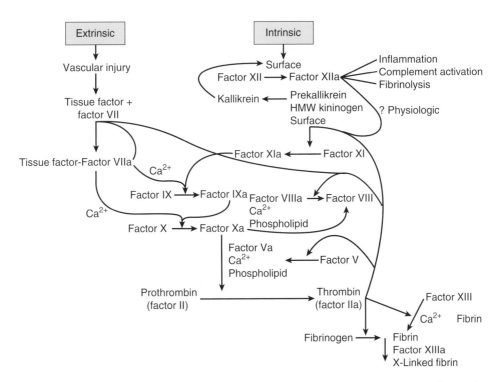

FIGURE 2-1. Schematic of the coagulation system. HMW, high molecular weight. *(Reproduced from Brunicardi FC, Andersen DK, Billiar TR, et al. Schwartz's Principles of Surgery. 9th ed. http://www.accessmedicine.com. Copyright © The McGraw-Hill Companies, Inc. All rights reserved.)*

Sequence of the extrinsic pathway of coagulation:
Factor VII + tissue factor → activates Factor X, combines with Factor V → converts prothrombin into thrombin. Thrombin converts fibrinogen into fibrin.

Which factor is the convergence point and common to both the extrinsic and intrinsic pathways of coagulation?
Factor X

What does the prothrombin complex consist of?
Factor V, X, platelet factor 3, and prothrombin catalyzes the formation of thrombin

What function does thrombin have?
Activates factors V and VIII, activates platelets, and converts fibrinogen into fibrin and fibrin split products. It is instrumental in coagulation

Which factor has the shortest half-life?
Factor VII

What factor can be used to differentiate a consumptive coagulopathy from hepatocellular disease?
Factor VIII:C; consumptive coagulopathy will have reduced levels of all factors and hepatocellular disease will have reduced levels of all factors except factor VIII

Which factors are known as the labile factors (activity lost in stored blood)?
Factors V and VIII

What function does factor XIII have?
Cross-links fibrin

What does protein C do?
Degrades fibrinogen and Factors V and VIII (vitamin K dependent)

What does protein S do?
Acts as protein C cofactor (vitamin K dependent)

What does Von Willebrand factor (vWF) do?
Links collagen to the GpIb receptor on platelets

What is the function of antithrombin III?
Binds heparin, inhibits Factors IX, X, XI, and thrombin

Where does tissue plasminogen activator come from and what does it do?
Released from endothelium and it converts plasminogen into plasmin

What does plasmin do?
Degrades fibrinogen, fibrin, and Factors V and VIII

What is the natural inhibitor of plasmin called and where does it come from?
Alpha-2 antiplasmin; comes from the endothelium

What are the vitamin K–dependent factors?
Factors II, VII, IX, and X and proteins C and S

What function does tissue factor pathway inhibitor have?
Inhibits factor X

LABORATORY TESTS AND DATA

PT measures the function of these factors:
Factors II, V, VII, and X and fibrinogen

What 2 factors are not measured by the PTT?
Factors VII and XIII

PTT measures the function of these factors:
Factors II, V, VIII, IX, X, XI, and XII and fibrinogen

What is the normal value for bleeding time and what does it imply?
Normal bleeding time ranges from 3 to 9 minutes and implies platelet counts >50,000/mL and normal platelet function

What test aids in detecting circulating anticoagulants, qualitative abnormalities of fibrin, inhibition of fibrin polymerization, and measures the clotting time of plasma?
Thrombin time

Patients bleeding after a large number of blood transfusions should be considered to have:
Dilutional thrombocytopenia (vs hemolytic transfusion reaction)

What factors are common to both the PT and PTT?
Factors II, V, and X and fibrinogen

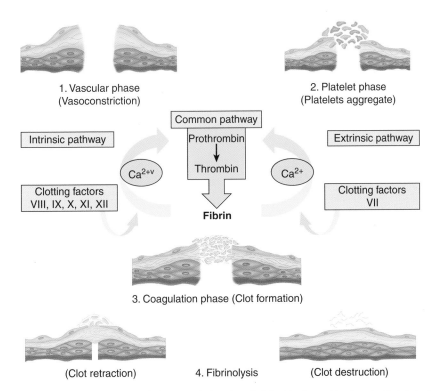

FIGURE 2-2. Biology of hemostasis. The 4 physiologic processes that interrelate to limit blood loss from an injured vessel are illustrated and include vascular constriction, platelet plug formation, fibrin clot formation, and fibrinolysis. *(Reproduced from Brunicardi FC, Andersen DK, Billiar TR, et al. Schwartz's Principles of Surgery. 9th ed. http://www.accessmedicine.com. Copyright © The McGraw-Hill Companies, Inc. All rights reserved.)*

How many hours must elapse after the last dose of IV heparin before the PT can be reliably measured?
Minimum of 5 hours

Sequence of physiologic reactions that mediate hemostasis following vascular injury?
1. Vasoconstriction
2. Platelet activation/adherence/aggregation
3. Thrombin generation

HYPERCOAGULABILITY DISORDERS

What is Virchow triad?
Stasis, endothelial injury, and hypercoagulability

What is the most common cause of acquired hypercoagulability?
Smoking

What is the most common inherited hypercoagulable state?
Factor V Leiden

What is the treatment for hyperhomocysteinemia?
Vitamin B-12 and folate

Name the prothrombin gene defect causing spontaneous venous thrombosis.
Prothrombin gene defect G20210A

PLATELET FUNCTION AND DYSFUNCTION

What is the normal life span of a platelet?
7 to 10 days

Formation of a platelet plug requires these 2 electrolytes:
Calcium and magnesium

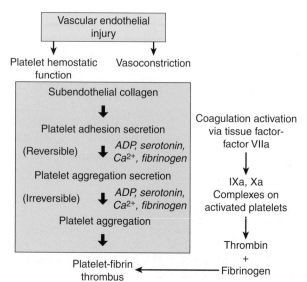

FIGURE 2-3. Schematic of platelet activation and thrombus function. ADP, adenosine diphosphate. *(Reproduced from Brunicardi FC, Andersen DK, Billiar TR, et al. Schwartz's Principles of Surgery. 9th ed. http://www.accessmedicine.com. Copyright © The McGraw-Hill Companies, Inc. All rights reserved.)*

Platelet count needed before surgery:
>50,000/mL

Platelet count associated with spontaneous bleeding:
<20,000/mL

Platelet count when prophylactic platelet transfusions should be given:
<10,000/mL

Time to formation of a platelet plug is measured by this test:
Bleeding time

Inhibits platelet aggregation by inhibiting prostaglandin synthesis (PGG_2, $PGGH_2$) from arachidonic acid:
NSAIDs (ASA, ibuprofen, etc)

Uremia leads to a downregulation of:
GpIb, GpIIb/IIIA, and vWF

Initial treatment of choice for uremic coagulopathy:
Dialysis

Drug that can be given to help correct platelet dysfunction from uremia, bypass, or ASA:
Desmopressin (DDAVP)

DDAVP and conjugated estrogens stimulate the release of:
Factor VII and vWF

RED BLOOD CELL/BLOOD PRODUCTS

Cause of microcytic anemia in a man or postmenopausal woman until proven otherwise:
Colon cancer

What is the normal life span of a red blood cell?
120 days

The electrolyte most likely to fall after infusion of stored blood:
Ionized calcium (citrate in stored blood binds serum calcium)

How long can PRBCs be stored?
~42 days or 6 weeks

Most common blood product to contain bacterial contamination:
Platelets

What type of bacteria is usually found in contaminated platelets?
Gram-positive organisms

Most common bacteria found with blood product contamination:
Gram-negative rods (*Escherichia coli*)

What types of infectious diseases can be transmitted by transfusion?
Hepatitis B and C, HIV, HTLV I and II, Chagas disease, malaria, and "theoretical risk" of Creutzfeldt-Jacob disease

True or False: Washed red blood cells can be given safely to patients who have had severe allergic/anaphylactic reactions to plasma.
True, because there are barely any plasma proteins in washed red blood cells.

The use of transfusion with leukocyte reduced packed red blood cells are justified in:
Patients with multiple reactions despite premedication with antipyretics, needing long-term platelet support, and transplant candidates in order to prevent formation of HLA antibodies.

What are the laboratory criteria for diagnosis of a hemolytic transfusion reaction?
Hemoglobinuria with free hemoglobin concentrations >5 mg/dL, serologic confirmation of incompatibility, and positive direct antiglobulin test results

Approximate formula to convert Hct into Hgb:
Hct/3 = Hgb

1 U PRBC should increase the Hgb and Hct by:
1 g/dL and Hct by ~3% to 4%

Which blood type is the universal donor?
O negative

What happens during a type and screen?
Patient's blood is screened for antibodies and blood type is determined.

What happens for a type and cross?
Recipient's serum is checked for preformed antibodies against donor's antigens in PRBC.

What fluid cannot be infused with PRBC and why?
Lactated Ringer's; calcium in LR may result in coagulation within the IV line.

What is the most common cause of transfusion hemolysis?
Clerical error leading to ABO incompatibility.

Symptoms of transfusion reaction:
Fever, chills, nausea, hypotension, lumbar/chest pain, abnormal bleeding, and pain at infusion site.

Treatment of transfusion hemolysis:
Stop transfusion; fluids; Lasix; alkalinize urine with bicarbonate; pressors as needed.

CLOTTING DISORDERS AND TREATMENT

How long does it take for vitamin K to take effect?
6 hours

How long do the effects of FFP last?
6 hours

How long does it take for FFP to work?
Immediately

What does cryoprecipitate contain?
vWF, Factor VIII, and fibrinogen

What does FFP contain?
All factors including labile Factors V and VIII, AT-III, proteins C and S

What is the best method for detecting patients at risk for bleeding?
A complete history and physical examination

True or False: A normal circumcision rules out a bleeding disorder.
False. Newborns may not bleed at circumcision because of clotting factors from the mother (Factor VIII crosses the placenta).

What percentage of patients with a bleeding disorder is picked up by abnormal bleeding from tonsillectomy or tooth extraction?
99%

What is the most common congenital bleeding disorder?
Von Willebrand disease

This factor is deficient in hemophilia A:
Factor VIII

Preoperative treatment for hemophilia A:
Factor VIII infusion to 100% normal preoperative levels

Coagulation study that is elevated in hemophilia A:
PTT

Factor deficient in hemophilia B:
Factor IX

Inheritance of hemophilia A and B:
Sex-linked recessive

What is the treatment for hemarthrosis in a patient with hemophilia A?
Initial therapy includes Factor VIII, joint rest, cold packs (3–5 days), and a compression dressing (3–5 days), followed by active range of motion exercised 24 hours after Factor VIII therapy.

How long does it take for desmopressin to reach its maximal procoagulant effect?
1 to 2 hours

Deficiency in Von Willebrand disease:
vWF and factor VIII:C

Inheritance of Von Willebrand disease:
Autosomal dominant

Treatment of Von Willebrand disease:
DDAVP or cryoprecipitate

What type of Von Willebrand disease is desmopressin or DDAVP specifically contraindicated?
Type 2B

Name of syndrome for deficiency of factor XI? Treatment?
Rosenthal syndrome; plasma

What is the eponym for the deficiencies of Factors VII and X? Treatment?
Stuart-Prower deficiency; plasma

What receptor deficiency is found in Glanzmann thrombocytopenia?
GpIIb/IIIa receptor deficiency. The platelets cannot bind to each other.

What is the treatment for Glanzmann thrombocytopenia?
Platelets

What receptor deficiency is found in Bernard Soulier disease?
GpIb receptor deficiency. The platelets cannot bind to collagen

What is the treatment for Bernard Soulier disease?
Platelets

Mechanism by which DIC occurs:
Thromboplastic materials are introduced into the circulation that leads to activation of the coagulation system with protective or secondary fibrinolysis.

What is the most important component in the treatment of DIC?
Correcting the underlying cause

Examples of fast DIC:
Amniotic fluid embolus, placenta abruption, septic abortion, septicemia, massive tissue injury, incompatible blood transfusion, purpura fulminans

Examples of slow DIC:
Liver disease, Kasabach-Merritt syndrome, acute promyelocytic leukemia, dead fetus syndrome, transfusion of activated prothrombin complex concentrates, carcinomas

Postoperative patients with untreated polycythemia vera are at risk for:
Postoperative thrombosis, bleeding, combination of thrombosis and bleeding, or infection

What are the desired platelet counts and hematocrit in a patient with polycythemia vera before an elective operation?
Plt < 400,000/mL and Hct < 48%

ANTICOAGULATION

Heparin binds to this protein for its anti-coagulation effects:
Anti-thrombin III; heparin-antithrombin III complex then binds Factor IX, X, and XI

What is the half-life of heparin?
90 minutes

What is the dose of protamine to reverse 100 U or 1 mg of heparin?
1 to 1.5 mg

What are signs seen in a protamine reaction?
Bradycardia, hypotension, and decreased heart function

Name the diagnosis: A patient is given Coumadin for a PE; 3 days later his skin sloughs off his arms and legs:
Warfarin-induced skin necrosis.

Reason that warfarin-induced skin necrosis occurs:
Proteins C and S have a shorter half-life than Factors II, VII, IX, and X. Coumadin leads to a decrease in proteins C and S before the other factors leading to a hypercoagulable state

Patients with this deficiency are at increased risk for warfarin-induced skin necrosis:
Protein C deficiency

Mechanisms where extracorporeal circulation may lead to bleeding?
Inadequate reversal of heparin, overadministration of protamine, or thrombocytopenia

Mechanism where extracorporeal circulation may lead to clotting?
Activation of Factor XII

What is the desired activated clotting time for routine anticoagulation?
150 to 200 seconds

What is the desired activated clotting time for cardiopulmonary bypass?
400 seconds

What surgical procedures require an INR < 1.2?
Neurosurgical procedures, operations on the prostate or eye, or blind needle aspiration

What INR is a contraindication to intramuscular injection?
INR > 1.5

What are the absolute contraindications to the use of thrombolytics?
Recent CVA (<2 months), intracranial pathology, and active internal bleeding

What is Argatroban?
A synthetic direct thrombin inhibitor derived from L-arginine

What is Hirudin?
An irreversible direct thrombin inhibitor derived from leeches

What is Ancrod?
Malayan pit viper venom that stimulates tPA release

What is the length of anticoagulation treatment for first, second, or third episode of DVT? For significant PE?
Coumadin for 6 months, 1 year, and lifetime, respectively; lifetime anticoagulation for those who had a significant PE.

What are the indications for an IVC filter?
Patients who have undergone a pulmonary embolectomy; patients with documented PE while anticoagulated; patients with free-floating femoral, iliofemoral, IVC DVT; patients with contraindication to anticoagulation; patients at high risk for DVT (head injured/orthopedic injured on prolonged bed rest)

MULTIPLE CHOICE QUESTIONS

1. **What is the first step in hemostasis?**
   A. Platelet aggregation
   B. Vascular vasodilation
   C. Vascular vasoconstriction
   D. Fibrin formation

2. **What is the most common congenital hypercoagulability disorder?**
   A. Prothrombin gene defect G20210 A
   B. Protein C deficiency
   C. Protein S deficiency
   D. Factor V Leiden

3. **What blood product listed below does not carry the risk of HIV and hepatitis B or C?**
   A. Whole blood
   B. Albumin
   C. Platelets
   D. Fresh frozen plasma

4. **The drug that can be used to treat bleeding with transurethral prostate resection?**
   A. Hirudin
   B. Ancrod
   C. Aminocaproic acid
   D. Urokinase

5. **A 45-year-old male with the diagnosis of antithrombin III deficiency develops a DVT. What do you have to administer to the patient prior to starting heparin?**
   A. Cryoprecipitate
   B. Platelets
   C. Fresh frozen plasma
   D. DDAVP

6. **A 55-year-old male was placed on a heparin drip for a lower extremity DVT. Three days later he had a platelet count of 52,000 (decreased from 180,000). You suspect heparin-induced thrombocytopenia (HIT). What antibody has he developed?**
   A. IgG PF4 Ab
   B. IgM PF4 Ab
   C. IgG PAF Ab
   D. IgM PAF Ab

7. **All of the following are relative contraindications to thrombolytic therapy except:**
   A. Pregnancy
   B. Recent surgery (<10 days)
   C. Recent trauma
   D. Recent CVA (<2 months)
   E. Liver disease

8. **A 36-year-old female is 32 weeks pregnant and has been diagnosed with a lower extremity DVT. The treatment that is absolutely contraindicated is:**
   A. IV heparin only
   B. Arixtra (Fondaparinux)
   C. Fragmin (Dalteparin)
   D. IV heparin transitioned to Coumadin
   E. Lovenox (Enoxaparin)

9. **This class of antibiotics can induce a platelet disorder:**

   A. Fluoroquinolones
   B. Cephalosporins
   C. Carbapenems
   D. Aminoglycosides

10. **Of the following scenarios, which patient has indication for an IVC filter?**

    A. A 36-year-old male who has a recurrent DVT while on Coumadin with an INR 1.5
    B. A 42-year-old female with an upper extremity DVT
    C. A 28-year-old female who is 27 weeks pregnant
    D. A 67-year-old male with a PE while on therapeutic Coumadin
    E. A 50-year-old male who has Factor V Leiden

ANSWERS

1. **Answer: C.** When there is disruption at the endothelium causing bleeding, the first step in hemostasis is vasoconstriction followed by the adherence of platelets to the injured site by the link of glycoprotein receptor 1b (platelet surface) to the vessel wall by circulation vWF. This expresses the surface receptor glycoprotein IIb/IIIa on the platelet. Platelets aggregate forming a platelet plug and this is followed by ultimately fibrin formation.

2. **Answer: D.** Factor V Leiden (resistance to activated Protein C) is reportedly present in 20% to 60% of cases of venous thrombosis. It is present in 1% to 2% of the population. Compared to other hypercoagulable disorders, it is of lower risk in forming thrombus and more likely the thrombus will be venous rather than arterial.

3. **Answer: B.** Albumin carries the theoretical risk of Creutzfeldt-Jakob disease.

4. **Answer: C.** Aminocaproic acid is a lysine analogue that inhibits fibrinolysis. It competitively binds to the lysine-binding sites of a fibrin clot blocking the binding of plasminogen.

5. **Answer: C.** Fresh frozen plasma is needed to be administered with patients who are antithrombin III deficient so that the mechanism of heparin (ie, activating antithrombin III, thereby inactivating Factor Xa and thrombin) is effective.

6. **Answer: A.** HIT develops when the body forms antibodies, usually IgG, against heparin when it is bound to platelet Factor 4 protein. With HIT, arterial and venous thromboses can both form.

7. **Answer: D.** Absolute contraindications to thrombolytic therapy include active internal bleeding, recent CVA (<2 months), and intracranial pathology.

8. **Answer: D.** Coumadin is teratogenic and crosses the placenta.

9. **Answer: B.** Pencillins and cephalosporins can bind platelets and increase bleeding time.

10. **Answer: D.** Indications for an IVC filter include patients who have a contraindication to anticoagulation; a pulmonary embolus while on therapeutic anticoagulation; free-floating iliofemoral, IVC or femoral DVT; and patients who have had a pulmonary embolectomy.

CHAPTER 3
Transplant and Immunology

Arjumand Ali

INTERLEUKINS

Name the cells of origin and functions of the following interleukins:

Interleukin-1
- Mononuclear phagocytes, T and B cells, NK, cells fibroblasts, neutrophils, smooth muscle cells
- Proliferation of T and B cells; fever, inflammation; endothelial cell activation; increases liver protein synthesis

Interleukin-2
- Activated T cells
- T-cell growth factor, cytotoxic T-cell generation; B-cell proliferation/differentiation; growth/activation of NK cells

Interleukin-4
- CD4+ T cells, mast cells
- B-cell activation/differentiation, T- and mast cell growth factor

Interleukin-5
- T cells
- Eosinophil proliferation/activation

Interleukin-6
- Mononuclear phagocytes, T cells, endothelial cells
- B-cell proliferation/differentiation; T-cell activation; increases liver acute phase reactants; fever, inflammation

Interleukin-8
- Lymphocytes, monocytes, multiple other cell types
- Stimulates granulocyte activity, chemotactic activity; potent angiogenic factor

Interleukin-10
- Mononuclear phagocyte, T cells
- B-cell activation/differentiation, inhibition, mononuclear phagocytes

Interleukin-12
- Mononuclear phagocytes, dendritic cells
- IFN-γ synthesis, T-cell cytolytic function, CD4+ T-cell differentiation

INTERFERONS AND OTHER CHEMOKINES

What cells produce interferon-γ and what are its functions?
- NK and T cells
- Increases expression of class I and class II MHC, activates macrophages and endothelial cells, augments NK activity, antiviral

What cells produce interferon-α, β and what are their functions?
- Mononuclear phagocyte-α; fibroblast-β
- Mononuclear phagocyte increases class I MHC expression, antiviral, NK-cell activation

What cells produce tumor necrosis factor-α, β and what are their functions?
- NK and T cells, mononuclear phagocyte
- B-cell growth/differentiation, enhances T-cell function, macrophage activator, neutrophil activator

What cells produce transforming growth factor-β and what are its functions?
- T cells, mononuclear phagocyte
- T-cell inhibition

What cells produce lymphotoxin and what are its functions?
- T cells
- Neutrophil activator, endothelial activation

IMMUNOSUPPRESSANTS

What was the first effective clinical immunosuppressive regimen for the transplantation of solid organs? (It was introduced in 1962.)
Azathioprine and corticosteroids

What are the 2 commercially available antilymphocyte globulins used for induction immediately after transplantation?
Horse antithymocyte globulin; rabbit antithymocyte globulin (most commonly used)

What is OKT3?
A monoclonal antibody that binds to CD3, a site associated with the TCR, that blocks cell-mediated cytotoxicity by inhibiting the function of naive T cells and established cytotoxic lymphocytes

What may be seen with the first or second dose of OKT3?
Acute cytokine release syndrome; avoid with concomitant administration of steroids or indomethacin

What 2 monoclonal antibodies that became available in 1998 decrease rejection by leaving cells with no free receptors for IL-2 to bind by binding to the IL-2R without activating it?
Basiliximab; daclizumab

Table 3-1 Summary of the Main Immunosuppressive Drugs

Drug	Mechanism of Action	Adverse Effects	Clinical Uses	Dosage
Cyclosporine (CSA)	Binds to cyclophilin	Nephrotoxicity	Improved bioavailability of microemulsion form	Oral dose is 8–10 mg/kg/d (given in 2 divided doses)
	Inhibits calcineurin and IL-2 synthesis	Tremor	Used as mainstay of maintenance protocols	
		Hypertension		
		Hirsutism		
Tacrolimus (FK506)	Binds to FKBP	Nephrotoxicity	Improved patient and graft survival in (liver) primary and rescue therapy	IV 0.05–0.1 mg/kg/d
	Inhibits calcineurin and IL-2 synthesis	Hypertension		PO 0.15–0.3 mg/kg/d (given q12h)
		Neurotoxicity		
		GI toxicity (nausea, diarrhea)	Used as mainstay of maintenance, like CSA	
Mycophenolate mofetil	Antimetabolite	Leukopenia	Effective for primary and rescue therapy (kidney transplants)	1 g bid PO (may need 1.5 g in black recipients)
	Inhibits enzyme necessary for de novo purine synthesis	GI toxicity	May replace azathioprine	
Sirolimus	Inhibits lymphocyte effects driven by IL-2 receptor	Thrombocytopenia	May allow early withdrawal of steroids and decreased calcineurin doses	2–4 mg/d, adjusted to trough drug levels
		Increased serum cholesterol/LDL		
		Vasculitis (animal studies)		
Corticosteroids	Multiple actions	Cushingoid state	Used in induction, maintenance, and treatment of acute rejection	Varies from mg to several grams per day
	Anti-inflammatory	Glucose intolerance		Maintenance doses, 5–10 mg/d
	Inhibits lymphokine production	Osteoporosis		
Azathioprine	Antimetabolite	Thrombocytopenia	Used in maintenance protocols	1–3 mg/kg/d for maintenance
	Interferes with DNA and RNA synthesis	Neutropenia		
		Liver dysfunction		

FKBP, FK506-binding protein; IL, interleukin; LDL, low-density lipoprotein.
Brunicardi FC, Andersen DK, Billiar TR, Dunn DL, Hunter JG, Matthews JB, Pollock RE. *Schwartz Principles of Surgery*. 9th ed. www.accessmedicine.com. Copyright © The McGraw-Hill Companies, Inc. All rights reserved.

What is rituximab?
An anti-CD20 monoclonal antibody; CD20 is a surface molecule expressed on B cells

What is alemtuzumab?
A humanized anti-CD52 monoclonal antibody (Campath 1H)

What are the anti-inflammatory effects of glucocorticoids?
Inhibition of cytokine gene transcription in macrophages; inhibition of cytokine secretion (IL-1, IL-6, TNF); suppression of the production and effect of T-cell cytokines; inhibition of the ability of macrophages to respond to lymphocyte-derived signals (migration inhibition factor, macrophage activation factor); suppression of prostaglandin synthesis

RENAL TRANSPLANT

What are the indications for kidney transplant?
Irreversible renal failure from: glomerulonephritis; pyelonephritis; polycystic kidney disease; malignant HTN; reflux pyelonephritis; Goodpasture syndrome; congenital renal hyperplasia; Fabry disease; Alport syndrome; renal cortical necrosis; damage from DM I

Define renal failure.
Glomerular filtration rate (GFR) < 20% to 25% normal; GFR drops to 5% to 10% of normal; uremic symptoms begin (lethargy, seizures, neuropathy, electrolyte disorders)

What is the most common reason for kidney transplant?
Diabetes (25%)

What are the 3 anastomoses of a heterotopic kidney transplant?
Renal artery to iliac artery; renal vein to iliac vein; ureter to bladder

If the choice of a left or right donor kidney is available, which one is preferred and why?
The left kidney; longer renal vein allows for an easier anastomosis

Why is the external iliac artery preferred over the internal iliac artery for vascular anastomosis during a renal transplantation?
The external iliac artery requires less dissection and there is less of a chance for anastomotic narrowing over the internal iliac artery

What might happen if accessory renal arteries are ligated in a renal allograft used for transplantation?
Renal infarcts/necrosis; ureteral necrosis; urinary fistula formation

What is the expected time period for return of normal renal function after renal transplantation?
Living related 3 to 5 days; cadaveric 7 to 15 days

What drug is used routinely by most centers for prophylaxis against urinary tract infections and *Pneumocystis jiroveci* (*carinii*)?
Trimethoprim-sulfamethoxazole

What is the most common cause of sudden cessation of urinary output in the immediate postoperative period following a renal transplant?
The presence of a blood clot in the bladder or urethral catheter; can be relieved by irrigation

How is the definitive diagnosis of a primary infection with polyomavirus (type BK) made in a patient with a kidney transplant?
Allograft biopsy to demonstrate nuclear inclusions in tubular epithelial cells and the absence of rejection or drug toxicity

What is the mainstay of treatment of posttransplant lymphoproliferative disorder (PTLD)?
Decreasing the level of immunosuppression

REJECTION AFTER RENAL TRANSPLANT

What kind of rejection results from preformed antibodies against the donor organ characterized by the transplanted kidney turning blue within minutes of revascularization?
Hyperacute rejection

When does acute cellular rejection after renal transplantation occur?
The first few weeks-months after transplantation, and occasionally years later

What is the red flag that indicated rejection following renal transplantation?
Increasing creatinine

What are the classic signs and symptoms of acute cellular rejection after renal transplantation?
Malaise, fever, oliguria, hypertension, tenderness, swelling of the allograft, elevated creatinine

When does chronic allograft nephropathy occur?
Often after years of stable function; may be accelerated in allografts that have had multiple or incompletely treated episodes of acute rejection

GRAFT AND PATIENT SURVIVAL AND COMPLICATION RATES

What is the 1-year graft survival for a living donor kidney compared to a standard criteria cadaveric kidney?
95% for a living donor kidney; 91% for a standard-criteria cadaveric kidney

What is the 5-year graft survival for a living donor kidney compared to a standard criteria cadaveric kidney?
80% for a living donor kidney; 69% for a standard criteria cadaveric kidney

What is the 1-year patient survival rate after a living donor kidney transplant compared to a standard criteria cadaveric kidney transplant?
98% for a living donor kidney transplant; 96% for a standard criteria cadaveric kidney transplant

What is the 5-year patient survival rate after a living donor kidney transplant compared to a standard criteria cadaveric kidney transplant?
91% for a living donor kidney transplant; 84% for a standard criteria cadaveric kidney transplant

Table 3-2 Causes of Increased Serum Creatinine Early after Kidney Transplant

Cause	Characteristics	Diagnosis	Treatment
Hypovolemia	• Decreased CVP • Decreasing urine output • Low blood pressure • Low Hgb if due to bleeding	• Check Hgb and CVP	• Rehydrate with appropriate fluids
Vascular thrombosis	• Sudden drop in urine output • Dark hematuria • Tender, swollen graft	• Ultrasound with Doppler	• Re-explore for thrombectomy or nephrectomy
Bladder outlet obstruction	• Clots in urinary catheter • Sudden drop in urine output	• Distended bladder on examination or by ultrasound	• Irrigate or change bladder catheter —
Ureter obstruction	—	• Euvolemic • Ultrasound showing hydroureter • Possible lymphocele on ultrasound	• Do percutaneous nephrostogram • Drainage of lymphocele (if it is the cause of ureter obstruction)
Drug toxicity	• High CSA or FK506 level	• Check drug levels	• Decrease dosage of drugs
Acute rejection	• May have risk factors such as low drug levels, high PRA	• Kidney biopsy	• Administer bolus steroid or antilymphocyte treatment • Begin plasmapheresis (and IVIG if humoral rejection)

CSA, cyclosporin A; CVP, central venous pressure; Hgb, hemoglobin; IVIG, intravenous immunoglobulin; PRA, panel reactive antibody.

LIVER TRANSPLANT

What is the most frequent vascular complication with liver transplantation?
Hepatic artery thrombosis; can manifest as rapid or indolent worsening of graft function or as necrosis of the bile duct and dehiscence of the biliary-enteric anastomosis

What is the treatment for a post-op bile leak seen in a patient after liver transplantation?
Surgical exploration and revision of the anastomosis or stenting of the anastomosis by ERCP; if leak secondary to ischemic bile duct injury as a result of early hepatic artery thrombosis treatment if urgent retransplantation

What is the MELD score?
Model for end-stage liver disease is the formula currently used to assign points for prioritizing position on the waiting list for cadaveric liver transplant; MELD is based on INR, bilirubin, creatinine, with extra points for presence of liver cancer

What 3 laboratory values is the MELD (model for end-stage liver disease) score based on?
Total bilirubin; international normalized ratio; creatinine

What are the indications for a liver transplant?
Liver failure from: cirrhosis; Budd-Chiari; biliary atresia; neonatal hepatitis; chronic active hepatitis; fulminant hepatitis with drug toxicity; sclerosing cholangitis; Caroli disease; subacute hepatic necrosis; congenital hepatic fibrosis; inborn errors of metabolism; fibrolamellar hepatocellular carcinoma

How is the liver transplant placed (orthotopic, heterotopic)?
Orthotopic

What are the options for biliary drainage for liver transplantation?
Donor common bile duct to recipient common bile duct end-to-end; Roux-en-Y choledochojejunostomy

What Child-Turcotte-Pugh score is needed before a patient can be placed on the liver transplant waiting list?
>7 points

What is chronic liver rejection called?
Vanishing bile duct syndrome

What are the red flags indicating rejection of a liver transplant?
Decreasing bile drainage; increased serum bilirubin; increased LFTs

Where is the site of rejection with a liver transplant?
The biliary epithelium is involved with rejection first, followed by vascular endothelium

True or False: Renal function in a patient with hepatorenal syndrome does not improve after liver transplantation?
False; renal function improves in patients with hepatorenal syndrome after liver transplantation

What must be excluded on imaging on initial workup in all liver transplant candidates?
Extrahepatic metastases; macrovascular invasion of the liver

Hepatic portoenterostomy is otherwise known as?
The Kasai procedure

What are indications for liver transplantation in a patient with biliary atresia?
Failure of the Kasai procedure; failure to thrive; recurrent cholangitis; typical signs of end-stage liver disease

CHILD-TURCOTTE-PUGH SCORE OF THE SEVERITY OF LIVER DISEASE

Number of points given to the following conditions …

Encephalopathy
None—1 point
Grade I-II—2 points
Grade III-IV encephalopathy—3 points

Ascites
None—1 point
Slight—2 points
Moderate—3 points

Total bilirubin
Total bilirubin level <2 mg/dL—1 point
Total bilirubin level 2 to 3 mg/dL—2 points
Total bilirubin >3 mg/dL—3 points

PANCREAS TRANPLANT

What are the indications for pancreas transplant?
Type 1 diabetes associated with severe complications (renal failure, blindness, neuropathy) or very poor glucose control

What are the options for placement of a pancreas transplant?
Heterotopic, in iliac fossa or paratopic

What is the associated electrolyte complication with a heterotopic pancreas transplant?
Loss of bicarbonate

Where is the anastomosis of the exocrine duct with a paratopic pancreas transplant?
To the jejunum; advantage endocrine function drains from portal vein directly to liver and pancreatic contents stay within GI tract (no need to replace bicarb)

What are the red flags indicating rejection of a pancreas transplant?
Graft tenderness

Why should a kidney and pancreas be transplanted together if possible?
Kidney function is a better indicator of rejection; better survival of graft associated with kidney-pancreas than pancreas alone

Why is hyperglycemia not a good indicator for rejection surveillance?
Appears relatively late with pancreatic rejection

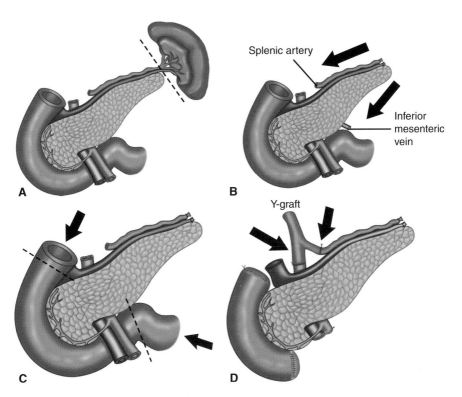

FIGURE 3-1. Bench preparation of pancreas graft. Steps include the following: (**A**) removal of the spleen; (**B**) removal of tissue along the superior and inferior aspect of the tail of the pancreas; (**C**) trimming of excess duodenum; and (**D**) ligation of vessels at the root of the mesentery and placement of arterial Y-graft. *(Reproduced from Brunicardi FC, Andersen DK, Billiar TR, et al. Schwartz's Principles of Surgery. 9th ed. http://www. accessmedicine.com. Copyright © The McGraw-Hill Companies, Inc. All rights reserved.)*

If a combined kidney-pancreas transplant is performed, which organ is usually transplanted first?
The pancreas is usually transplanted first to minimize ischemia time for the pancreas

What is the most commonly used transplant site for pancreatic islet transplantation?
The liver (via portal vein embolization)

HEART TRANSPLANT

What are the indications for heart transplant?
Age birth-65 years with terminal acquired heart disease-class IV of New York Heart Association classification (inability to do any physical activity without discomfort = 10% of surviving 6 months)

What are contraindications for heart transplant?
Active infection; poor pulmonary function; increased pulmonary artery resistance

What are the red flags of rejection of a heart transplant?
Fever, hypotension or hypertension, increased T4/T8 ratio

What are the tests for rejection of a heart transplant?
Endomyocardial biopsy

LUNG TRANSPLANT

What are the indications for lung transplant?
Disease that substantially limits activities of daily living and is likely to result in death within 12 to 18 months: pulmonary fibrosis, COPD, eosinophilic granuloma, primary pulmonary HTN, Eisenmenger syndrome, cystic fibrosis

What are the contraindications for lung transplant?
Current smoking; active infection

What are the donor requirements for lung transplant?
55 years of age or younger; clear CXR, PA oxygen tension = 300 on 100% oxygen and 5 cm PEEP; no purulent secretions on bronchoscopy

What are the necessary anastomoses in a lung transplant?
Anastomoses of the bronchi, pulmonary artery, and pulmonary veins; bronchial artery is not necessary

What are the postoperative complications following lung transplantation?
Bronchial necrosis/stricture; reperfusion; pulmonary edema; rejection

What are the red flags of rejection for a lung transplant?
Decreased arterial oxygen tension; fever; increased fatigability, infiltrate on x-ray

What is chronic lung rejection called?
Obliterative bronchiolitis

INTESTINAL TRANSPLANT

What are the transplant anastomoses in an intestinal transplantation?
Donor SMA to recipient aorta; donor SMV to recipient portal vein

What is the most common indication for intestinal transplant?
Inability to sustain successful TPN because of lack of IV access sites or severe complications from chronic TPN (liver failure)

Name another common immunologic problem other than rejection following intestinal transplantation?
Graft-versus-host disease from large lymphoid tissue in transplanted intestines

What is the most common cause of death after small bowel transplantation?
Sepsis and multiorgan failure

How is rejection surveillance conducted on transplanted intestine?
Endoscopic biopsies

What is the largest lymphoid organ in the human body?
The intestine

POTPOURRI

What is the leading cause of chronic rejection and subsequent graft loss?
Inadequately treated acute rejection

What is the primary cause of late renal allograft loss?
Chronic rejection

What is the most common cause of renal failure in African Americans?
Hypertensive nephrosclerosis

How long is the projected extension in life in a patient with a kidney transplant compared to the same patient on dialysis?
10 years

What are the 3 most common causes of renal failure treated by kidney transplantation?
Diabetes mellitus (27%); glomerular diseases (21%); hypertension (20%)

Absolute contraindication to transplantation?
Infection or malignancy that cannot be eradicated

After the successful treatment of cancer, what is the usual required time period without evidence of disease before transplantation?
2 years

What GFR is required before a patient can become eligible to be listed for a cadaveric kidney?
GFR < 20 mL/min

What does a positive cross-match signify?
The presence of donor-reactive antibodies, detected by incubation of recipient serum with donor cells in the presence of complement

What does a high panel-reactive antibody signify?
A lower likelihood of being cross-match-compatible with a donor

MULTIPLE CHOICE QUESTIONS

1. Pancreatic transplantation is considered a lifesaving procedure in which of the following patients?

   A. 32-year-old F on dialysis secondary to diabetic nephropathy
   B. 46-year-old M with high insulin requirements to maintain normoglycemia
   C. 37-year-old F with episodes of severe hypoglycemic unawareness
   D. 21-year-old F with brittle diabetes

2. Which virus is associated with PTLD?

   A. EBV
   B. HSV
   C. RSV
   D. HIV

3. Which of the following is a complication of calcineurin inhibitors that is LESS pronounced in sirolimus?

   A. Hyperlipidemia
   B. Thrombocytopenia
   C. Rash
   D. Nephrotoxicity

4. **If a patient has tertiary hyperparathyroidism, when should he/she undergo total parathyroidectomy with autotransplantation?**

   A. In 3 months if moderate hypercalcemia persists

   B. In 12 months if hypercalcemia and elevated PTH levels persist

   C. In 6 months if PTH levels are twice normal

   D. Immediately after transplant if PTH levels are greater than normal

5. **Which of the following are the most common indications for liver transplantation in adults and children, respectively?**

   A. Autoimmune hepatitis and inborn errors of metabolism

   B. Malignant neoplasms and biliary atresia

   C. Cholestatic cirrhosis and viral hepatitis

   D. Noncholestatic cirrhosis and biliary atresia

6. **In the Child-Turcotte-Pugh Score, which of the following would be assigned the highest point value in a patient with cryptogenic cirrhosis?**

   A. INR—2.2

   B. Ascites—moderate

   C. Albumin—2.7

   D. Encephalopathy—none

7. **Which of the following is the active component of azathioprine?**

   A. 12-mercaptoprimer

   B. 3-mercaptopurine

   C. 6-mercaptopyrimidine

   D. 6-mercaptopurine

8. **In a patient who has recently undergone a cadaveric renal transplant, which of the following is a correct pairing between a virus and the appropriate medication to treat it?**

   A. HSV—ritonavir

   B. CMV—ganciclovir

   C. EBV—lamivudine

   D. CMV—acyclovir

9. **What is the number one cause of early mortality after lung transplantation?**

   A. Pneumonia

   B. Acute rejection

   C. Bronchopleural fistula

   D. Reperfusion injury

10. **What is the disease most likely to recur in a new liver allograft?**

    A. Hepatitis B

    B. Hepatitis C

    C. Hepatitis D

    D. CMV

ANSWERS

1. **Answer: C.** 37-year-old F with episodes of severe hypoglycemic unawareness. Over time, patients with multiple episodes of hypoglycemia may not experience typical symptoms. Therefore, hypoglycemia can become severe resulting in neurologic injury.

2. **Answer: A.** EBV. Immunosuppression allows B cells that are infected with EBV to proliferate.

3. **Answer: D.** Nephrotoxicity. Sirolimus can be used for immunosuppression in patients with renal transplants if there is evidence of caclineurin inhibitor induced nephropathy on biopsies.

4. **Answer: B.** In 12 months if hypercalcemia and elevated PTH levels persist. A diagnosis of tertiary hyperparathyroidism warrants surgical correction so that consequences (osteomalacia and renal osteodystrophy) of the disease do not ensue.

5. **Answer: D.** Noncholestatic cirrhosis (65%) in adults—includes viral hepatitis (B and C), alcoholic and cryptogenic cirrhosis; biliary atresia (58%) in children.

   Although the diseases listed above are the most common indications for liver transplants, there are many others. They include:

   - Cholestatic liver disease/cirrhosis (eg, primary biliary cirrhosis, primary sclerosing cholangitis, Caroli disease, and biliary atresia)
   - Fulminant liver failure (eg, acetaminophen overdose or other drug-induced toxicity, hepatitis, ischemia)
   - Metabolic diseases (eg, α1-antitrypsin deficiency, Crigler-Najjar disease, etc)
   - Malignant neoplasms
   - Budd-Chiari syndrome
   - Benign neoplasms
   - TPN

6. **Answer: C.** Albumin—2.7—would get 3 points

Child-Turcotte-Pugh Score			
	Points		
	1	2	3
Encephalopathy	None	1–2	3–4
Ascites	Absent	Slight	Moderate
Bilirubin (g/dL)	<2	2–3	>3
For PBC/PSC	<4	4–10	>10
Albumin (g/dL)	>3.5	2.8–3.5	<2.8
PT (INR)	<1.7	1.7–2.3	>2.3

7. **Answer: D.** 6-MP (6-mercaptopurine)

   - (Hepatic conversion) Azathioprine → 6-mercaptopurine (6-MP) → 6-thioinosine monophosphate (6-tIMP)
   - 6-MP and 6tIMP cause alkylation of DNA precursors and also deplete cells of adenosine by inhibiting conversion of IMP to adenosine monophosphate and guanosine monophosphate.

8. **Answer: B.** CMV—ganciclovir. Acyclovir and ganciclovir are used to treat herpesviruses. Although acyclovir has some activity against CMV, ganciclovir is more effective against CMV. Acyclovir is more effective in treating HSV, herpes zoster, and EBV.

9. **Answer: D.** Reperfusion injury. The most common cause of early death (within 90 days from transplant) is primary graft failure. Infection is the second most common cause of early death, followed by heart failure, then hemorrhage and airway dehiscence, and less commonly rejection. Infection is the most common cause of late deaths following pulmonary transplantation.

10. **Answer: B.** Hepatitis C. HCV has universal recurrence after transplant. Compared with HCV-negative donors, graft and patient survival are comparable when HCV-positive donors are used for HCV-positive recipients.

CHAPTER 4
Infection and Antibiotics

Dale A. Dangleben, James Lee, and Firas Madbak

Familiarize yourself with the table below for wound classification and general indication for antibiotic therapy.

WOUNDS

Name factors that influence the development of infection:
Poor approximation of tissue, hematoma/seroma, hypothermia, long operation
(>2 hours), excessive local tissue destruction/necrotic tissue, low blood flow, foreign body, dead space, and strangulation of tissues by tight sutures

Wound Class	Definition	Infection Rate
Clean	Nontraumatic, elective wound without acute inflammation	2%
Clean-contaminated	Wounds associated with operation on biliary, GU tract, or respiratory or GI tract without gross contamination	3%–5%
Contaminated	Traumatic wound, GI tract spillage, acute inflammation, or a major break in sterile technique	5%–10%
Dirty	Dirty traumatic wound, perforated viscous, or presence of pus	30%

Most common nosocomial infection:
Urinary tract infection (UTI)

How many colony-forming units (CFUs) are needed on urine culture to confirm a diagnosis of UTI?
>100,000 CFU

Most common nosocomial infection causing death:
Pneumonia

Overall most common organism in surgical wound infections:
Staphylococcus aureus

Most common anaerobe in surgical wound infections:
Bacteroides fragilis

When do wound infection classically arise?
Postoperative day 5 to 7

Treatment for a wound infection:
Remove sutures/staples, culture wound, examine to rule out fascial dehiscence, leave wound open and pack, start antibiotics

Bacteria that will cause wound infection and fever within 24 hours after surgery:
Group A β-hemolytic *Streptococcus* and *Clostridium perfringens*

Organisms that can cause necrotizing soft tissue infections:
Group A β-hemolytic *Streptococcus* and *Clostridium perfringens*

Usual organism to cause necrotizing fasciitis:
Polymicrobial (anaerobes with gram-negative organisms)

Time period to wait before obtaining a CT scan to look for postoperative abscess:
>POD no. 7 (otherwise abscess may look like normal post-op fluid collection)

Findings on CT scan to indicate abscess:
Gas in fluid collection, fibrous ring surrounding fluid collection

Usual initial treatment for intraabdominal abscess:
Percutaneous drainage

Most common bacteria to cause a line infection:
Staphylococcus epidermidis

How many CFUs are needed from a central line culture to indicate line infection?
>15 CFU

In what instance should a central line be changed over a guidewire?
Fever without obvious external signs of infection (catheter tip culture should be sent)

A line changed over a guidewire can be left in place with what catheter tip culture result:
<15 CFU from previous line culture

A line change over a guidewire should be discontinued and a new line should be placed at a new site with this culture result:
>15 CFU from previous line culture

Term for blanching erythema from superficial epidermal/dermal infection:
Cellulitis

Name the classic signs and symptoms of infection/inflammation:
Rubor (redness), calor (heat), dolor (pain), tumor (swelling)

Most common pathogen to cause bacterial meningitis in a patient with cerebrospinal fluid rhinorrhea:
Streptococcus pneumoniae

True or false: Prophylactic antibiotics have proven benefit to prevent bacterial meningitis in a patient with cerebrospinal fluid rhinorrhea?
False. Prophylactic antibiotics have shown no proven benefit and may predispose to meninigitis with antibiotic-resistant bacteria.

Empiric treatment for a patient with cerebrospinal fluid rhinorrhea who develops bacterial meningitis:
Vancomycin and an extended-spectrum cephalosporin (ceftriaxone, cefepime, or cefotaxime)

Term for infection/abscess formation in apocrine sweat glands:
Suppurative hidradenitis

Name the locations at which suppurative hidradenitis may occur:
Any site with apocrine glands: axilla, buttocks/perineum, and inguinal area

Most common organism involved in suppurative hidradenitis:
Staphylococcus aureus

What is the treatment for suppurative hidradenitis:
Antibiotics, incision and drainage, excision of skin for chronic infections

Microscopic finding associated with *Actinomyces* infection:
Sulfur granules

Antibiotic of choice for *Actinomyces* infection:
Penicillin G

ANTIFUNGAL

Name clinical situations that require systemic antifungal therapy:
Candida endophthalmitis, osteomyelitis, septic arthritis, and endocarditis, or any patient with a single positive blood culture from an indwelling intravascular catheter

Treatment for mucocutaneous candidiasis:
Local clotrimazole or nystatin

Treatment for *Candida* isolated from a surgical drain:
Nothing, most likely represents colonization

Mechanism of action of voriconazole:
Prevents the production of ergosterol by acting as a selective inhibitor of the fungal cytochrome P-450 system

Mechanism of action of caspofungin:
Inhibits the synthesis of an essential fungal cell wall component; β-(1-3)-D-glycan

Mechanism of action of amphotericin B:
Increases permeability of the fungal cell membrane by binding ergosterol, which causes leakage of macromolecules and intracellular ions leading to cell death

SPONTANEOUS BACTERIAL PERITONITIS

True or false: Spontaneous bacterial peritonitis (SBP) is usually a polymicrobial infection?
False. SBP is a monomicrobial infection.

Most frequent organism responsible for SBP:
Escherichia coli followed by *Klebsiella pneumoniae*

True or false: SBP results from translocation of gut flora?
False. It is thought to be from the combination of impaired bactericidal activity of ascitic fluid, abnormal host defense, and intrahepatic shunting, which leads to prolonged bacteremia.

The ascitic fluid protein concentration associated with 10-fold increased risk of SBP:
<1 g/100 mL

Who should be admitted and treated for SBP?
All symptomatic patients with a peritoneal fluid polymorphonuclear count of 250 to 500 cells/µL

Current antibiotic regime for SBP:
Third-generation cephalosporin (cefotaxime)

What does cefotaxime not cover?
Enterococci

HEPATITIS/HIV/TB

Which is the most likely blood-borne organism to be transmitted after a hollow bore needle stick?
Hepatitis B

Recommendation for a nonimmune health care worker exposed to hepatitis B:
Begin hepatitis B vaccination series and give hepatitis B immunoglobulin within 7 days of the exposure

Recommendation for a health care worker vaccinated against hepatitis B but whose immune status is unknown and is exposed to a patient with active hepatitis B infection:
Determine immune status. If anti-hep B antibody–positive—no intervention; If anti-hep B antibody–negative—hep B vaccine booster with hep B immunoglobulin

Prophylaxis for a nonimmune health care worker exposed to hepatitis C:
No postexposure prophylaxis for hepatitis C

Method to diagnose and the treatment for lymphogranuloma venereum:
Serologic testing and treatment with oral doxycycline 100 mg BID × 21 days

Name risk factors that increase the risk of transmission of HIV after percutaneous injury:
Deep puncture injury, visible blood present on a sharp object causing injury, injury from object present within a blood vessel of the source patient, and injury involving a source patient with advanced HIV (CD4 count <50 cells/mm^3)

Time period to start postexposure prophylaxis for HIV in a high-risk injury:
Within 72 hours

Most common intestinal manisfestation of AIDS:
Cytomegalovirus (CMV) colitis

Most common cause of upper gastrointestinal (GI) bleed in AIDS:
Kaposi sarcoma

Most common cause of lower GI bleed in AIDS:
CMV

Most common anorectal lesion in a patient with HIV:
Anal condylomata

Normal CD4 count:
800 to 1200 cells/mm^3

CD4 count associated with symptomatic disease:
300 to 400 cells/mm^3

CD4 count associated with opportunistic infections:
<200 cells/mm^3

Prophylaxis is given to this organism when an HIV-infected patient has a CD4 count <200 cells/mm^3:
Pneumocystis carinii

Recommended prophylaxis for *Pneumocystis carinii*:
Bactrim (trimethoprim/sulfamethoxazole)

Prophylaxis is given to this organism when an HIV-infected patient has a CD4 count <50 cells/mm^3:
Mycobacterium avium

Recommended prophylaxis for *Mycobacterium avium*:
Azithromycin

Greatest known risk factor for the reactivation of latent tuberculosis infection:
HIV infection

Recommended 4 drug treatments for patients with active pulmonary tuberculosis:
Isoniazid, rifampin, pyrazinamide, and ethambutol for 2 months; if drug-susceptible and negative sputum cultures can complete treatment with isoniazid and rifampin for 4 months

ANTIBIOTICS/MECHANISM OF ACTION

Name bactericidal antimicrobial agents:
Aminoglycosides, bactrim, β-lactams, carbapenems, cephalosporins, daptomycin, metronidazole, monobactams, nitrofurantoin, quinolones, vancomycin

Name bacteriostatic antimicrobial agents:
Chloramphenicol, clindamycin, erythromycin, lincosamides, linezolid, macrolides, spectinomycin, sulfonamides, tetracyclines, trimethoprim

Mechanism of action of aminoglycosides:
Interferes with ribosomal protein synthesis and disrupts cell wall cation homeostasis affecting the integrity of the bacterial cell membrane

Mechanism of action of bactrim:

Sulfamethoxazole is an analogue of *p*-aminobenzoic acid and acts as a false-substrate inhibitor of dihydropteroate synthetase ultimately inhibiting the production of dihydropteroic acid.

Trimethoprim interferes with dihydrofolate reductase inhibiting the synthesis of tetrahydrofolic acid.

Mechanism of action of β-lactams:

Interferes with cross-linking of peptidoglycan (primary component in the cell wall of a Gram-positive bacteria) by covalently binding to and inactivating a bacterium's transpeptidase enzymes

What are carbapenems?

A class of β-lactam antibiotics that are highly resistant to β-lactamases with a broad spectrum of antibacterial activity

The only β-lactams capable of inhibiting L,D-transpeptidases:

Carbapenems

Mechanism of action of cephalosporins:

Disrupt the synthesis of the peptidoglycan layer of the bacterial cell wall

Mechanism of action of daptomycin:

Binds to the membrane and causes rapid depolarization resulting in a loss of membrane potential leading to inhibition of protein, DNA, and RNA synthesis, resulting in bacterial cell death

Mechanism of action of metronidazole:

Once taken up by anaerobes, it is nonenzymatically reduced by reacting with reduced ferredoxin, resulting in the production of toxic products, which are taken up into bacterial DNA and form unstable molecules.

Mechanism of action of nitrofurantoin:

Rapid reduction of nitrofurantoin inside the bacterial cell by flavoproteins (nitrofuran reductase) leads to multiple reactive intermediates that attack DNA, pyruvate metabolism, respiration, ribosomal proteins, and other macromolecules within the cell

Mechanism of action of quinolones:

Inhibits bacterial DNA gyrase and topoisomerase IV, leading to inhibition of DNA replication and transcription

Mechanism of action of vancomycin:

Prevents incorporation of *N*-acetylmuramic acid and *N*-acetylglucosamine peptide subunits into the peptidoglycan matrix (major structural component of Gram-positive cell wall)

Mechanism of action of chloramphenicol:

Inhibits peptidyl transferase activity by binding to A2451 and A2452 residues in the 23S rRNA of the 50S ribosomal subunit, thus preventing peptide bond formation and protein synthesis

Mechanism of action of clindamycin:
Inhibits ribosomal translocation by binding preferentially to the 23S rRNA of the large bacterial ribosome subunit, thus preventing protein synthesis

Mechanism of action of erythromycin:
Interferes with aminoacyl translocation (prevents transfer of tRNA bound at A site of rRNA complex to P site) and inhibits protein synthesis by binding to the 50S subunit of the bacterial 70S rRNA complex

Mechanism of action of lincosamides:
Causes premature dissociation of the peptidyl-tRNA from the ribosome by binding to the 23S portion of the 50S subunit of bacterial ribosomes

Mechanism of action of linezolid:
Binds to the 23S portion of the 50S subunit and prevents the formation of the initiation complex (30S and 50S subunits of the ribosome, tRNA, and mRNA)

Mechanism of action of spectinomycin:
Binds to the 30S ribosomal subunit and disrupts protein synthesis

Mechanism of action of sulfonamides:
Competitive inhibitor of the enzyme dihydropteroate synthetase

Mechanism of action of tetracyclines:
Prevents the docking of aminoacylated tRNA by binding the 30S ribosomal subunit, which interacts with 16S rRNA

The only tissue that cefazolin does not penetrate well:
Central nervous system

What are the appropriate vancomycin peak and trough values?
Peak 20 to 40 μg/mL and trough 5 to 10 μg/mL

What are the appropriate gentamicin peak and trough values?
Peak 5 to 10 μg/mL and trough <1 μg/mL

Mechanism of acquired vancomycin resistance:
Alteration to the terminal amino acid residues of the NAM/NAG peptide subunits that vancomycin binds

Name the 3 known mechanisms of fluoroquinolone resistance:
1. Efflux pumps that decrease intracellular quinolone concentration
2. Plasmid-mediated resistance genes that produce proteins, which bind to and protect DNA gyrase
3. Decreased binding affinity from mutations at key sites in DNA gyrase or topoisomerase IV

Usual mechanism of penicillin resistance:
Plasmids that code for β-lactamase

Mechanisms for aminoglycoside resistance:
Enzymatic modification (most common), reduced uptake or decreased cell permeability, and altered ribosome-binding sites

MULTIPLE CHOICE QUESTIONS

1. **You are preparing your patient for a colostomy reversal. The procedure is scheduled for 9 AM. The junior resident asks you about the timing of giving prophylactic antibiotics to the patient. Your response is:**
   A. Six hours prior to incision
   B. One hour to making incision
   C. One hour after making the incision
   D. At the time of incision

2. **A 65-year-old female is readmitted 3 weeks after being admitted for pneumonia and treated with antibiotics for a week. Her major complaint is worsening diarrhea. *Clostridium difficile* is sent and comes back positive. Which antibiotic would you choose?**
   A. IV vancomycin
   B. Metronidazole
   C. Clindamycin
   D. Cefepime

3. **What is one of the usual mechanism of penicillin resistance?**
   A. Dissociation of the peptidyl-tRNA
   B. Efflux pumps
   C. Plasmids that code for β-lactamase
   D. Cross-linking of peptidoglycan

4. **During the repair of an incisional hernia, you inadvertently create 2 enterotomies. Some intestinal content has spilled into the incision. The circulating nurse asks you for the wound classification.**
   A. Clean
   B. Clean contaminated
   C. Contaminated
   D. Dirty

5. **A 44-year-old male is found to have a mycotic aneurysm. Which of the following is the most likely bacteria involved?**
   A. *Salmonella*
   B. *Klebsiella*
   C. *Streptococcus*
   D. *Staphylococcus*

6. **Abscess with yellow-brown particles resembling sulphur granules is associated with which of the following?**
   A. Actinomycosis
   B. Histoplasmosis
   C. Blastomycosis
   D. Listeriosis

7. **Which of the following antibiotics is associated with gallbladder sludge and cholestatic jaundice?**
   A. Vancomycin
   B. Metronidazole
   C. Clindamycin
   D. Cefepime
   E. Ceftriaxone

8. **Fluconazole is ineffective against which of the following *Candida* species?**
   A. *Candida kefyr*
   B. *Candida krusei*
   C. *Candida marina*
   D. *Candida tropicalis*
   E. *Candida rugosa*

9. **A 50-year-old farmer stepped on a nail approximately 5 hours ago. He now presents with pain and redness around the puncture site in his right foot. Initial gram stain shows large pleomorphic Gram-positive rods and an x-ray of the right foot shows air in the soft tissues. Which of the following would provide the best initial antibiotic coverage?**
   A. Tigecycline
   B. Daptomycin
   C. Linezolid and metronidazole
   D. Combination therapy with penicillin G 10 to 24 million U/d and clindamycin

10. **Which portion of endotoxin, found in the outer membrane of Gram-negative bacteria, is responsible for its toxic effects?**
    A. O-antigen
    B. Outer core
    C. Inner core
    D. Lipid A

ANSWERS

1. **Answer: B.** It has been shown that antibiotic administration 30 minutes to an hour to skin incision is adequate. At the time of incision, adequate tissue concentration of the antibiotic should be achieved. This will not occur if given at the time of incision and definitely not after an hour after making incision.

2. **Answer: B.** The treatment for *Clostridium difficile* infection is IV metronidazole or oral vancomycin. Clindamycin and cephalosporins are actual offenders.

3. **Answer: C.** The usual mechanism of penicillin resistance is through plasmids that code for β-lactamase. Most β-lactam antibiotics work by inhibiting cell wall synthesis. Some bacteria produce β-lactamase, which hydrolyzes the β-lactam ring within the antibiotic, making it ineffective. One known mechanism of fluoroquinolone resistance is via efflux pumps that decrease intracellular quinolone concentration.

The mechanism of action of lincosamides is through the premature dissociation of the peptidyl-tRNA from the ribosome by binding to the 23S portion of the 50S subunit of bacterial ribosomes. The interference of cross-linking of peptidoglycan is the mechanism of action of β-lactams where there is cross-linking of peptidoglycan by covalently binding to and inactivating a bacterium's transpeptidase enzymes.

4. **Answer: C.** A nontraumatic, elective wound without acute inflammation such as a thyroidectomy is a clean wound with a 2% infection rate. Anyway wound associated with surgery on the biliary tree, genitourinary tract, respiratory, and GI tract without gross contamination is considered a clean contaminated wound and has an infection rate of 3% to 5%. A contaminated wound has an infection rate of more than 10%. Traumatic wound, GI tract spillage, acute inflammation, or a major break in sterile technique are considered contaminated. A dirty traumatic wound, perforated viscus, or presence of pus is a dirty wound and has an infection rate of 30%.

5. **Answer: D.** A mycotic aneurysm is bacterial infection of the aorta. Currently, the most common bacteria associated with mycotic aneurysms is *Staphylococcus aureus*. *Salmonella* used to be the most common organism but that is no longer the case.

6. **Answer: A.** Actinomycosis infections present with granulomas and abscess (sinus tracts). It can be caused by any of the *Actinomyces* species (eg, *A israelii*). It is Gram-positive and part of the normal flora primarily in the nose and oropharyngeal area. Most infections are in the head and neck. The purulence is yellow and resembles sulphur granules. Histoplasmosis is fungal, found primarily in river valleys, (eg, Mississippi) and diagnosis is made by antibody complement fixation. *Blastomyces* is a dimorphic soil fungus that can be demonstrated with standard KOH preparations. Listeriosis is an infection caused by the Gram-positive bacteria *L monocytogenes* from the ingestion of infected food. Severe infections result in meningitis.

7. **Answer: E.** Ceftriaxone is known to precipitate particularly when administered with calcium-containing solutions. The ceftriaxone-calcium complex can mimic cholelithiasis and gallbladder sludge, which usually resolves when the antibiotic is discontinued.

8. **Answer: B.** In general, fluconazole is active against most *Candida* species with the exception of *C krusei* and *C glabrata*. *Candida krusei* can be successfully treated with voriconazole and amphotericin B and caspofungin.

9. **Answer: D.** This patient has necrotizing myositis, or gas gangrene, from infection with *Clostridium perfringens*. The most widely used antibiotic regimen is a combination of penicillin and clindamycin. The combination of clindamycin and metronidazole can be used for penicillin-allergic patients. The newer antibiotics used for treating complicated skin and soft tissues infections, such as tigecycline, linezolid, and daptomycin, have not been studied in patients with gas gangrene.

10. **Answer: D.** Lipid A is responsible for the toxic effects of endotoxin. The O-antigen is a repetitive glycan polymer. The outer and inner core connect the O-antigen to lipid A.

CHAPTER 5
Pharmacology

Peter Bechtel

MECHANICS

What are some basic drug properties?
Absorption, distribution, metabolism, elimination

What is first-order kinetics?
Drug dose determines quantity eliminated (dose-dependent elimination)

What is zero-order kinetics?
Also known as Hoffman elimination: constant drug quantity eliminated per unit time

What is the primary role of the P450 system?
Primary drug oxidizers

What are some of the inducers of the P450 system?
Cigarette smoke, phenobarbital, rifampin, ethanol, INH, phenytoin, etc

What are some of the inhibitors of the P450 system?
Grapefruit, erythromycin, nelfinavir, itraconazole, etc

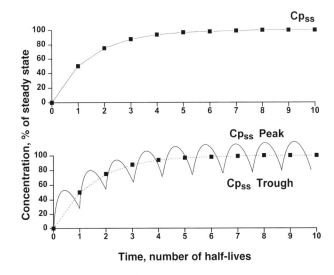

FIGURE 5-1. Drug administration by continuous intravenous infusion (upper panel) or intermittent intravenous bolus (lower panel). Attainment of steady-state plasma concentration (Cp_{ss}) occurs after 3 to 5 half-lives, regardless of the dosing regimen. Peak and trough fluctuations around Cp_{ss} are aimed to each be within the therapeutic range (therapeutic but subtoxic plasma levels). *(Reproduced from Hall JB, Schmidt GA, Wood LDH. Principles of Critical Care. 3rd ed. http://www.accessmedicine.com. Copyright © The McGraw-Hill Companies, Inc. All rights reserved.)*

What is half-life of a drug?
Purpose of dosing by half-life is to achieve steady-state concentration. Typical drugs reach steady state after 5 half-lives

What is a Phase I reaction?
Nonsynthetic reaction, for example, oxidation/reduction, *NOT* conjugation

What is a Phase II reaction?
Synthetic reaction, for example, conjugation, methylation, sulfation, etc

GASTROINTESTINAL

ESOPHAGUS

What are some treatments for achalasia?
Calcium channel blockers, long-acting nitrates, botulinum toxin injections

What is the management for esophageal varices bleeding?
Vasopressin (splanchnic vasoconstrictor at V1 receptors, increases factor VIII and VWF via extrarenal V2 receptors). Propanolol/Nadolol (preventative role; inhibits B2 adrenergic splanchnic vasodilation). Nitrates (reduce portal venous pressure)

What are some treatment options for reflux disease?
Selective H_2 blockers (cimetidine, ranitidine, etc) = 24-hour acid reduction by 70%. Proton pump inhibitors (pantoprazole, omeprazole, etc) = 10% rebound hyperacidity after discontinuing due to hypergastrinemia

STOMACH

What are the D_2 agonists motility agents and how do they work?
Domperidone and metoclopramide, they increase lower esophageal sphincter (LES) tone, increase antrum contraction, increase small bowel peristalsis (beware of extrapyramidal symptoms [EPS] and tardive side effects)

How does erythromycin work as motility agent?
Motilin agonists, it amplifies Phase III activity via migrating motor complex

What are the general categories of antiemetics?
Serotonin receptor antagonist (ondansetron)
Compazine (ill-defined μ-opiate agonists [MOA])
Nonselective antihistamine/H_1 blocker (Phenergan)
Substance P antagonist (aprepitant)

How do you treat peptic ulcer disease?
See H_2 blockers and proton pump inhibitors (PPIs) above
Misoprostol (prostaglandin E_2) increases mucin production, decreases intracellular cyclic AMP (cAMP), and therefore acid reduction—used in "type 5" ulcers
Sucralfate = sucrose plus aluminum hydroxide (coats gastric lining, resists pepsin)
Bismuth (adjunct to antibiotics in setting of *Helicobacter pylori*)

What is the treatment for *Helicobacter pylori*?
PPI plus 2 antibiotics (usually Clarithromycin plus either amoxicillin or metronidazole) Bismuth occasionally used as adjunct. (*Note:* Gastric mucosa-associated lymphoid tissue [MALT] can be treated by *Helicobacter pylori* eradication)

What chemotherapeutic agent is used for gastrointestinal stromal tumors (GIST)?
Imatinib (Gleevec): tyrosine kinase inhibitor at Philadelphia chromosome

SMALL BOWEL

List of medications used in the management of inflammatory bowel disease.
Corticosteroids, Sulfasalazine, Mesalamine, Metronidazole, immunosuppression (azathioprine, 6-mercaptopurine, cyclosporine, methotrexate)

COLON

Bowel preparations

- Magnesium based (mag-citrate, mag-hydroxide, mag-sulfate, etc)
- Phosphate based (fleets phospha-soda, sodium phosphate, etc)
- Both exert main mechanism of action by osmotic draw of fluid into bowel lumen phosphate preparations moderately absorbed, caution in renal impairment
- Lactulose, sorbitol, mannitol: all act by osmotic MOA
- Polyethylene glycol (Golytely, Miralax): nonabsorbable long-chain polyethylene glycol molecules. Bowel mixed with isotonic electrolyte solutions to prevent metabolic derangement

INTRA-OP

Used to relax the sphincter of Oddi in setting of common bile duct stones and also for intestinal smooth muscle relaxation to accommodate sizers/staplers:
Glucagon

What dyes can be used to evaluate integrity of viscus, ureter, etc?
Methylene blue, indigo carmine

This can be used as an adjunct to determine intestinal perfusion:
Fluorescein

This agent aids in sentinel lymph node biopsy (some patients have severe anaphalytic reaction, risk less than 1%):
Lymphazurin

PANCREAS

Pancreatic enzyme replacement:
Pancreatin
Lipase, protease, amylase formulations (viokase, ku zyme, pancrease, Creon, Ultrase)

What prophylaxis may be used in the setting of necrotizing pancreatitis (controversial)?
Adequate penetrance of pancreas tissue: imipenem, third-generation cephalosporins, piperacillin, mezlocillin, fluoroquinolones, metronidazole

What drugs are implicated in pharmacologic pancreatitis?
Anti-inflammatories: Sulfasalazine, Sulindac, Salicylates
Immunosuppressants: Azathioprine, 6-mercaptopurine
Diuretics: diazoxide, ethacrynic acid, furosemide, thiazides
Antibiotics: Didanosine, metronidazole, tetracycline, nitrofurantoin, pentamidine, Trimethoprim-sulfamethoxazole

ENDOCRINE

List the antihyperthyroid agents:
Thionamides: Methimazole and Propothiouracil: inhibit oxidation of iodide to iodine. PTU, as well, prevents T_4 to T_3 conversion
>Agranulocytosis most common serious adverse side effect of thionamides
Ionic inhibitors: Lugol iodine (potassium iodide): inhibits thyroglobulin proteolysis as well as TH release. May reduce gland vascularity if resection planned
Radioactive ablation (I^{131}) electron-generating concentration of isotope leads to cytotoxicity
Imaging
Technetium 99, Iodine^{123}, PET (fluorodeoxyglucose), SestaMIBI
Hormone replacement
Levothyroxine, liothyronine
advantage of liothyronine is lessened suppression of TRH/TSH axis

What is the treatment of hypercalcemia?
IVF rehydration
Loop diuretic
Bisphosphonates (Pamidronate, Zoledronic acid)
Vitamin D analogues (calcitriol, doxercalciferol, cinacalcet)

How do you treat hypoparathyroid tetany (severe hypocalcemia)?
IV calcium gluconate, oral calcium, vitamin D, magnesium

What is the Cosyntropin test?
0.25 mg Cosyntropin IV, after 30 minutes rise in cortisol to minimum 20 mcg/dL

What is the treatment of adrenal insufficiency?
Glucocorticoid = hydrocortisone
Mineralocorticoid = fludrocortisone
Sex steroid replacement: DHEA (primarily in women)

Which medications may suppress ACTH secretion?
Metyrapone, octreotide, ketoconazole

Treatment includes administration of K^+ sparing diuretic (spironolactone):
Hyperaldosteronism

Treated preoperatively with α-adrenergic blockade (phenoxybenzamine) calcium channel blockers can be used as adjunct but avoid β-blockers:
Pheochromocytoma

VASCULAR

Medications indicated for claudication:
Cilostazol: cellular phosphodiesterase inhibitor
Pentoxyfylline: increases RBC pliability/flexibility

List the antiplatelets:
Aspirin: irreversible block of thromboxane production
Dipyridamole: increases platelet cAMP
Ticlodipine and Clopidogrel: inhibits ADP-induced aggregation
Glycoprotein IIb/IIIa inhibitors (abciximab, eptifibatide, tinofiban)

List the anticoagulants:
Heparin-inhibits antithrombin—dose-dependent half-life: 100, 400, 800 u/kg = 1, 2.5, 5 hours
Low-molecular-weight heparin (enoxaparin, dalteparin, etc)
Direct thrombin inhibitor (lepirudin, bivalirudin, argatroban). Caution lepirudin in renal failure (use argatroban), dose reduces argatroban in liver failure (use lepirudin). Ximelagatran = first approved oral thrombin inhibitor
Factor Xa inhibitors (danaparoid, fondaparinux) 24-hour half-life
Warfarin—inhibits Vitamin K-dependent cofactors: II, VII, IX, X, C, and S

List the available thrombolytics and their functions:
Plasminogen: enhances fibrinolysis
Streptokinase: binds plasminogen enhancing conversion to plasmin
Tissue plasminogen activator: self-explanatory
Aminocaproic acid: potential antidote in case of overdose. Competes for lysine-binding sites and blocks interaction of plasmin with fibrin

How does protamine work? Dosage?
Binds heparin ionically. Dose = 1 to 1.5 mg/100 units reduce as time after heparin administration increases. Half-life is unknown.

CENTRAL NERVOUS SYSTEM/ANESTHESIA

Functions via the GABA receptor (agonists):
Benzodiazepines/Barbiturates

It induces hypnotic state, has a caloric content of 1.1 kcal/mL (lipid), and is contraindicated in patients with egg allergy:
Propofol

Opioids work via which receptors?
μ, κ, δ

What are the conscious altering medications?
Ketamine—increases intracerebral pressure; do not use in head injury
Etomidate—large infusions adrenal suppressing

Name the depolarizing paralytic agent:
Succinylcholine (risk of malignant hyperthermia—stop drug, give dantrolene. Patients with atypical pseudocholinesterases can have unusual prolonged duration of action)

What are the nondepolarizing agents?
Competitive acetylcholine inhibitors (rocuronium, pancuronium, mivacurium, cis-atracurium, etc). Cis-atracurium undergoes Hoffman elimination, making it safe in patients with liver/renal dysfunction

What is the role of a "reversal" agent and how do they work?
Intended to curb effect of paralytics (neostigmine, edrophonium) act by blocking acetylcholinesterase, leaving more acetylcholine to overcome original competing drug

Used preoperatively (antimuscarinic) to reduce salivary, tracheobronchial, and pharyngeal secretions:
Glycopyrrolate, atropine

List the inhaled agents:
Nitrous oxide halothane, enflurane, isoflurane, sevoflurane

What is minimal alveolar concentration (MAC)?
Lowest degree of drug concentration causing 50% of patients to not respond to noxious stimuli. High MAC is less potent. Low MAC is highly lipid soluble (think brain tissue) and highly potent

What is the mechanism of action of most local anesthetics?
Blocks sodium channel ATPase increasing threshold for action potential.
(*Note:* general maximum dose of lidocaine is 7 mg/kg if using with epinephrine, 4.5 mg/kg if using preparation without epinephrine

MULTIPLE CHOICE QUESTIONS

1. **Rank the following compounds in decreasing order of antisecretory efficacy (going from most efficacious to least efficacious).**
   A. Atropine, famotidine (Pepcid), omeprazole (Prilosec)
   B. Famotidine, atropine, omeprazole
   C. Famotidine, omeprazole, atropine
   D. Omeprazole, atropine, famotidine
   E. Omeprazole, famotidine, atropine

2. **Which of the following should be used for treatment of severe diarrhea in an infant, until the cause of the diarrhea can be treated adequately?**
   A. Attapulgite suspension (Kaopectate)
   B. Cholestyramine (Questran)
   C. Doxycycline (Vibramycin)
   D. An electrolyte replenisher (such as Pedialyte)
   E. An opiate such as loperamide (Imodium)

3. **A patient presents with 15 lb of unintentional weight loss in the last 3 months, tremor, tachycardia, hot skin, and protruding eyeballs. The drug of choice for long-term (months) treatment of this condition would be:**
   A. Levothyroxine (Synthroid)
   B. Liothyronine (Cytomel)
   C. Potassium iodide
   D. Propranolol (Inderal)
   E. Propylthiouracil (PTU)

4. **Corticosteroids produce their effects by binding to:**
   A. Cytoplasmic receptors that affect nuclear expression of genes
   B. G-protein-coupled receptors that activate adenylate cyclase
   C. G-protein-coupled receptors that activate phospholipase C
   D. Ion channels that promote depolarization of cells
   E. Membrane receptors that activate tyrosine kinase

5. **A male patient known to have adrenal insufficiency (Addison disease) has been involved in an automobile accident. Although there is no obvious physical injury, he complains of weakness and nausea. His blood pressure is 85/50 mm Hg, and he is hypoglycemic. Treatment of his condition should include:**
   A. IV administration of cortisol
   B. IV administration of dexamethasone (Decadron)
   C. IV administration of prednisone
   D. IV administration of spironolactone (Aldactone)

6. **A postmenopausal woman desires the benefits of estrogen therapy in the reduction or prevention of osteoporosis, but is concerned about the possibility of increased risk of breast cancer. An appropriate agent for treating this patient may be:**
   A. Estradiol
   B. Ethinyl estradiol
   C. Mifepristone (RU 486)
   D. Raloxifene (Evista)
   E. Testosterone

7. **A broad-spectrum antibiotic such as doxycycline may reduce the effectiveness of oral contraceptive preparations by:**
   A. Increasing levels of free LH and FSH
   B. Increasing the viscosity of cervical mucus
   C. Reducing levels of free estrogen
   D. Reducing levels of free progestin
   E. Reducing transit time of ova in the Fallopian tube

8. **A patient with prolonged renal failure requiring hemodialysis requires surgery. Which of the following is the best choice of paralytic for the prolonged duration of the procedure?**
   A. Vecuronium
   B. Rocuronium
   C. cis-atricurium
   D. Succynlcholine

9. **After upper endoscopy reveals a submucosal tumor in the distal stomach, a 56-year-old patient undergoes surgical resection. Post-op chemotherapy is indicated based on tumor stage. Which of the following is the best choice?**
   A. 5-flourouracil
   B. Imatinib
   C. Cisplatin
   D. None of the above

10. **After upper endoscopy is performed on a 46-year-old patient, biopsies confirm MALT lymphoma. Which of the following is the best initial chemical treatment of this lesion?**

   A. 5-fluorouracil with cisplatin
   B. Imatinib with sucralfate
   C. Esomeprazole, clarithromycin, amoxicillin
   D. Bismuth with vincristine

ANSWERS

1. **Answer: E.** Proton pump inhibitors virtually completely block acid secretion; histamine-2 blockers reduce acid secretion by 70% to 95% (usually); muscarinic blockers typically reduce secretion by 25% to 50%.

2. **Answer: D.** The priority is to prevent serious fluid and electrolyte imbalance until source of diarrhea can be eradicated.

3. **Answer: E.** A and B are incorrect because the patient is already hyperthyroid. C would have a short-term effect but is not effective over several months or more. D would treat some of the symptoms of hyperthyroidism but E is the superior choice because it blocks conversion of peripheral thyroid hormone.

4. **Answer: A.** G-protein-coupled receptors are abundantly present in human physiology but not used by corticosteroids. Ion channels are important for nerve conduction but not used by steroids. Tyrosine kinases are part of cell proliferation signaling but not used by steroids.

5. **Answer: A.** Need both mineralocorticoid and glucocorticoid effects, and of the listed choices, cortisol is more potent than prednisone or dexamethasone. Spironolactone is a K^+ sparing diuretic, not a steroid.

6. **Answer: D.** A SERM that is antagonist at receptors in breast but agonist at receptors in bone. A and B would increase breast cancer risk. Answer C is a form of contraceptive. E is not a good option for this woman.

7. **Answer: C.** Most oral contraceptives rely on enterohepatic cycle and doxycycline reduces hydrolysis of conjugated estrogens by enteric bacteria.

8. **Answer: C.** Of the listed choices, cis-atricurium is the only drug that undergoes Hoffman elimination by plasma cholinesterase.

9. **Answer: B.** A GIST tumor is described. Imatinib is a tyrosine kinase inhibitor indicated in the treatment of GIST.

10. **Answer: C.** The eradication of *Helicobacter pylori* is the first-line treatment for MALT lymphoma. Biopsies for determination of *Helicobacter pylori* should be performed at the time of endoscopic evaluation for MALT.

CHAPTER 6
Anesthesia

Patty T. Liu

What is the optimal distance above the carina for an endotracheal tube (ETT)?
2 cm above the carina

What are the steps of rapid sequence induction?
Oxygenation and short-acting induction agent → muscle relaxant → cricoid pressure → intubation → inhalational anesthetic

What is the most commonly used technique for induction of general anesthesia in children?
Inhalational

What are the steps that both the surgeon and anesthesiologist should take during an airway fire?
Stop all gas and oxygen flow → extinguish fire with water/saline → remove ET tube and any foreign body in airway → perform mask ventilation until patient is reintubated → perform bronchoscopy to assess extent of airway damage.

What factors affect the accuracy of pulse oximetry?
Decreased reading—intense environmental lighting, motion, methylene blue dye, hypothermia, low cardiac output, hypotension, peripheral edema, nail polish
Increased reading—bilirubin, carbon monoxide

Define minimum alveolar concentration (MAC):
The smallest concentration of gas at which 50% of patients will not move to painful stimuli such as incision

Relate lipid solubility, speed of induction, and potency for an inhalational agent with a low MAC:
Low MAC means that the agent is more lipid-soluble and more potent but slower speed of induction

What inhalational agent has the fastest speed of induction, high minimal alveolar concentration, and low potency?
Nitrous oxide (NO_2)

Name contraindications to the use of nitrous oxide:
Middle ear occlusion, pneumothorax, small bowel obstruction, and any other instance where there is an air-filled body pocket

Which inhalational agent can cause eosinophilia, fever, increased liver function tests, and jaundice and is associated with the highest degree of cardiac depression and arrhythmias?
Halothane

Which inhalational agent has a pleasant smell and is ideal for mask induction in children?
Sevoflurane

What induction agent should not be used in patients with an egg allergy?
Propofol

What induction agent is contraindicated in head injury?
Ketamine

Which induction agent can cause adrenocortical suppression with continuous infusion?
Etomidate

First muscle to be paralyzed after administration of a paralytic? Last muscle?
Face and neck muscles
Diaphragm

First muscle to recover after administration of a paralytic? Last muscle?
Diaphragm
Face and neck muscles

Triggering agents for malignant hyperthermia:
Volatile anesthetics (halothane, enflurane, isoflurane, sevoflurane, desflurane) and depolarizing paralytic succinylcholine

What is the mechanism leading to malignant hyperthermia?
Mutation of the ryanodine receptors located on the sarcoplasmic reticulum resulting in a drastic increase in intracellular calcium levels inducing an uncontrolled increase in skeletal muscle oxidative metabolism

First sign seen with malignant hyperthermia? Other signs?
Increase in end-tidal CO_2
Acidosis, fever, hyperkalemia, rigidity, tachycardia

Treatment for malignant hyperthermia:
First stop offending agent, cooling blankets, dantrolene (10 mg/kg IV), glucose, HCO_3, IV fluids, supportive care

Name the only depolarizing paralytic
Succinylcholine

Use of succinylcholine should be avoided in which patients?
Patients with extensive burns, crush injuries/extensive trauma, eye trauma or glaucoma (raises intraocular pressure), neurologic disorders/injury, spinal cord injury, acute renal failure with increased potassium

How long does succinylcholine last? Metabolized by? Antidote?
<6 minutes, hydrolyzed by plasma cholinesterase (pseudocholinesterase), time

How is cisatracurium metabolized?
Hofmann elimination

How is mivacurium metabolized?
Hydrolyzed by plasma cholinesterase

What is the most common side effect of pancuronium?
Tachycardia (vagolytic effect)

What can be used to reverse nondepolarizing paralytics?
Acetylcholinesterase inhibitors (neostigmine, edrophonium, pyridostigmine)

Mechanism of action of local anesthetics:
Blocks transmission of neural impulses by stabilizing Na channels, thus preventing propagation of action potential

Where is lidocaine with epinephrine contraindicated?
Fingers, penis, nose, pinna of ear, and toes (vasoconstriction can lead to ischemia/necrosis)

Maximum dose of lidocaine without epinephrine? Lidocaine with epinephrine (1:100,000)?
5 mg/kg (remember 1% of drug = 10 mg/mL)
7 mg/kg

Maximum dose of bupivacaine:
3 mg/kg

Earliest symptom of lidocaine toxicity:
Perioral numbness or tingling of the tongue are early symptoms. This may progress to lightheadedness and visual disturbances. CNS-related symptoms are more common and occur before cardiovascular-related symptoms such as cardiac arrhythmias and arrest.

Severe signs seen with a large overdose of lidocaine:
Tonic-clonic seizures, unconsciousness, and eventually coma (cardiovascular toxicity less common)

Duration of lidocaine without epinephrine? Lidocaine with epinephrine?
30 to 60 minutes
Up to 4 hours

Type of local anesthetic that is more likely to cause an allergic reaction secondary to a *p*-aminobenzoic acid analogue:
Ester-type anesthetics (cocaine, procaine, tetracaine)

Most feared side effect of bupivacaine (Marcaine) after intravascular injection:
Fatal refractory dysrhythmia

In patients on monoamine oxidase inhibitors, the concurrent use of narcotics can cause:
Hyperpyrexic coma

Histamine release is characteristic of this narcotic:
Morphine

Name of the metabolite of demerol that can cause seizures:
Normeperidine

Overdose of narcotic can be treated with this drug:
Narcan

Which benzodiazepine (BZ) is contraindicated in pregnancy because it crosses the placenta?
Versed (midazolam)

Competitive inhibitor of BZs that can be given to treat an overdose:
Flumazenil

True or false: Flumazenil can also reverse the CNS effects of other GABAergic-acting drugs such as barbiturates and ethanol?
False, only works with BZs

Contraindications to use of flumazenil:
Patients with serious signs of tricyclic antidepressant overdose and when BZs are used for life-threatening conditions (status epilepticus, increased intracranial pressure)

Initial treatment for a postdural puncture headache:
Conservative measures with analgesics, bed rest, and fluids

Treatment to relieve severe symptoms associated with postdural puncture headache persisting after 24 hours after ineffective conservative measures:
Epidural blood patch

Name some side effects of epidural anesthesia:
Decreased motor function, orthostatic hypotension, urinary retention

Treatment for hypotension from epidural anesthesia:
Turn down epidural dose, IV fluids, and phenylephrine

Major advantage of epidural anesthesia:
Analgesia without decreased cough reflex

Morphine in an epidural can contribute to this untoward effect:
Respiratory depression

Lidocaine in an epidural can contribute to these untoward effects:
Bradycardia and hypotension

When should the foley be taken out with an epidural catheter?
Several hours after the epidural catheter is removed (epidural can cause urinary retention)

What is the best determinant of esophageal versus tracheal intubation?
End-tidal CO_2

Most common postanesthesia care unit complication from anesthesia:
Nausea and vomiting

List the greatest risk factors for postop myocardial infarction (MI):
Age >70, congective heart failure, diabetes mellitus (DM), previous MI, and
unstable angina

Most common cause of sudden transient rise in end-tidal CO_2 in intubated patient?
Other causes of rise in end-tidal CO_2?
Alveolar hypoventilation (increase tidal volume or respiratory rate to correct)
Malignant hyperthermia, release of tourniquet, pneumothorax, mucus plug, faulty
equipment

Causes for sudden decrease in end-tidal CO_2 in the intubated patient?
Disconnection from ventilator, kinking of ETT, pulmonary embolism (PE), significant
hypotension, CO_2 embolus

MULTIPLE CHOICE QUESTIONS

1. **Which of the following drugs should be avoided in patients with inherited
   atypical pseudocholinesterase?**

   A. Succinylcholine
   B. Cisatracurium
   C. Pancuronium
   D. Rocuronium

2. **Which of the following drugs may trigger malignant hyperthermia?**

   A. Sevoflurane
   B. Midazolam
   C. Etomidate
   D. Ketamine

3. **While providing local anesthesia in a 60-kg patient, what is the maximum volume
   of lidocaine 1% that can be used?**

   A. 20 cc
   B. 30 cc
   C. 60 cc
   D. 80 cc

4. **Local anesthetics act on which of the following to block nerve conduction?**

   A. $Na^+ K^+ 2Cl^-$ transporter
   B. $H^+ K^+$ ATPase
   C. Calcium channel
   D. Sodium channel

5. **Spinal and epidural block all of the following nerves except which of the
   following?**

   A. Parasympathetic nerves
   B. Sympathetic nerves
   C. Sensory nerves
   D. Motor nerves

6. **What is the common mechanism for neuromuscular blockade reversal agents?**
   A. Increased metabolism of the neuromuscular blocking agent
   B. Increased resistance to the neuromuscular blocking agent
   C. Increased concentration of acetylcholine at the neuromuscular junction
   D. Efflux of the neuromuscular blocking agent from the axon

7. **Select the inhalational agent with the lowest potency and fastest onset from among the following:**
   A. Desflurane
   B. Sevoflurane
   C. Nitrous oxide
   D. Halothane

8. **Which of the following local anesthetic agents is least likely to cause an allergic reaction?**
   A. Chloroprocaine
   B. Lidocaine
   C. Cocaine
   D. Benzocaine

9. **Which of the following is associated with an abrupt drop in exhaled carbon dioxide to zero in an intubated patient?**
   A. Atelectasis
   B. Flash pulmonary edema
   C. Circuit disconnection
   D. Hypoxia

10. **A 54-year-old male is intubated and general anesthesia is induced. After 2 minutes, his pulse oximeter reads 93%, systolic blood pressure decreases to 40 mm Hg, and his heart rate decreases to 35 bpm. Which of the following is the next best step?**
    A. Synchronized cardioversion
    B. Place the patient in Trendelenberg position with the left side down
    C. Assess ETT placement
    D. Rapid IV push of α agonist
    E. Administer atropine followed by epinephrine

11. **A 60-year-old man undergoes an elective right carotid endarterectomy under a cervical plexus block with bupivacaine. Five seconds after injecting lidocaine 0.5% into the carotid bulb to decrease blood pressure lability, the patient becomes unresponsive and experiences a generalized tonic-clonic seizure particularly of the right side lasting 30 seconds. What is the most likely cause for the seizure?**
    A. Overdose from bupivacaine cervical plexus block
    B. Cerebral ischemia from embolized plaque
    C. Intraarterial injection of lidocaine
    D. Development of new-onset seizure disorder

ANSWERS

1. **Answer: A.** Both succinylcholine and mivacurium are hydrolyzed by pseudocholinesterase. For example, a single dose of succinylcholine may last hours rather than minutes. Mivacurium is the only nondepolarizing paralytic to be hydrolyzed by pseudocholinesterase. Cisatracurium is broken down in the plasma by Hoffmann elimination.

2. **Answer: A.** Succinylcholine, a depolarizing muscle relaxant, and all volatile anesthetics (halothane, enflurane, desflurane, isoflurane, and sevoflurane) may trigger malignant hyperthermia.

3. **Answer: B.** Calculation of the toxic dose of lidocaine requires the knowledge of 2 things:

   The toxic dose of lidocaine is ~5 mg/kg (toxic dose of lidocaine with epinephrine 7 mg/kg; toxic dose of bupivacaine ~3mg/kg).

   1% = 10 mg/mL = 1000 mg/100 mL = 1 g/100 mL for any drug or solution.

   So, the toxic dose of lidocaine for a 60-kg patient is: 60 kg × 5 mg/kg = 300 mg.

   To calculate the volume of lidocaine 1% that can be given: 300 mg/(10 mg/mL) = 30 mL.

4. **Answer: D.** Local anesthetics prevent action potentials from propagating along the nerve by crossing the plasma membrane and stabilizing sodium channels in their closed state. This is a reversible process.

5. **Answer: A.** Sympathetic, sensory, and motor nerves are all bathed with local anesthetic when it is injected into the epidural space. This results in hypotension from sympathetic nerve blockade, muscle relaxation from motor nerve blockade, and analgesia from sensory nerve blockade. The parasympathetic nerves are not affected.

6. **Answer: C.** Acetylcholinesterase inhibitors such as edrophonium, pyridostigmine, and neostigmine can be used to reverse the effects of nondepolarizing agents. They raise the concentration of acetylcholine by preventing further breakdown of acetylcholine at the neuromuscular junction.

7. **Answer: C.** Potency is inversely related to MAC. The higher the MAC, the lower the potency. Nitrous oxide has the highest MAC of all of the inhalational agents (105%), and therefore the lowest potency. Nitrous oxide also has low lipid solubility, which accounts for its rapid onset and offset compared to other agents with higher lipid solubility, which would demonstrate higher potency with longer induction and emergence times.

8. **Answer: B.** Amide local anesthetics such as bupivacaine, prilocaine, lidocaine, mepivicaine, and ropivicaine are distinguished from esters by having 2 "i's" in their names rather than 1 "i," respectively. Esters are generally metabolized by plasma cholinesterases and yield metabolites with a slightly higher allergic potential than the metabolites from amides. Amides are generally metabolized by the liver.

9. **Answer: C.** A circuit disconnect can account for an exhaled carbon dioxide of zero. Other causes include PE and significant hypotension.

10. **Answer: C.** The first step of action is to confirm ETT placement by expired carbon dioxide and auscultation.

11. **Answer: C.** The temporal relationship between the lidocaine injection and the onset of seizure activity is highly suggestive of direct injection into the internal carotid artery. Lidocaine toxicity begins with numbness of the tongue, lightheadedness, and visual disturbances and progresses to muscle twitching, unconsciousness, and seizures, then coma, respiratory arrest, and cardiovascular depression.

CHAPTER 7
Fluids/Electrolytes/Nutrition

Firas Madbak

FLUIDS

Name the 2 major body fluid compartments:
Intracellular and extracellular

Extracellular fluid is divided into these 2 subcompartments:
Interstitial fluid and intravascular fluid

Mnemonic for the composition of body fluid:
60, 40, 20; 60% total body weight fluid, 40% total body weight intracellular, 20% total body weight extracellular

Approximate percentage of body weight that is fluid:
60%

Approximate percentage of body fluid that is extracellular:
33%

Approximate percentage of body weight that is intracellular:
66%

Percentage of extracellular fluid within the vascular compartment in the venous system:
85%

Percentage of extracellular fluid within the vascular compartment in the arterial system:
15%

The approximate percentage of body weight that blood accounts for in an adult:
7% (so to estimate how many liters of blood in a 70-kg man; 0.07×70 kg = 5 liters)

Requirement of water per 24-hour period:
~30 to 35 mL/kg

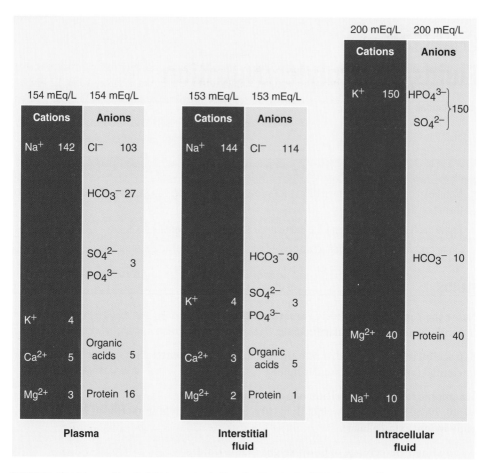

FIGURE 7-1. Chemical composition of body fluid compartments. *(Reproduced form Brunicardi FC, Anderson DK, Billiar TR, et al. Schwartz's Principles of Surgery. 9th ed. http://www.accessmedicine.com. Copyright © The McGraw-Hill Companies, Inc. All rights reserved.)*

Requirement of sodium per 24-hour period:
~1 to 2 mEq/kg

Requirement of chloride per 24-hour period:
~1.5 mEq/kg

Requirement of potassium per 24-hour period:
~1 mEq/kg

Name the sources and the amount of normal daily water loss:
Respiratory losses: 500 to 700 cc
Sweat: 200 to 400 cc
Urine: 1200 to 1500 cc
Feces: 100 to 200 cc

Name the sources and the amount of insensible fluid loss:
Skin: ~300 cc/24 h
Breathing: 500 to 700 cc/24 h
Feces: 100 to 200 cc/24 h

General rate of fluid loss during an open abdominal procedure in the absence of measurable blood loss:
0.5 to 1.0 L/h

Name the sources and the amount of normal daily electrolyte loss:
Chloride: 150 mEq, sodium: 100 mEq, potassium: 100 mEq

Name the sources and the amount of daily secretions:
Saliva: ~1500 cc/24 h
Gastric: ~2000 cc/24 h
Small intestine: ~3000 cc/24 h
Bile: ~1000 cc/24 h
Pancreatic: ~600 cc/24 h

State the electrolyte composition of sweat:
30 to 50 mEq sodium, 5 mEq potassium, 45 to 55 mEq hydrogen

State the electrolyte composition of gastric secretions:
40 to 65 mEq sodium, 90 mEq hydrogen, 100 to 140 mEq chloride

State the electrolyte composition of biliary secretions:
135 to 155 mEq sodium, 5 mEq potassium, 80 to 110 mEq chloride, 70 to 90 mEq bicarbonate

State the electrolyte composition of pancreatic secretions:
135 to 155 mEq sodium, 5 mEq potassium, 55 to 75 mEq chloride, 70 to 90 mEq bicarbonate

State the electrolyte composition of ileostomy output:
120 to 130 mEq sodium, 10 mEq potassium, 50 to 60 mEq chloride, 50 to 70 mEq bicarbonate

State the electrolyte composition of diarrhea:
25 to 50 mEq sodium, 35 to 60 mEq potassium, 20 to 40 mEq chloride, 30 to 45 mEq bicarbonate

Define the "third space."
Fluid accumulation in the interstitium of tissues (first 2 spaces: intravascular and intracellular)

When does third-spaced fluid tend to mobilize back into the intravascular space?
Postoperative day #3

What is the earliest sign of volume excess during the postoperative period?
Weight gain

Classic finding with overaggressive nasogastric tube suctioning or long-standing vomiting:
Hypokalemic hypochloremic metabolic alkalosis

Name the various mechanisms that loop diuretics employ to decrease pulmonary edema:
Inhibit active sodium absorption in the thick ascending loop of Henle, increase venous capacitance, stimulate vasodilatory prostaglandins leading to increased renal blood flow

Formula to calculate serum osmolality:
$2 \times$ sodium + urea/2.8 + glucose/18

How much sodium and chloride are in normal saline?
154 mEq Na^+ and 154 mEq Cl^-

Composition of lactated Ringer's:
130 mEq Na^+, 109 mEq Cl^-, 4 mEq K^+, 28 mEq lactate, and 3 mEq calcium

How many grams of dextrose in a liter of D5W?
50 g; D5W is a 5% solution of dextrose (5 g dextrose/100 cc $\times$ 1000 cc/1 L = 50 g dextrose)

The 2 "rules" for the calculation of maintenance fluids:
100/50/20 rule and 4/2/1 rule; for both rules cc/kg for first 10 kg/cc/kg for next 10 kg/cc/kg for every kg >20 kg

Name the standard maintenance fluid used in an adult:
D5 1/2 normal saline (NS) with 20 mEq KCl

Name the standard maintenance fluid used in a pediatric patient:
D5 1/4 NS with 20 mEq KCl

Usual minimal urine output for an adult:
~30 mL/h or 0.5 mL/kg/h

How much of a 1-L NS bolus will stay intravascular in a 5-hour period?
~200 cc or 20%

ELECTROLYTES

Normal range for sodium:
135 to 145 mEq/L

Define pseudohyponatremia and list causes:
Spuriously low lab result for sodium; hyperglycemia, hyperlipidemia, hyperproteinemia

Name the 3 types of hyponatremia:
Hypovolemic, euvolemic, hypervolemic

Name surgical causes of hypovolemic hyponatremia:
Burns, diaphoresis, diuretics, hypoaldosteronism, NG suctioning, pancreatitis, vomiting

Name surgical causes of euvolemic hyponatremia:
CNS abnormalities, drugs, syndrome of inappropriate secretion of antidiuretic hormone (SIADH)

Name surgical causes of hypervolemic hyponatremia:
Congestive heart failure, cirrhosis, iatrogenic, renal failure

Signs and symptoms of hyponatremia:
Coma/confusion, ileus, lethargy, nausea/vomiting, seizure, weakness

Treatment of hypovolemic hyponatremia:
Correct the underlying cause, give IV NS

Treatment of euvolemic hyponatremia (SIADH):
Acute treatment with furosemide and normal saline; fluid restriction

Treatment of hypervolemic hyponatremia (dilutional):
Fluid restriction and diuretics

Grave consequence of correcting hyponatremia too quickly:
Myelinolysis (formerly known as central pontine myelinolysis)

Formula to calculate the sodium deficit:
(normal sodium concentration – observed sodium concentration) × total body water;
Remember: total body water = 0.6 × weight (kg)

Approximately how much does the apparent serum sodium concentration fall for each 100 mg/dL rise in blood glucose level above normal?
1.6 to 3.0 mEq/L

Maximal rate of sodium correction for acute hyponatremia:
1 to 2 mEq/L/h for 3 to 4 hours until neurologic symptoms subside or until plasma Na is >120 mEq/L

Maximal rate of sodium correction for chronic hyponatremia:
0.5 to 1 mEq/L/h or no faster than 10 to 12 mEq/L in the first 24 hours and 18 mEq/L in the first 48 hours

Name surgical causes of hypernatremia:
Dehydration, diabetes insipidus, diaphoresis, diarrhea, diuresis, iatrogenic, vomiting

Signs and symptoms of hypernatremia:
Confusion, peripheral/pulmonary edema, respiratory paralysis, stupor, seizures, tremors

Treatment of hypernatremia:
Slow supplementation of 1/4 NS or 1/2 NS over days

Formula to calculate the free water deficit:
Total free water deficit = $0.6 \times$ weight (kg) $\times [(Serum\ Na^+/140) - 1]$

What is the normal range for potassium:
3.5 to 5.0 mEq/L

Critical values for potassium:
K^+ <2.8 mEq/L or >6.0 mEq/L

Name some surgical causes of hypokalemia:
Alkalosis, diuretics, drugs (steroids/antibiotics), diarrhea, iatrogenic, insulin, intestinal fistula, NG suctioning, vomiting

Signs and symptoms of hypokalemia:
Ileus, weakness, tetany, nausea/vomiting, paresthesia

EKG findings of hypokalemia:
Flattened T waves, U waves, ST segment depression, atrial fibrillation, premature atrial complexes/premature ventricular complexes

Acute treatment for hypokalemia:
IV KCl

Maximum amount of potassium that can be administered through a peripheral IV:
10 mEq/h

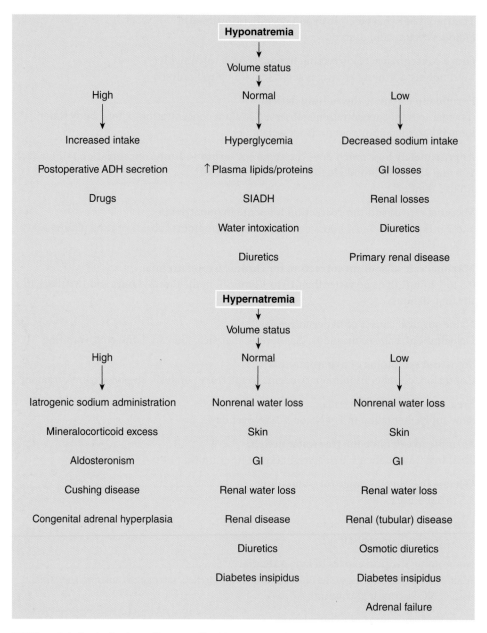

FIGURE 7-2. Evaluation of sodium abnormalities. ADH, antidiuretic hormone; SIADH, syndrome of inappropriate secretion of antidiuretic hormone. (Reproduced form Brunicardi FC, Anderson DK, Billiar TR, et al. Schwartz's Principles of Surgery. 9th ed. http://www.accessmedicine.com. Copyright © The McGraw-Hill Companies, Inc. All rights reserved.)

Maximum amount of potassium that can be administered through a central line: 20 mEq/h

Most common cause for an electrolyte mediated ileus in a surgical patient: Hypokalemia

Digitalis toxicity is worsened by this electrolyte condition:
Hypokalemia

Name surgical causes of hyperkalemia:
Iatrogenic, diuretics, acidosis, trauma, hemolysis, renal failure, blood transfusion

Signs and symptoms of hyperkalemia:
Areflexia or decreased deep tendon reflexes, paresthesia, paralysis, weakness, and respiratory failure

EKG findings of hyperkalemia:
Peaked T waves, prolonged PR, wide QRS, depressed ST segment, ventricular fibrillation, bradycardia

What is the treatment for hyperkalemia?
IV calcium, sodium bicarbonate, dextrose and insulin (1 amp 50% dextrose and 10 U insulin), albuterol, kayexalate, furosemide, dialysis

Most of the calcium in the body is contained within:
Bone

Percentage of serum calcium that is nonionized and bound to plasma protein:
~50%

Percentage of serum calcium that is nonionized and bound to substances other than plasma protein in the plasma:
5%

How much does a 1-g drop in protein decrease the measured total serum calcium?
0.8 mg/dL

In the setting of rapid transfusion, how much calcium should be given per 500 cc of transfused blood?
0.2 g/500 cc transfused blood

Name some surgical causes of hypocalcemia:
Acute pancreatitis, aminoglycosides, diuretics, hypomagnesemia, intestinal bypass, osteoblastic metastasis, renal failure, rhabdomyolysis, sepsis, short bowel syndrome, vitamin D deficiency

Formula to determine the calcium level with hypoalbuminemia:
Serum calcium + [(4 − measured albumin) × 0.8]

Signs and symptoms of hypocalcemia:
Abdominal cramping, Chvostek signs, confusion, depression, hallucinations, increased deep tendon reflexes, laryngospasm, paranoia, perioral paresthesia, seizures, stridor, tetany, Trousseau sign

Define Chvostek sign:
Tapping of facial nerve with resultant facial muscle spasm

Define Trousseau sign:
Utilization of a blood pressure cuff to occlude blood flow to the forearm with resultant latent tetany evidenced by carpal spasm

EKG findings hypocalcemia:
Peaked T waves, prolonged QT and ST intervals

Acute treatment of hypocalcemia:
IV calcium supplementation

Chronic treatment of hypocalcemia:
PO calcium and vitamin D supplementation

Mnemonic for hypercalcemia:
Chimpanzees: Calcium supplementation, hyperparathyroidism (primary/tertiary)/
hyperthyroidism, iatrogenic/immobility, milk alkali syndrome/mets, Paget disease,
Addison disease/acromegaly, neoplasm, Zollinger-Ellison syndrome, excessive
vitamin A, excessive vitamin D, sarcoid

Signs and symptoms of hypercalcemia:
Polydipsia, polyuria, and constipation and the classic "stones, bones, abdominal groans,
and psychiatric overtones"

EKG findings of hypercalcemia:
Prolonged PR interval and shortened QT interval

Acute treatment for hypercalcemic crisis:
Normal saline volume expansion with furosemide diuresis

Additional options for treating hypercalcemia:
Bisphosphonates, calcitonin, mithramycin, steroids, and dialysis

What kind of diuretic should be avoided in the face of hypercalcemia?
Thiazide diuretics (calcium-sparing diuretic)

Normal range for magnesium:
1.5 to 2.5 mEq/L

**Electrolyte abnormality associated with "impossible to correct" hypokalemia and
hypocalcemia:**
Hypomagnesemia

Name surgical causes of hypomagnesemia:
Aminoglycosides, diarrhea, gastric suctioning, hypocalcemia, renal failure, total
parenteral nutrition (TPN), vomiting

Signs and symptoms of hypomagnesemia:
Asterixis, Chvostek sign, dysrhythmias, increased deep tendon reflexes, tachycardia,
tetany, tremor, ventricular ectopy, vertigo

Treatment for acute hypomagnesemia:
IV magnesium sulfate (or magnesium chloride)

Treatment for chronic hypomagnesemia:
PO magnesium oxide

Name surgical causes of hypermagnesemia:
Iatrogenic, renal failure, TPN

Signs and symptoms of hypermagnesemia:
IV calcium, dextrose and insulin, dialysis, Lasix

Normal range for phosphorus:
2.5 to 4.5 mg/dL

Critical value for phosphorus:
<1.0 mg/dL

Name surgical causes of hypophosphatemia:
Alcohol abuse, gastrointestinal losses, inadequate supplementation, medications, renal loss, sepsis

Signs and symptoms of hypophosphatemia:
Ataxia, cardiomyopathy, hemolysis, poor response to pressors, rhabdomyolysis, neurologic dysfunction, weakness

Treatment for acute hypophosphatemia:
IV sodium phosphate or potassium phosphate

Treatment for chronic hypophosphatemia:
PO replacement (Neutra phos)

Name surgical causes of hyperphosphatemia:
Chemotherapy, hyperthyroidism, renal failure, sepsis

Signs and symptoms of hyperphosphatemia:
Calcification, heart block

List the disturbances seen with tumor lysis syndrome:
Hypocalcemia, hyperkalemia, hyperuricemia, hyperphosphatemia

Name the important intracellular buffer:
Phosphate buffer system and proteins

Name the primary extracellular buffering system:
Bicarbonate-carbonic acid system

Henderson-Hasselbalch equation:
$pH = pK + \log [HCO_3^-]/[CO_2]$

Formula to calculate the anion gap:
Anion gap = Sodium – (bicarbonate + chloride)

Mnemonic for anion gap acidosis:
Mudpiles: methanol, uremia, diabetic ketoacidosis, paraldehyde, isoniazid, lactic acidosis, ethylene glycol, salicylates

Formula for functional excretion of sodium (FeNa):
FeNa = (urine sodium/urine creatinine)/(plasma sodium/plasma creatinine)

List some common laboratory values seen in a prerenal state:
BUN/Cr ratio >20, FeNa <1%, urine sodium <20, urine osmolality >500 mOsm

NUTRITION

The term for the initial period during the activation of stress hypermetabolism where there is a decrease in oxygen consumption, cellular shock, and fluid imbalance lasting 24 to 36 hours:
Ebb phase

The term for the adaptation of the body to the ebb phase of stress hypermetabolism where body temperature, metabolic rate, and nitrogen loss are increased:
Flow phase

Sepsis/surgery/trauma can increase the kcal requirement by:
20% to 40%

The percentage increase of the basal metabolic rate for every degree above 38°C:
10%

General method to calculate the calorie requirement for a burn patient:
25 kcal/kg/d + (30 kcal/d × %burn)

General method to calculate the protein requirement for a burn patient:
1 to 1.5 g/kg/d + (3 g × %burn)

Level of albumin that is a strong risk factor for morbidity/mortality after surgery:
<3.0 g/dL

Pregnancy can increase the kcal requirement by:
300 kcal/d

What fuel source does the brain use during progressive starvation?
Ketones

Most efficient form for the storage of calories:
Triglycerides

Amino acid that is the primary substrate for gluconeogenesis:
Alanine

Only amino acids to increase during stress:
Alanine and phenylalanine

Primary enzyme responsible for the transamination of amino acids (ammonia, α-ketoglutarate):
Glutamate dehydrogenase

Where does gluconeogenesis occur during late starvation?
Kidney

Name the places where glycogen is stored and the rough percentages:
One-third in liver and two-thirds in skeletal muscle

How long does it take to deplete glycogen stores during starvation?
24 to 36 hours

List obligate glucose users in the body:
Adrenal medulla, peripheral nerves red blood cells, white blood cells

Carbohydrate digestion begins with this enzyme:
Salivary amylase

What is the protein requirement for an average healthy adult male?
1 g protein/kg/d; 20% from essential amino acids

Protein digestion begins with this enzyme:
Pepsin

1 g of nitrogen is contained in how many grams of protein:
6.25 g of protein contains 1 g nitrogen

Formula to calculate the nitrogen balance:
$(N_{in} - N_{out}) = [(protein/6.25) - (24 \text{ hour urine } N + 4 \text{ g})]$

Name the branched chain amino acids:
Isoleucine, leucine, valine

Where are branched chain amino acids metabolized?
Muscle

List the nutrients included in immune-enhancing formulas:
Arginine, glutamine, ω-3 fatty acids, ω-6 fatty acids

Where is iron absorbed?
Most in duodenum and some in jejunum

Where is Vitamin B12 (cobalamin) absorbed?
Terminal ileum

Where are bile salts absorbed?
Terminal ileum

Where are fat soluble vitamins absorbed?
Terminal ileum

Name the fat soluble vitamins:
Vitamin A, D, E, K

Where is calcium absorbed?
Actively in the duodenum and passively in the jejunum

What vitamin increased the oral absorption of iron?
Vitamin C

Fuel for colonocytes:
Short-chain fatty acids (butyrate)

Fuel for small bowel enterocytes:
Glutamine

Primary fuel for cancer cells:
Glutamine

Term for an acute form of childhood protein-energy malnutrition characterized by anorexia, edema, enlarged liver with fatty infiltrates, irritability, and ulcerating dermatoses:
Kwashiorkor

Term for severe protein-energy malnutrition characterized by energy deficiency and characterized by extensive tissue/muscle wasting and variable edema:
Marasmus

How many kcal are there in a gram of dextrose?
3.4 kcal/g

How many kcal are there in a gram of oral carbohydrates?
4 kcal/g

How many kcal are there in a gram of protein?
4 kcal/g

How many kcal are there in a gram of fat?
9 kcal/g

List metabolic complications from TPN:
Acid-base abnormalities
Excessive glucose resulting in hyperosmolar nonketotic coma with resultant dehydration
Increase in CO_2 production
Lipogenesis with resulting fatty liver/hepatic abnormalities

Maximal glucose administration for TPN delivered through a central line:
3 g/kg/h

For an average healthy adult male, what percentage of calories should come from fat?
30%

Rate that should not be exceeded with fat infusion:
2.5 g/kg/d

Name an amino acid solution that contains an increased percentage of branched chain amino acids that is used in patients with encephalopathy:
Hepatamine 8% amino acid solution

The caloric value from the lipid propofol is stored in:
1 kcal/cc

Formula to calculate the ideal body weight for a man:
106 lb + 6 lb for every inch over 5 ft

Formula to calculate the ideal body weight for a woman:
105 lb + 5 lb for every inch over 5 ft

List the rough percentage of calories from carbohydrates in TPN:
50% to 60%

List the rough percentage of calories from proteins in TPN:
10% to 20%

List the rough percentage of calories from lipids in TPN:
20% to 30%

Electrolyte abnormalities found with refeeding syndrome:
Hypokalemia, hypomagnesemia, hypophosphatemia; occurs when feeding after prolonged malnutrition/starvation

The best parameter to check for adequate nutritional status:
Prealbumin

Half-life of retinol-binding protein:
~12 hours

Half-life of prealbumin:
2 to 3 days

Half-life of transferrin:
8 to 9 days

Half-life of albumin:
14 to 20 days

Formula for the respiratory quotient:
$RQ = CO_2 \text{ produced}/O_2 \text{ consumed}$

Respiratory quotient for carbohydrate:
1

Respiratory quotient for ethanol:
0.67

Respiratory quotient for fat:
0.7

Respiratory quotient during hyperventilation:
>1.1

Respiratory quotient to indicate lipogenesis or overfeeding:
>1.0

Respiratory quotient in starvation:
0.6 to 0.7 (fat is fuel source during starvation)

Ideal respiratory quotient during mixed substrate oxidation:
0.85 to 0.95

Respiratory quotient <0.82 indicates:
Occurrence of protein oxidation; increase total energy intake by increasing carbohydrates and caloric intake

Respiratory quotient >1 indicates:
Excessive calorie load; decrease carbohydrate intake and caloric intake

List the effects seen with chromium deficiency:
Encephalopathy, hyperglycemia, neuropathy

List the effects seen with cobalamin (B_{12}) deficiency:
Beefy tongue, megaloblastic anemia, peripheral neuropathy

List the effects seen with copper deficiency:
Pancytopenia

List the effects seen with essential fatty acids deficiency:
Dermatitis, hair loss, thrombocytopenia

List the effects seen with folate deficiency:
Glossitis, megaloblastic anemia

List the effects seen with niacin deficiency:
Diarrhea, dermatits, dementia (Pellagra)

List the effects seen with phosphate deficiency:
Encephalopathy, decreased phagocytosis, weakness

List the effects seen with pyridoxine (B_6) deficiency:
Glossitis, peripheral neuropathy, sideroblastic anemia

List the effects seen with thiamine (B_1) deficiency:
Cardiomyopathy, peripheral neuropathy, Wernicke encephalopathy

List the effects seen with zinc deficiency:
Hair loss, rash, poor healing

List the effects seen with vitamin A deficiency:
Night blindness

List the effects seen with vitamin D deficiency:
Rickets, osteomalacia

List the effects seen with vitamin E deficiency:
Neuropathy

List the effects seen with vitamin K deficiency:
Coagulopathy

MULTIPLE CHOICE QUESTIONS

1. A 55-year-old female underwent a Hartmann procedure for Hinchey III perforated diverticulitis. On postoperative day 8, she had failed 3 attempts at extubation and was still on mechanical ventilator support. One possible reason to explain her difficult weaning is a respiratory quotient of:

   A. 0.67
   B. 0.7
   C. 0.8
   D. 0.9
   E. 1.1

2. Which electrolyte and acid-base abnormality is present in a neonate with intractable projectile vomiting from hypertrophic pyloric stenosis?

   A. Hyperkalemic hypochloremic metabolic alkalosis
   B. Hypokalemic hypochloremic metabolic acidosis
   C. Hypokalemic hyperchloremic metabolic alkalosis
   D. Hypokalemic hypochloremic metabolic alkalosis
   E. Hypernatremic metabolic acidosis

3. What is the major primary nutrient of colonocytes?

   A. Acetoacetate
   B. β-transferrin
   C. Glutamine
   D. Arginine
   E. Butyrate

4. A 25-year-old female driver of an automobile sustained severe multiple traumatic injuries. She had an altered sensorium and required intubation. Etomidate was used for induction. A noted side effect of this agent is associated with what electrolyte abnormality?

   A. Hypomagnesemia
   B. Hypokalemia
   C. Hyperphosphatemia
   D. Hyponatremia and hyperkalemia
   E. Hypernatremia and hypokalemia

5. Which of the following conditions is associated with hypovolemic hyponatremia?

   A. Cirrhosis
   B. Congestive heart failure
   C. Nephrotic syndrome
   D. Enterocutaneous fistula
   E. SIADH

6. Hypernatremia in a volume-depleted patient is best treated with what initial fluid choice?

   A. Normal saline
   B. 0.25% saline
   C. 3% saline
   D. Lactated Ringer's
   E. No fluid should be given

7. A 60-year-old cancer patient has gastric outlet obstruction and presents with refractory vomiting. Which intravenous fluid is most appropriate for volume repletion?

   A. Normal saline
   B. 0.45% saline
   C. 3% saline
   D. Lactated Ringer's
   E. Free water

8. Routine lab work on a patient with small bowel obstruction shows refractory hypocalcemia causing perioral numbness that is uncorrectable with calcium supplementation. What other electrolyte level must be checked and corrected?

   A. Sodium
   B. Phosphate
   C. Bicarbonate
   D. Magnesium
   E. Chloride

9. A patient with Crohn disease undergoes an ileocecectomy for perforation and subsequently has a prolonged postoperative ileus. What is the most common electrolyte abnormality associated with starting TPN?
   A. Hypernatremia
   B. Hypokalemia
   C. Hypophosphatemia
   D. Hypomagnesemia
   E. Hypochloremia

10. The best nutrition access method for a critically ill burn patient is:
   A. Nasogastric
   B. Nasojejunal
   C. Parenteral
   D. Percutaneous gastrostomy
   E. Witzel jejunostomy

ANSWERS

1. **Answer: E.** The RQ is defined as ratio of volume of carbon dioxide produced to the volume of oxygen used on oxidation of a nutrient. The RQ is nearly 1 for carbohydrates, 0.7 for fat, 0.8 for protein, and 0.67 for alcohol. Respiratory failure requiring mechanical ventilation and difficulty with weaning patients can occur if excess glucose is provided, hence raising the RQ to greater than 1.

2. **Answer: D.** Persistent emesis causes progressive loss of fluids rich in hydrochloric acid, which causes the kidneys to retain hydrogen ions in favor of potassium. Electrolyte abnormalities depend on the duration of symptoms in the affected infant. The dehydration may result in hypernatremia or hyponatremia and prerenal renal failure.

3. **Answer: E.** Compared with common fuels, butyrate is the principal fuel for colonocytes, followed by acetoacetate, glutamine, and glucose.

4. **Answer: D.** Etomidate has minimal effects on the cardiovascular system, making it an attractive induction agent in trauma patients. However, even a single dose of etomidate is a major risk factor for the development of relative adrenal insufficiency for at least 24 hours after its administration. Mineralocorticoid deficiency can cause sodium excretion and potassium retention as a result of hypoaldosteronism.

5. **Answer: D.** Cirrhosis, congestive heart failure, and nephrotic syndrome are all associated with hypotonic hypervolemia hyponatremia. A variety of factors can contribute to the development of hyponatremia in patients with cirrhosis. The most important factor is systemic vasodilation, which leads to activation of endogenous vasoconstrictors including antidiuretic hormone (ADH); ADH promotes the water retention that is responsible for the fall in serum sodium. Neurohumoral stimulation as a result of atrial underfilling causes ADH release in heart failure leading to hyponatremia as well. Intrinsic renal disease leads to salt wasting and impaired water balance in nephrotic syndrome. SIADH is associated with euvolemia, by definition. GI fistulas cause loss of fluid and electrolytes causing hypovolemic hyponatremia.

6. **Answer: A.** The main priority in this patient is volume replacement. After this is accomplished, the sodium concentration can be decreased in the intravenous fluids. Hypernatremia associated with hypovolemia occurs with Na loss accompanied by a relatively greater loss of total body water. Common extrarenal causes include most of those that cause hyponatremia and volume depletion. Either hypernatremia or hyponatremia can occur with severe volume loss, depending on the relative amounts of Na and water lost and the amount of water ingested before presentation.

Renal causes of hypernatremia and volume depletion include therapy with diuretics.

Loop diuretics inhibit Na reabsorption in the concentrating portion of the nephrons and can increase water clearance. Osmotic diuresis can also impair renal concentrating capacity because of a hypertonic substance present in the tubular lumen of the distal nephron. The most common cause of hypernatremia due to osmotic diuresis is hyperglycemia in patients with diabetes.

In patients with hypernatremia and hypovolemia, particularly in patients with diabetes with nonketotic hyperglycemic coma, 0.45% saline can be given as an alternative to a combination of 0.9% normal saline and 5% D/W to replenish Na and free water. Alternatively, extracellular fluid volume and free water can be replaced separately, using the formula given to estimate the free water deficit.

7. **Answer: A.** This is favorite. Similar to neonatal pyloric stenosis, the metabolic alkalosis of GOO response to the administration of chloride is important; therefore, sodium chloride solution should be the initial IV fluid of choice. Potassium deficits are corrected after repletion of volume status and after replacement of chloride.

8. **Answer: D.** Low magnesium concentrations may impair adenylate cyclase activity, leading to refractory hypocalcemia secondary to impaired secretion of PTH. Remember to check and correct magnesium levels in the hypocalcemic patient as in postparathyroidectomy or postthyroidectomy.

9. **Answer: C.** The serum phosphorous level falls precipitously with refeeding, due to a shift of phosphate from the extracellular to intracellular compartment, due to the huge demands for this ion for synthesis of phosphorylated compounds. The result of this sudden massive reduction in phosphorous levels is a multitude of life-threatening complications involving multiple organs: respiratory failure, cardiac failure, cardiac arrhythmias, rhabdomyolysis, seizures, coma, red cell, and leukocyte dysfunction.

10. **Answer: B.** Guidelines published by a multitude of burn associations that are based on several trials recommend nasojejunal feeding in severely burned patients due to complications associated with early enteral feeding by the nasogastric route. Percutaneous and surgical feeding tubes are premature and usually unnecessary.

CHAPTER 8
Surgical Oncology

Ryan Lawless

CELL CYCLE

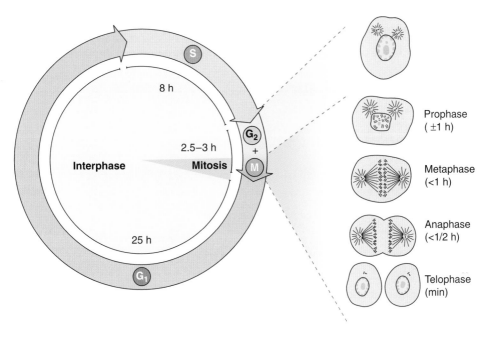

FIGURE 8-1. The cell cycle. The ability to recognize microscopically cells during both mitosis and DNA replication (by autoradiography after administering radiolabeled thymidine) led to the concept of the cell "cycle." In this concept new interphase cells undergo a period after leaving mitosis and before starting DNA synthesis called the first gap or G1. Another gap, G2, occurs after DNA replication and before the next mitotic prophase. After mitosis both new cells repeat this cycle. In rapidly dividing cells, G1 is a period in which cells accumulate the enzymes and nucleotides required for DNA replication, S is the period devoted primarily to DNA replication, G2 is a usually short period of preparation for mitosis, and M includes all phases of mitosis itself. In rapidly growing human tissues the cell cycle varies from 24 to 36 hours. The length of G1 depends on many factors and is usually the longest and most variable period; the length of S is largely a function of the genome size. G2 and mitosis together normally last only 2 to 3 hours. *(Reproduced from Mescher A. Junqueira's Basic Histology: Text and Atlas. 12th ed. www.accessmedicine.com Copyright © The McGraw-Hill Companies, Inc. All rights reserved.)*

In what phase of mitosis does the nucleus disappear?
Prophase

In what phase of mitosis does chromosome alignment occur?
Metaphase

In what phase of mitosis do chromosomes separate?
Anaphase

In what phase of mitosis do nuclei form around replicated DNA?
Telophase

Name the purines:
Guanine, adenine

Name the pyrimidines:
Cytosine, thymidine, uracil

What is translation as it refers to the cell cycle?
Protein synthesis using an mRNA template by ribosomes

What is transcription as it refers to the cell cycle?
Synthesis of mRNA from DNA template by RNA polymerase

In what phase of the cell cycle do protein synthesis and chromosomal duplication occur?
S phase

In what phase of the cell cycle does mitosis occur?
M phase

TUMOR MARKERS

What tumor marker is associated with choriocarcinoma/testicular cancer?
β-Human chorionic gonadotropin (HCG)

What tumor marker is associated with colon cancer?
Carcinoembryonic antigen

What tumor marker is associated with liver cancer?
α-Fetoprotein

What tumor marker is associated with ovarian cancer?
CA-125

What tumor marker is associated with pancreatic cancer?
CA 19-9

What tumor marker is associated with melanoma?
S-100

Chromogranin A is elevated in what adrenal tumor?
Carcinoid tumor

What tumor marker is associated with prostate cancer?
Prostate-specific antigen (PSA)

Table 8-1 Genes Associated with Hereditary Cancer

Gene	Location	Syndrome	Cancer Sites and Associated Traits
APC	17q21	Familial adenomatous polyposis	Colorectal adenomas and carcinomas, duodenal and gastric tumors, desmoids, medulloblastomas, osteomas
BMPR1A	10q21-q22	Juvenile polyposis coli	Juvenile polyps of the GI tract, GI and colorectal malignancy
BRCA1	17q21	Breast-ovarian syndrome	Breast cancer, ovarian cancer, colon cancer, prostate cancer
BRCA2	13q12.3	Breast-ovarian syndrome	Breast cancer, ovarian cancer, colon cancer, prostate cancer, cancer of the gall bladder and bile duct, pancreatic cancer, gastric cancer, melanoma
p16; CDK4	9p21; 12q14	Familial melanoma	Melanoma, pancreatic cancer, dysplastic nevi, atypical moles
CDH1	16q22	Hereditary diffuse gastric cancer	Gastric cancer
hCHK2	22q12.1	Li-Fraumeni syndrome and hereditary breast cancer	Breast cancer, soft tissue sarcoma, brain tumors
hMLH1; hMSH2; hMSH6; PMS1; hPMS2	3p21; 2p22-21; 2p16; 2q31-33; 7p22	Hereditary nonpolyposis colorectal cancer	Colorectal cancer, endometrial cancer, transitional cell carcinoma of the ureter and renal pelvis, and carcinomas of the stomach, small bowel, ovary, and pancreas
MEN1	11q13	Multiple endocrine neoplasia type 1	Pancreatic islet cell cancer, parathyroid hyperplasia, pituitary adenomas
MET	7q31	Hereditary papillary renal cell carcinoma	Renal cancer
NF1	17q11	Neurofibromatosis type 1	Neurofibroma, neurofibrosarcoma, acute myelogenous leukemia, brain tumors
NF2	22q12	Neurofibromatosis type 2	Acoustic neuromas, meningiomas, gliomas, ependymomas
PTC	9q22.3	Nevoid basal cell carcinoma	Basal cell carcinoma
PTEN	10q23.3	Cowden disease	Breast cancer, thyroid cancer, endometrial cancer
rb	13q14	Retinoblastoma	Retinoblastoma, sarcomas, melanoma, and malignant neoplasms of brain and meninges
RET	10q11.2	Multiple endocrine neoplasia type 2	Medullary thyroid cancer, pheochromocytoma, parathyroid hyperplasia

(continued)

Table 8-1 Genes Associated with Hereditary Cancer (*Continued*)

Gene	Location	Syndrome	Cancer Sites and Associated Traits
SDHB; SDHC; SDHD	1p363.1-p35; 11q23; 1q21	Hereditary paraganglioma and pheochromocytoma	Paraganglioma, pheochromocytoma
SMAD4/DPC4	18q21.1	Juvenile polyposis coli	Juvenile polyps of the GI tract, GI and colorectal malignancy
STK11	19p13.3	Peutz-Jeghers syndrome	GI tract carcinoma, breast carcinoma, testicular cancer, pancreatic cancer, benign pigmentation of the skin and mucosa
p53	17p13	Li-Fraumeni syndrome	Breast cancer, soft tissue sarcoma, osteosarcoma, brain tumors, adrenocortical carcinoma, Wilms tumor, phyllodes tumor of the breast, pancreatic cancer, leukemia, neuroblastoma
TSC1; TSC2	9q34; 16p13	Tuberous sclerosis	Multiple hamartomas, renal cell carcinoma, astrocytoma
VHL	3p25	von Hippel-Lindau disease	Renal cell carcinoma, hemangioblastomas of retina and central nervous system, pheochromocytoma
WT	11p13	Wilms tumor	Wilms tumor, aniridia, genitourinary abnormalities, mental retardation

Schwartz's Principles of Surgery. Chapter 10. Oncology.
Reprinted and modified with permission from Marsh DJ, Zori RT. Genetic insights into familial cancers–update and recent discoveries. *Cancer Lett.* 2002; 181(2):125–164, Copyright © 2002, with permission from Elsevier.

What tumor marker is associated with neuroblastoma/small cell lung CA?
Neuron-specific enolase

What tumor marker is associated with nonseminomatous testicular cancer?
α-Fetoprotein

CARCINOGENESIS

What is the term for an increased number of cells?
Hyperplasia

What is the term for replacement of one tissue with another?
Metaplasia

What is the term for altered shape, size, or organization of cells?
Dysplasia

What is the most sensitive stage of the cell cycle for radiation?
M phase

What is the term for human genes with malignant potential?
Proto-oncogenes

What cancer are aflatoxins associated with?
Hepatocellular carcinoma

What organism produces aflatoxins?
Aspergillus flavus

What cancer is associated with *Schistosoma haematobium*?
Urinary bladder cancer

What cancer is associated with *Opisthorchis viverrini*?
Cholangiocarcinoma

What cancer was associated with chimney sweeps (due to soot)?
Scrotal cancer

What cancer is associated with benzene?
Leukemia

What is the primary cause of skin cancer in humans?
Ultraviolet radiation

How do viruses cause cancer?
Insertion of foreign DNA into the human genome

What is the first phase of chemical carcinogenesis?
Initiation. A carcinogen reacts with DNA irreversibly without enzymatic activity or specificity

What is the second phase in chemical carcinogenesis?
Promotion. Cells that were initiated are then stimulated to develop into cancer cells. This process is slow and reversible

What is the last phase of chemical carcinogenesis?
Progression. This involves the maturation of cancer cells

What cancers are associated with the Epstein-Barr virus?
Nasopharyngeal carcinoma and Burkitt lymphoma

What viruses are associated with adult T-cell leukemia?
Human immunodeficiency virus and human T-lymphotropic virus type 1

What is the major fuel source for tumor cells?
Glutamine

What are small circular rings of DNA capable of autonomous replication?
Plasmids

BREAST CANCER

What hormone receptors are commonly tested for in breast cancer?
Estrogen receptor and progesterone receptor

What hormonal therapy is used for estrogen- and progesterone receptor–positive breast tumors?
Hormone receptor–positive tumors are targeted by tamoxifen and aromatase inhibitors. Tamoxifen has shown survival benefit as adjuvant treatment and for metastatic disease in both premenopausal and postmenopausal women. Aromatase inhibitors (anastrozole, letrozole, and exemestane) have shown a survival benefit as adjuvant therapy and for metastatic disease in postmenopausal women.

What cancers are associated with estrogen replacement therapy?
Endometrial and breast

What is the mechanism of action of Tamoxifen?
Selective estrogen receptor modulator, which binds to and inhibits estrogen receptors

What tumor markers are associated with breast cancer?
BRCA I and II

What is the lifetime risk of cancer in a woman with BRCA I mutation?
Ninety percent lifetime risk of breast cancer and 40% lifetime risk of ovarian cancer

What is the lifetime risk of cancer in a woman with BRCA II mutation?
Eighty percent lifetime risk of breast cancer and 35% lifetime risk of ovarian cancer; 60% lifetime risk of breast cancer in men.

What tumor characteristics are associated with BRCA I and II mutations?
BRCA I tumors are poorly differentiated invasive ductal carcinoma and usually hormone receptor–negative, whereas RCA II tumors are well-differentiated invasive ductal carcinoma and more likely to be hormone receptor–positive.

What other tumors are associated with the BRCA II mutation?
Prostate, colon, stomach, pancreatic, gall bladder, and bile duct tumors

What type of receptor is the human epidermal growth factor receptor 2 (HER-2)/neu receptor?
HER-2/neu is an epidermal growth factor receptor

What does overexpression of HER-2/neu in breast cancer portend?
Overexpression of HER-2/neu is associated with increased tumor invasiveness and metastatic potential.

Overexpression of HER-2/neu is used to identify patients who would benefit from this drug:
Trastuzumab (Herceptin)

What is the mechanism of action of Herceptin (trastuzumab)?
Herceptin (trastuzumab) is a murine monoclonal antibody, which targets the HER-2/neu receptor. Its use as adjuvant therapy was associated with a 50% reduction in recurrence after 1 year.

COLON CANCER

What is the second leading cause of cancer death in the United States?
Colon cancer

What is the sequence of tumorigenesis of colon cancer?
Mutation/loss in APC (chromosome 5q) → K-ras mutation (chromosome 12p) → loss of DCC (chromosome 18q) → loss of p53 (chromosome 17p)

What is the recommended screening for colon cancer in the average risk population?
Starting at age 50, fecal occult blood test (FOBT) annually with flexible sigmoidoscopy every 5 years or flexible colonoscopy every 10 years or air/contrast barium enema every 5 to 10 years as recommended by the American Cancer Society. Annual FOBT alone has been given as an option for colon and rectal cancer screening; however, small tumors may be missed.

What are the Amsterdam criteria?
At least 3 relatives with colorectal cancer, 1 of whom is a first-degree relative of the other, at least 2 successive generations involved, and 1 or more relative diagnosed before the age of 50 years

What percentage of patients who develop colon cancer has no identifiable risk factors?
75%

SKIN CANCER

What 3 carcinomas account for 95% of all skin cancers?
Basal cell and squamous cell carcinoma and melanoma

What is the most common form of skin cancer?
Basal cell carcinoma

Where are melanocytes located?
Dermoepidermal junction

What is the most carcinogenic portion of the UV spectrum?
UVB

How are melanomas described on physical examination?
ABCDE: **A**symmetric, irregular/blurred **B**order, more than a single **C**olor, **D**iameter >6 mm, **E**levated

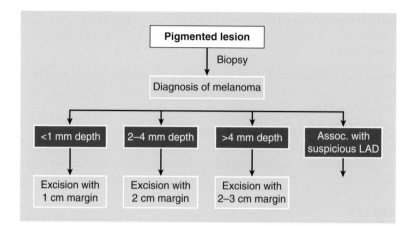

FIGURE 8-2. The diagnosis of melanoma should be made via excisional biopsy. Based on tumor depth, appropriate margins may be planned. Indications for lymph node evaluation continue to advance as our understanding of tumor behavior improves and outcome data become available. LAD, lymphadenopathy. *(Reproduced from Brunicardi FC, Anderson DK, Billar TR, et al. Schwartz's Principles of Surgery. 9th ed. http://www. accessmedicine.com. Copyright © The McGraw-Hill Companies, Inc. All rights reserved.)*

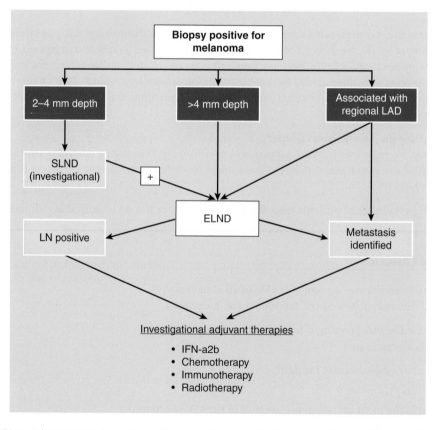

FIGURE 8-3. Melanoma treatment algorithm. The algorithmic approach to melanoma has taken many forms throughout the last several decades. However, as our diagnostic technology, therapeutic approaches, and ability to assess outcome improve, the current algorithm incorporates these advances. ELND, elective lymph node dissection; IFN-a2b, interferon alfa-2b; LAD, lymphadenopathy; LN, lymph node; SLND, sentinel lymph node dissection. *(Reproduced from Brunicardi FC, Andersen DK, Billiar TR, et al. Schwartz's Principles of Surgery. 9th ed. http://www.accessmedicine. com. Copyright © The McGraw-Hill Companies, Inc. All rights reserved.)*

What are the subtypes of melanoma?
Superficial spreading, nodular, lentigo maligna, acral lentiginous

What is the most common type of melanoma?
The most common form of melanoma is the superficial spreading variant (70%).

What type of melanoma has the worst prognosis?
The variant with the worst prognosis is nodular melanoma.

What is the eponym for squamous cell carcinoma?
Bowen disease

What is the eponym for squamous cell carcinoma in situ of the glans penis?
Erythroplasia of Queyrat

CHEMOTHERAPEUTICS

What is the mechanism of action of taxanes?
Disruption of microtubule function (mitotic inhibitor)

Doxorubicin and daunorubicin fall under which class of chemotherapeutic agent?
Anthracycline

Screen for virilization in suspected adrenal carcinoma:
Androstenedione, dehydroepiandrosterone, serum testosterone, and 24-hour urinary 17 ketosteroids

What chemotherapeutic agent is used for the management of adrenocortical carcinoma?
Mitotane

Etoposide is what type of chemotherapeutic agent?
Topoisomerase II inhibitor

Cyclophosphamide is what type of chemotherapeutic agent?
Alkylating agent

What is the mechanism of action for 6-mercaptopurine?
Inhibition of purine nucleotide synthesis.

What medication inhibits xanthine oxidase, the enzyme that breaks down 6-MP?
Allopurinol

Vinblastine and Vincristine are examples of what class of chemotherapeutic agents?
Vinca alkaloids

What chemotherapeutic agents are antimetabolites?
5-Fluorouracil (5-FU), 6-mercaptopurine

What common chemotherapeutic agent is a pyrimidine analog?
5-FU through noncompetitive inhibition of thymidylate.

Pulmonary fibrosis is a serious side effect of what chemotherapeutic?
Bleomycin

What chemotherapeutic agent is used in the treatment of carcinoid syndrome?
Streptozocin

Alkylating Agents	*Purine analogues*
Classic alkylating agents	Azathioprine
Busulfan	Mercaptopurine
Chlorambucil	Thioguanine
Cyclophosphamide	Cladribine (2-chlorodeoxyadenosine)
Ifosfamide	Fludarabine
Mechlorethamine (nitrogen mustard)	Pentostatin
Melphalan	*Pyrimidine analogues*
Mitomycin C	Capecitabine
Triethylenethiophosphoramide (thiotepa)	Cytarabine
Nitrosoureas	Floxuridine
Carmustine (BCNU)	Gemcitabine
Lomustine (CCNU)	*Ribonucleotide reductase inhibitors*
Semustine (MeCCNU)	Hydroxyurea
Streptozocin	**Plant Alkaloids**
Miscellaneous DNA-binding agents	*Vinca alkaloids*
Carboplatin	Vinblastine
Cisplatin	Vincristine
Dacarbazine (DTIC)	Vindesine
Hexamethylmelamine	Vinorelbine
Procarbazine	*Epipodophyllotoxins*
Antitumor Antibiotics	Etoposide
Bleomycin	Teniposide
Dactinomycin (actinomycin D)	*Taxanes*
Daunorubicin	Paclitaxel
Doxorubicin	Docetaxel
Idarubicin	**Miscellaneous Agents**
Plicamycin (mithramycin)	Asparaginase
Antimetabolites	Estramustine
Folate analogues	Mitotane
Methotrexate	

Table 8-2 Classification of Chemotherapeutic Agents

What is CHOP regimen?
Cyclophosphamide, Hydroxydaunorubicin, Oncovin, Prednisone

CHOP regimen is used in treatment of:
Non-Hodgkin lymphoma

MISCELLANEOUS

What are the recommendations for prostate cancer screening?
PSA and digital rectal examination annually beginning at age 50.

HCG is present in about 20% of this tumor?
Seminoma

What is the primary test to detect the overproduction of serotonin in carcinoid tumors?
Urinary 5-hydroxyindoleacetic acid

What are the 3 most common sarcomas?
Liposarcoma, malignant fibrous histiocytoma, and leiomyosarcoma

What are the most common sarcomas of the extremity?
Liposarcoma and malignant fibrous histiocytoma

What are the most common sarcomas of the retroperitoneum?
Liposarcoma and leiomyosarcoma

What is the most common sarcoma in childhood?
Rhabdomyosarcoma

MOPP, for a long time, was the standard treatment for Hodgkin disease. What is MOPP?
Mustargen, Oncovin, Procarbazine, Prednisone

MOPP has been replaced by ABVD as the treatment of Hodgkin disease. What is ABVD?
Adriamycin, Bleomycin, Vinblastine, Dacarbazine

What are the cells with bilobed nuclei seen in Hodgkin lymphoma referred to as?
Reed-Sternberg cells

What mesenchymal neoplasm is derived from the interstitial cells of Cajal?
Gastrointestinal stromal tumor (GIST)

What is the gene mutation associated with gastrointestinal stromal tumors?
c-kit gene

What is the mechanism of Gleevec, the pharmacologic therapy for GIST?
Inhibition of tyrosine kinase

What syndrome is caused by p53 mutations and is associated with multiple cancers?
Li-Fraumeni syndrome

What rare genetic syndrome caused by *PTEN* mutations is associated with intestinal hamartomas, cutaneous lesions, and thyroid cancer?
Cowden disease

MULTIPLE CHOICE QUESTIONS

1. **What organ is not prophylactically resected to prevent cancer in patients with specific genetic mutations?**
   A. Colon
   B. Breast
   C. Thyroid
   D. Pancreas

2. **Which of the following is not associated with gastric cancer?**
   A. Virchow node
   B. Krukenberg tumor
   C. Male preponderance world-wide
   D. Associated with Menetrier disease

3. **Which of the following is the most important prognostic factor in patients with soft tissue sarcoma?**

    A. Histologic grade
    B. Tumor size
    C. Expression of tumor markers
    D. Tumor depth

4. **In which of the following cases should a sentinel lymph node biopsy be performed?**

    A. A 0.7-mm melanoma over the right tibia with a clinically negative right groin
    B. A 1.0-mm melanoma overlying the left groin
    C. A 1.5-mm melanoma of the right upper arm and clinically negative right axilla
    D. A 1.7- to 5-mm melanoma of the left thigh with palpable adenopathy of the left groin

5. **Which of the following chemotherapeutic agents is associated with hemorrhagic cystitis?**

    A. Cisplatin
    B. Methotrexate
    C. Cyclophosphamide
    D. 5-FU

6. **Which of the following constitutes the Nigro protocol?**

    A. CHOP
    B. MOPP
    C. 5-FU, mitomycin C, radiation
    D. Tamoxifen and Herceptin

7. **Which of the following side effects caused Lance Armstrong to forgo therapy with Bleomycin?**

    A. Pulmonary fibrosis
    B. Cardiomyopathy
    C. Weight loss
    D. Nausea/vomiting

8. **What is the mechanism of action of the chemotherapeutic treatment of a GIST?**

    A. Xanthine oxidase inhibition
    B. Tyrosine kinase inhibition
    C. Alkylating agent
    D. Topoisomerase II inhibition

9. **What phase of the cell cycle has radiation most effect in?**

    A. S phase
    B. M phase
    C. G1
    D. G2

10. **What is the sequence of mutations involved in colon cancer?**

    A. APC → p53 → DCC → k-ras
    B. P53 → APC → DCC → k-ras
    C. DCC → k-ras → APC → p53
    D. K-ras → APC → p53 → DCC

ANSWERS

1. **Answer: D.** In patients with familial adenomatous polyposis, the colon can be removed in order to prevent the development of colon cancer. Patients with an increased susceptibility to breast cancer, for example, women with the BRCA I or II mutation, can undergo prophylactic mastectomy. The thyroid is removed in patients with MEN II syndrome to prevent the development of medullary thyroid carcinoma.

2. **Answer: D.** Virchow node, a palpable enlarged lymph node in the left supraclavicular fossa, is often associated with gastric cancer. It is one of the first places in which gastric cancer metastasizes. Krukenberg tumor is a metastatic lesion to the ovary often arising from a gastrointestinal source, gastric most commonly. Gastric cancer, worldwide, is more common in men than in women.

3. **Answer: A.** Although tumor size, expression of tumor markers, and depth of tumor can be assessed in the prognosis of soft tissue sarcoma, the histologic grade of the tumor is the most important prognostic factor.

4. **Answer: C.** A melanoma less than 1.0 mm does not undergo a sentinel lymph node dissection. A melanoma overlying a draining lymph node basin should undergo lymph node dissection. The patient with palpable adenopathy should undergo lymph node dissection.

5. **Answer: C.** Cyclophosphamide (Adriamycin) is associated with hemorrhagic cystitis.

6. **Answer: C.** The Nigro protocol is the treatment for squamous cell carcinoma of the anus.

7. **Answer: A.** Bleomycin is a chemotherapeutic used in the treatment of testicular cancer. A major side effect of the medical can be pulmonary fibrosis, which is detrimental to any athlete.

8. **Answer: B.** The chemotherapeutic agent involved in the treatment of a GIST is imatinib mesylate (Gleevec). Gleevec is a tyrosine kinase inhibitor, which inhibits the duplication of cancer cells.

9. **Answer: B.** M phase is the most sensitive to radiation effects.

10. **Answer: A.** The correct sequence of mutations is loss of the *APC* gene followed by p53, DCC (deleted in colon cancer), and finally k-ras activation.

CHAPTER 9
Wound Healing

Ramon Garza III

Name the 3 phases of wound healing:
Inflammation (1–6 days), proliferation (3 days–3 weeks), maturation (3 weeks–1 year)

Name several factors that can inhibit wound healing:
Diabetes, infection, ischemia, malnutrition, radiation, steroids, neoplasia, anemia

What are the optimal nutrition parameters?
Albumin >3 g/dL and prealbumin >16 mg/dL

What is primary wound closure (primary intention)?
Immediate closure of a wound with suture or staples

Most important factor in healing closed wounds by primary intention:
Tensile strength

What is the most important layer to close for strength in skin lacerations?
Dermis

How long does it take a surgical incision become "water tight"?
24 to 48 hours

What is secondary wound closure?
Leaving a wound open and allowing it to heal by granulation, contraction, and epithelialization over time

Most important factor in the healing of open wounds by secondary intention:
Epithelial integrity

What causes contraction in wounds healing by secondary intention?
Myofibroblasts

What is delayed primary closure?
Closing a wound several days (3–5 days) after incision

Rate of regeneration of a peripheral nerve:
1 mm/d or 1 in./mo

Rate of epithelialization:
1 to 2 mm/d

The strongest layer of the bowel:
Submucosa

The time period that a small bowel anastomosis is at its weakest:
3 to 5 days

Name the 2 major events in the process of epithelialization:
Migration and mitosis

Name the process by which keratinocytes pile up on top of each other at the leading edge of a migration and tumble forward over the top of the heap:
Epiboly

What cell is the most essential for wound healing?
Macrophage

This cell is responsible for the movement and contraction of wound edges:
Myofibroblast

Name the order of arrival of the different cells involved in wound healing:
Platelets (not a true cell)
Neutrophils (predominant cell type from day 0–2)
Macrophages (predominant cell type from day 3–4)
Fibroblasts (predominant cell type from day 5 and so on)
Lymphocytes

Platelet factor 4, β-thrombomodulin, PDGF, and TGF-β are contained in this type of platelet granule:
α granule

Adenosine, serotonin, and calcium are contained in this type of platelet granule:
Dense granule

Name the predominant cell during days 0 to 2 of wound healing:
Neutrophils

Name the predominant cell during days 3 to 4 of wound healing:
Macrophages

Name the predominant cell present after day 5 of wound healing?
Fibroblasts

When does the maturation phase usually begin?
~3 weeks after the injury

What is the maximal tensile strength that a wound can reach?
80% of original tissue strength

Time period for maximum collagen accumulation in a wound:
2 to 3 weeks (mostly type III, then gets converted to type I with maturation)

Phases of healing

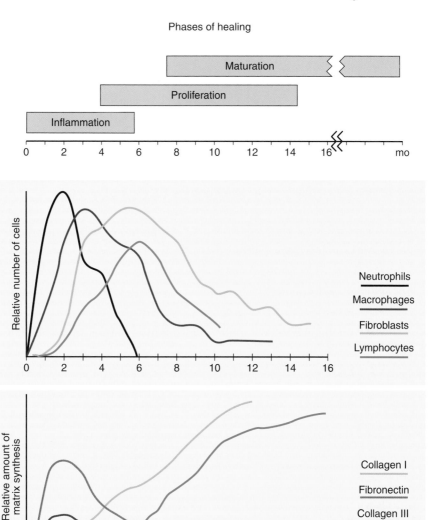

FIGURE 9-1. The cellular, biochemical, and mechanical phases of wound healing. *(Reproduced from Brunicardi FC, Anderson DK, Billiar TR, et al. Schwartz's Principles of Surgery. 9th ed. http://www.accessmedicine.com. Copyright © The McGraw-Hill Companies, Inc. All rights reserved.)*

Time period for a wound to reach its maximal tensile strength:
8 weeks

True or false: Denervation negatively affects epithelialization and wound contraction:
False; denervation has no effect on epithelialization/wound contraction

The number of organisms/cm² required to retard wound healing:
100,000 organisms/g (10^5 organisms/g)

What is the generally recommended period of time to wait for scar maturation before considering scar revision?
12 to 18 months

What can be given to combat the inhibitory effects of steroids on wound healing and epithelialization? Dose?
Vitamin A; 25,000 IU daily

Necessary cofactor for hydroxylation and cross-linking of proline and lysine in collagen synthesis:
Vitamin C (deficiency causes scurvy)

Type of scar that extends beyond the boundaries of the original wound:
Keloid

Type of scar that remains confined to the boundaries of the original wound and contains an overabundance of collagen:
Hypertrophic scar

The most common type of collagen is:
Type I collagen

Type of collagen predominantly synthesized in the first 48 hours of a healing wound:
Type III collagen

Type of collagen located in skin, bone, tendon, and is the primary collagen found in a healed wound:
Type I collagen

Type of collagen found in hyaline cartilage:
Type II collagen

Type of collagen in arteries, dermis, and increased in wound healing:
Type III collagen

Type of collagen that is predominant in the basement membrane:
Type IV collagen (type IV found on floor)

Type of collagen found in the cornea:
Type V collagen

Stage the pressure sore: nonblanchable erythema of intact skin:
Stage I (can be seen after 30 minutes, resolves after 1–2 hours)

Stage the pressure sore: partial-thickness skin loss involving epidermis/dermis:
Stage II (can present as blister, forms after 2–6 hours, erythema lasts >24 hours)

Stage the pressure sore: full-thickness skin loss with involvement of underlying subcutaneous tissue:
Stage III (does not extend through fascia)

Stage the pressure sore: full-thickness skin loss with tissue necrosis or extensive destruction of underlying structures (muscle/bone):
Stage IV

Areas at greatest risk for pressure sores:
Ischium 28%, Trochanter 19%, Sacrum 17%, Heel 9%, Occiput of scalp

Rules of operative management for pressure sores (name 4):
Debride all devitalized tissue
Excise entire bursa (can use methylene blue to identify entire bursa)
Identify and remodel bony prominences
Reliable tissue coverage with appropriate flap without burning bridges for future reconstruction

Name the amino acid that is found in every 3 residues in collagen:
Proline

Name the necessary cofactors for the hydroxylation of proline:
Vitamin C, oxygen, iron, and α-ketoglutarate

What enzyme is the rate-limiting step in collagen synthesis?
Propylhydroxylase

Albumin level that puts a patient at risk for poor wound healing:
<3.0 g/dL

Time period to wait for chemotherapy to have no effect on wound healing:
14 days

MULTIPLE CHOICE QUESTIONS

1. **What determines if a scar is hypertrophic or keloid?**
   A. Amount of scar elevation
   B. Borders of scar tissue extend beyond incision
   C. Associated erythema
   D. Results from biopsy

2. **What is the most abundant collagen in the body?**
   A. Type I
   B. Type II
   C. Type III
   D. Type IV

3. **Where do epithelial cells come from in wounds healing from secondary intention?**
   A. Base of wound
   B. Hair follicles, sebaceous glands, and skin edges
   C. Capillary ingrowth
   D. Basement membrane

4. **What nutritional parameter has a half-life of about 20 days?**
   A. Transferrin
   B. Albumin
   C. Prealbumin
   D. Retinal-binding protein

5. **What is the most common organism found in osteomyelitis?**
    A. *Staphylococcus aureus*
    B. *Staphylococcus epidermis*
    C. *Streptococcus pyogenes*
    D. *Escherichia coli*

6. **Wounds heal best in what type of environment?**
    A. Dry
    B. Moist
    C. Wet
    D. Warm

7. **A superficial surgical site infection (SSI) is considered when?**
    A. Purulent drainage from wound
    B. Occurs within 2 months from surgery
    C. Temperature >38°C
    D. WBC >12,000/mm³

8. **When does chemotherapy not affect wound healing?**
    A. Chemotherapy always affects wound healing
    B. 1 week after surgery
    C. 2 weeks after surgery
    D. 2 months after surgery

9. **Which nutritional factor is missing in scurvy?**
    A. Vitamin A
    B. Vitamin B
    C. Vitamin C
    D. Vitamin D

10. **Which factor(s) is/are important for management of foot ulcers in diabetic patients?**
    A. Glucose control
    B. Foot care/hygiene
    C. Frequent visits to a physician for inspection of feet
    D. All of the above

ANSWERS

1. **Answer: B.** Hypertrophic scars can be raised and erythematous, but do not extend beyond the borders of the incision laterally.
2. **Answer: A.** Type I collagen is the most abundant collagen in the body.
3. **Answer: B.** Epithelial cells from these structures migrate out and cover the wound bed.
4. **Answer: B.** Albumin has a long half-life compared to the other nutritional parameters and can give the clinician an idea of the nutritional status of patients.
5. **Answer: A.** *Staphylococcus aureus* is the most common pathogen in osteomyelitis; however, these infections are often polymicrobial.

6. **Answer: B.** A moist environment is best for wound healing; however, it is imperative that wounds are not frankly wet, as this can cause stagnant fluid to form, which is a great environment for bacteria.

7. **Answer: A.** SSI has to occur within 30 days of surgery, has redness, purulence, tenderness, positive wound cultures, or is diagnosed by the attending surgeon.

8. **Answer: C.** Two weeks is generally considered the safe amount of time postsurgery to perform chemotherapy, although some recommend 1 month.

9. **Answer: C.** Vitamin C is required as a cofactor for collagen hydroxylation in the synthesis of collagen.

10. **Answer: D.** All of these factors are important for diabetic patients with foot ulcers. These patients often have difficulty evaluating their own feet and frequently have poor sensation secondary to their peripheral neuropathy. These things in combination can lead to an unrecognized ulcer that can blossom into a wound requiring surgical intervention and possibly amputation.

CHAPTER 10
Head and Neck

Jonathan M. Lee and Margaret M. Moore

Test Taking Tips

- Know that the treatment for benign parotid tumors is superficial parotidectomy and that the treatment for malignant parotid tumors is total parotidectomy.
- Know the staging for squamous cell cancer of the head and neck. There is often a question about squamous cell cancer of the head and neck and the appropriate adjuvant treatment (in regards to the size of the primary tumor).

ANATOMY

Name the 3 auditory ossicle bones:
Malleus (hammer), incus (anvil), stapes (stirrup)

Name the nerve that crosses the internal carotid artery 1 to 2 cm above the carotid bifurcation:
Hypoglossal nerve

The hypoglossal nerve supplies motor innervation to all of the muscles of the tongue except:
Palatoglossus

The phrenic nerve lies on top of what muscle?
Anterior scalene

Name the branches of the facial nerve:
Temporal, zygomatic, buccal, marginal mandibular, cervical branches

Which branch of the facial nerve is most often injured in carotid surgery?
Marginal mandibular nerve

Name the branches of the trigeminal nerve:
Opthalmic (V1), maxillary (V2), mandibular (V3)

What nerve is found within the carotid sheath?
Vagus

The recurrent laryngeal nerve innervates all of the muscles of the larynx except:
Cricothyroid muscle

Which nerve is responsible for sensory innervation of the larynx above the level of the vocal folds?
Internal branch of the superior laryngeal nerve

Which nerve is responsible for sensory innervation of the larynx below the level of the vocal folds?
Recurrent laryngeal nerve

Name the branches of the thyrocervical trunk:
STAT
Suprascapular artery
Transverse cervical artery
Ascending cervical artery
Inferior thyroid artery

What is the first branch of the external carotid artery?
Superior thyroid artery

Name the blood supply to the nose:
Anterior/posterior ethmoidal arteries off the ophthalmic artery
Superior labial artery from the facial artery
Sphenopalatine artery off the internal maxillary artery

What nerve innervates the strap muscles?
Ansa cervicalis

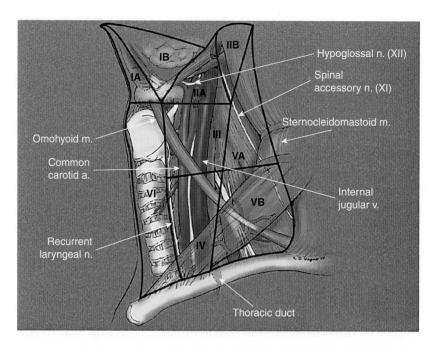

FIGURE 10-1. Lymph node compartments in the neck. The central compartment (level VI) is defined laterally by the carotid sheaths, superiorly by the hyoid bone, and inferiorly by the suprasternal notch. The lateral compartment contains superior jugular (level II), middle jugular (level III), and inferior jugular (level IV) lymph nodes, as well as the posterior triangle nodal tissue bound by the posterior border of the sternocleidomastoid, the anterior border of the trapezius, and the clavicle (level V). The division between levels II and III is a horizontal plane defined by the inferior body of the hyoid bone. The division between levels III and IV is a horizontal plane defined by the inferior border of the cricoid cartilage. Level I contains the submental and submandibular lymph nodes. a., artery; m., muscle; n., nerve; v., vein. *(Reproduced with permission from The University of Texas MD Anderson Cancer Center. Visual Art © 2008 The University of MD Anderson Cancer Center. All rights reserved.)*

Define the regions of the cervical lymph nodes:
Level I: submental and submandibular nodes
Level II: upper jugular nodes
Level III: middle jugular nodes
Level IV: lower jugular nodes
Level V: posterior triangle
Level VI: anterior compartment
Level VII: upper mediastinal nodes

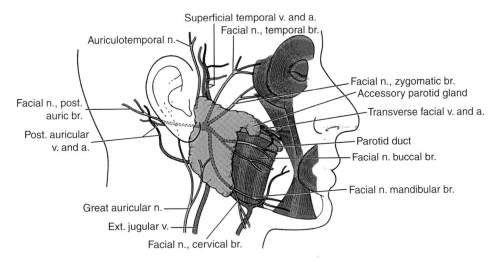

FIGURE 10-2. Diagrammatic representation of the relations of the parotid gland to the facial nerve and its branches. a., artery; m., muscle; n., nerve; v., vein. *(Modified from Skandalakis' Surgical Anatomy: The Embryologic Basis of Modern Surgery. Paschalidis Medical Publications; 2004, with permission.)*

What structure divides the parotid gland into superficial and deep lobes?
Facial nerve

What is the name of the duct in the parotid gland?
Stenson duct

What is the name of the duct in the submandibular gland?
Wharton duct

What is the most common nerve injured in parotid surgery?
Greater auricular nerve

TUMORS

What is the most common type of cancer of the oral cavity, pharynx, and larynx?
Squamous cell carcinoma

What is the biggest risk factor for head and neck cancer?
Tobacco

What is the most common location for an oral cavity cancer?
Lower lip

Oral cavity cancer is most likely to spread to which regional lymph nodes?
Submental and submandibular (level I)

What is the most common benign head and neck tumor in adults?
Hemangioma

What is the most common tumor of the nasopharynx in children?
Lymphoma

What is the most common benign neoplasm of the nose and paranasal sinuses?
Papilloma

What is the most common benign lesion of the larynx?
Papilloma

What is the treatment for an early glottic squamous cell carcinoma?
Primary radiation versus conservative surgical resection—laser versus endoscopic
(if recurs perform chordectomy)

What is the treatment for an advanced glottic squamous cell carcinoma?
Laryngectomy, modified radical neck dissection, and postoperative radiation

Where do head and neck tumors most often distantly metastasize?
Lung

Which disorder involves dysphagia, esophagitis, iron deficiency anemia, and an increased incidence of oral cavity cancer?
Plummer-Vinson syndrome

What are the indications for a radical neck dissection?
Clinically positive lymph nodes
Fixed cervical mass
High rate of suspicion for metastatic disease

In oral cavity cancer, when is a modified radical neck dissection indicated?
Clinically positive nodes
Tumor size >2cm

Which structures are taken in a radical neck dissection?
Accessory nerve, cervical branch of the facial nerve, internal jugular vein, ipsilateral
thyroid, omohyoid, sternocleidomastoid muscle, submandibular gland, sensory nerves
C2-C5

What is spared in a modified radical neck dissection?
Type I: spinal accessory nerve
Type II: spinal accessory nerve, internal jugular vein
Type III: spinal accessory nerve, internal jugular vein, sternocleidomastoid (SCM)

What percentage of salivary tumors are benign?
80%

What percentage of salivary tumors are in the parotid?
80%

What is the most common benign salivary tumor?
Pleomorphic adenoma

What percentage of pleomorphic adenomas undergo malignant degeneration?
5%

What is the second most common benign tumor of the salivary glands?
Warthin tumor

What percentage of Warthin tumor are bilateral?
10%

What is the most common salivary gland tumor in children?
Hemangioma

What is the most common malignant tumor of the salivary glands?
Mucoepidermoid carcinoma

What is the second most common malignant salivary gland tumor?
Adenoid cystic carcinoma

TRAUMA

What is the name of the vascular plexus located in the anterior portion of the nasal septum, which is responsible for 90% of epistaxis?
Kiesselbach plexus

What percentage of epistaxis can be controlled with anterior or combined anterior and posterior nasal packing?
95%

Which arteries can be ligated in order to control epistaxis?
Ethmoid artery, internal maxillary artery

Why does a nasal septal hematoma require emergent treatment?
The accumulation of blood in the nasal septum may deprive the septal cartilage of its blood supply from the perichondrium. It requires immediate incision and drainage, septal splinting, and antibiotics to prevent avascular necrosis of the septal cartilage and subsequent saddle nose deformity.

What is the initial management for a traumatic cerebrospinal fluid (CSF) leak?
Head elevation
Avoid nose blowing/straining
With/without antibiotics

Which diagnostic test can be used to confirm whether fluid is CSF?
B2-transferrin

What is the treatment for a persistent CSF leak (>4–6 weeks)?
Surgical repair

What is the treatment for a CSF leak associated with meningitis?
Surgical repair

What is the most common cause of laryngeal stenosis?
Trauma

Most common location for an esophageal foreign body:
Upper esophagus at the thoracic inlet

Above what level should a tracheostomy be placed to avoid the complication of a tracheo-innominate fistula?
Above the third tracheal ring

INFECTIONS

What is the initial treatment for a peritonsillar abscess?
IV antibiotics and needle aspiration

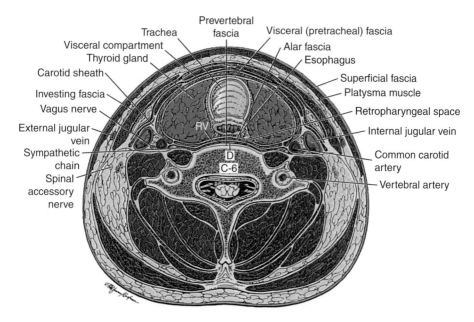

FIGURE 10-3. Cross-section of the neck showing fascial layers. D, the "danger space" within the prevertebral fascia. RV, retrovisceral or retropharyngeal space between the prevertebral fascia and the pretracheal (visceral) facial layers. *(Reproduced and modified from Skandalakis JE, Colburn GL. Clinical Gross Anatomy: A Guide for Dissection, Study, and Review, with permission of Informa Healthcare – Books via Copyright Clearance Center. Copyright 1993.)*

What is the treatment for a retropharyngeal abscess?
IV antibiotics and surgical drainage through the posterior pharynx or neck

What is the treatment for a parapharyngeal abscess?
IV antibiotics, incision and drainage through the lateral neck, and leave a drain in place

What is the initial treatment for acute suppurative parotitis?
Antibiotics, IV fluids, sialogogues, warm compresses

When is it necessary to operate on acute suppurative parotitis?
When there is no clinical improvement after 12 hours of treatment

MULTIPLE CHOICE QUESTIONS

1. **Which muscle is innervated by the external branch of the superior laryngeal nerve?**
   A. Posterior cricoarytenoid
   B. Lateral cricoarytenoid
   C. Thyroid arytenoid
   D. Cricothyroid
   E. Interarytenoid

2. **A 48-year-old male with massive head trauma does not have a gag reflex. Which nerve is responsible for the sensory nerve fibers that carry this reflex?**
   A. Marginal mandibular nerve
   B. Recurrent laryngeal nerve
   C. Facial nerve
   D. Glossopharyngeal nerve
   E. Vagus nerve

3. **The most common cause of a neck mass in males over the age of 60 is:**
   A. Laryngocele
   B. Metastatic carcinoma
   C. Brachial cleft cyst
   D. Bacterial adenitis
   E. Carotid aneurysm

4. **A 2nd year Internal Medicine resident stops you in the hall with a painless, 2-cm, slowly enlarging parotid mass. What does this most likely represent?**
   A. Hemangioma
   B. Warthin tumor
   C. Pleomorphic adenoma
   D. Mucoepidermoid carcinoma
   E. Adenoid cystic carcinoma

5. **A 14-year-old boy presents to the ER with epistaxis after being struck in the face with a baseball. Examination reveals a compressible, nontender mass involving the nasal septum. What is the most common complication resulting from this condition?**
   A. Delayed hemorrhage
   B. Cavernous sinus thrombosis
   C. Sepsis
   D. Osteomyelitis
   E. Saddle-nose deformity

6. **You are admitting a patient in the ER and previous records indicate she underwent a radical neck dissection. This means she has had:**
   A. An excisional biopsy of a neck mass
   B. Some of the lymph nodes removed in the anterior and posterior neck triangles
   C. All the lymph nodes removed but no vital structures removed from her neck
   D. All the lymph nodes removed and the spinal accessory nerve, the internal jugular vein, and the sternocleidomastoid removed
   E. All the lymph nodes removed and the spinal accessory nerve, the internal jugular vein, external carotid artery, and the sternocleidomastoid removed

7. **What is the treatment for a Warthin tumor?**

   A. Observation
   B. Surgical enucleation
   C. Total parotidectomy with resection of the facial nerve
   D. Total parotidectomy with postoperative radiation
   E. Superficial parotidectomy

8. **A 72-year-old man presents with a painless, gradually enlarging mass in the region of the left parotid with facial asymmetry and left-sided facial weakness. Following physical examination, what is the next step?**

   A. Superficial parotidectomy
   B. Total parotidectomy with modified radical neck dissection
   C. Fine-needle aspiration (FNA) of the mass and MRI of the head and neck
   D. Esophagogastroduodenoscopy and colonoscopy
   E. Complete metastatic work-up

9. **Following parotidectomy your patient has sweating in his retroauricular region while eating. This is most likely caused by:**

   A. Recurrent tumor
   B. Cross-innervation of the vagus and sympathetic nerves to the skin
   C. Cross-innervation of the auriculotemporal nerve and sympathetic nerves to the skin
   D. Cross-innervation to the glossopharyngeal nerve and sympathetic nerves to the skin

10. **A 10-year-old boy presents with a cyst and a cyst tract near the angle of his mandible. This cyst has had recurrent infections in it. This cyst most likely connects to the:**

    A. External auditory canal
    B. The tonsilar pillar
    C. The nasal septum
    D. Thoracic duct

ANSWERS

1. **Answer: D.** The cricothyroid muscle is the only muscle of the larynx innervated by the external branch of the superior laryngeal nerve. All other laryngeal muscles are innervated by the recurrent laryngeal nerve.

2. **Answer: D.** The afferent limb of the gag reflex comes from the glossopharyngeal nerve (cranial nerve IX).

3. **Answer: B.** Most neck masses in males over the age of 60 are as a result of metastatic spread from cancers in the chest and abdomen. These cancers frequently metastasize via lymphatic spread, and the most common location for the neck mass is within the supraclavicular fossa.

4. **Answer: C.** Pleomorphic adenomas are the most common benign salivary gland tumors, comprising 85% of all salivary gland neoplasms. Tumors of the parotid gland are the most common of the salivary gland tumors with a 5 × higher incidence than tumors of the minor salivary glands. The vast majority of tumors of the parotid gland are benign in nature.

5. **Answer: E.** The physical examination reveals findings consistent with a nasal septal hematoma. The most common complication of this condition is a saddle-nose deformity as a result of avascular necrosis from an infected septal hematoma.

6. **Answer: D.** A radical neck dissection includes removal of all the ipsilateral lymph nodes from levels I through V along with the spinal accessory nerve, the sternocleidomastoid muscle, and the internal jugular vein. A modified radical neck dissection removes all the lymph nodes but preserves one or all of the nonlymphatic structures.

7. **Answer: E.** A Warthin tumor is the second most common benign tumor of the parotid gland. It has an extremely low rate of malignant transformation (0.3%) as well as a low risk of recurrence (1.8% after local excision). The treatment is superficial parotidectomy, sparing the facial nerve. Simple enucleation is avoided because it increases the risk of recurrence and facial nerve injury.

8. **Answer: C.** The next step in the work-up includes an FNA and MRI of the head and neck. Given the patient's age and symptoms, tissue diagnosis is required for definitive diagnosis and MRI is necessary to evaluate the extent of disease. Local spread is common, but the incidence of metatatic disease with malignant salivary gland tumors is rare.

9. **Answer: C.** Gustatory sweating following parotidectomy is known as Frey's syndrome. Injury to the auriculotemporal nerve can occur during parotid surgery. The auriculotemporal nerve carries sympathetic fibers to the sweat glands of the scalp and parasympathetic fibers to the parotid gland. Following injury and subsequent regeneration, the fibers can cross-innervate leading to gustatory sweating.

10. **Answer: A.** First branchial cleft cysts typically originate at the angle of the mandible and often extend to the external auditory canal. Second branchial cleft cysts are found along the anterior border of the sternocleidomastoid muscle and connect with the tonsillar pillar.

CHAPTER 11
Breast

Christine Du and Daniel Barnas

ANATOMY/PHYSIOLOGY

The embryologic structure from which the breast forms:
Ectodermal thickenings termed mammary ridges or milk lines

Name the function of the following hormones:
Estrogen: branching differentiation and duct development in the breast
Progesterone: lobular development of the breast

Name the muscle the artery supplies:
Lateral thoracic artery
Serratus anterior muscle
Thoracodorsal artery
Latisimus dorsi

Name the nerve that innervates the following muscles:
Serratus anterior muscle
   Long thoracic nerve
   Latissimus dorsi
   Thoracodorsal nerve
Pectoralis minor
   Medial pectoral nerve
Pectoralis major
   Lateral and medial pectoral nerves

Name the complication if the following nerves were injured:
Long thoracic nerve: Winged scapula
Thoracodorsal nerve: Weak arm adduction/pull-ups

Name the arterial supply to the breast:
Branches derived from the intercostal arteries, internal thoracic artery, lateral thoracic artery, and thoracoacromial artery

The valveless venous plexus responsible for direct hematogenous spread of breast cancer to the spine:
Batson plexus

Suspensory ligaments that divide the breast into segments:
Cooper ligaments

What percentage of lymphatic drainage of the breast is to:
The axillary nodes: 97%
The internal mammary nodes: 1% to 2%

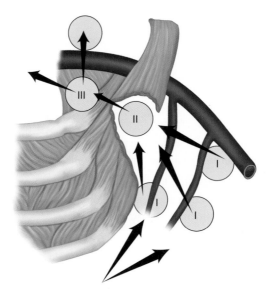

FIGURE 11-1. Axillary lymph node groups. Level I includes lymph nodes located lateral to the pectoralis minor (PM) muscle; level II includes lymph nodes located deep to the PM; and level III includes lymph nodes located medial to the PM. Arrows indicate the direction of lymph flow. The axillary vein with its major tributaries and the supraclavicular lymph node group are also illustrated. *(This article was published in Romrell LJ, Bland KI. Anatomy of the breast, axilla, chest wall, and related metastatic sites. In: Bland KI, Copeland EM III, eds. The Breast: Comprehensive Management of Benign and Malignant Diseases. Philadelphia: WB Saunders; 1998:19. Copyright © Elsevier 1998.)*

Anatomic description for Levels I, II, and III nodes in the breast?
Level I: Lateral to the pectoralis minor muscle
Level II: Beneath the pectoralis minor muscle
Level III: Medial to the pectoralis minor muscle

What are Rotter nodes?
Nodes between the pectoralis minor and major muscles

What are the boundaries of the axilla?
Superior: Axillary vein
Posterior: Long thoracic nerve
Lateral: Latissimus dorsi muscle
Medial: Pectoralis minor

Nerves to be aware of in an ALND:
Long thoracic nerve
Thoracodorsal nerve
Medial pectoral nerve
Lateral pectoral nerve
Intercostobrachial nerve

Potential complications of ALND:
Axillary vein thrombosis
Infection
Nerve injury
Lymphedema
Lymphatic fibrosis
Lymphangiosarcoma

Most likely cause of sudden, painful, early postop swelling of the ipsilateral arm after an axillary dissection:
Axillary vein thrombosis

Most likely cause of slow, painless, progressive swelling of the ipsilateral arm after an axillary dissection:
Lymphatic fibrosis

Most likely cause of hyperesthesia of the inner upper aspect of the ipsilateral arm after an axillary dissection:
Injury to the second intercostobrachiocutaneous nerve

Incidence of lymphedema after axillary node dissection:
15% to 30%

Incidence of lymphedema after sentinel node biopsy:
2% to 4%

SCREENING/IMAGING

Sensitivity and specificity of mammography:
90% for both

How large must a mass be to be detected on mammography?
5 mm or greater

Best time for a breast self-exam:
1 week after menstrual period

General population screening recommendations for breast cancer:
Initial screening mammogram at age 40 and annual mammograms after age 40

Screening recommendations for a patient at high risk for breast cancer:
Mammogram 10 years before the youngest age of diagnosis of breast cancer in a first-degree relative

What percentage of breast cancers have a negative mammogram and ultrasound?
10%

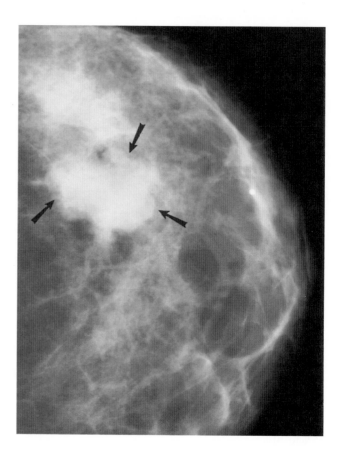

FIGURE 11-2. Breast cancer. Craniocaudal mammographic view of a palpable mass (arrows). *(Reproduced from Brunicardi FC, Andersen DK, Billiar TR, et al. Schwartz's Principles of Surgery. 9th ed. http://www. accessmedicine.com. Copyright © The McGraw-Hill Companies, Inc. All rights reserved.)*

Suspicious findings seen on mammography for breast cancer?
Asymmetric density
Distortion of architecture
Ductal asymmetry
Irregular borders
Multiple clusters
Linear, small, thin, and/or branching calcifications
Spiculation

What does BIRADS stand for?
Breast Imaging Reporting and Data System

What is the assessment and recommendation for each BIRADS category?
BIRADS 0: Incomplete; follow-up imaging necessary
BIRADS 1: Negative; routine screening
BIRADS 2: Definite benign finding; routine screening
BIRADS 3: Probably benign; 6-month short-interval follow-up
BIRADS 4: Suspicious abnormality; biopsy should be considered
BIRADS 5: Highly suspicious of malignancy; appropriate action should be taken
BIRADS 6: Known biopsy-proven malignancy; ensure that treatment is completed

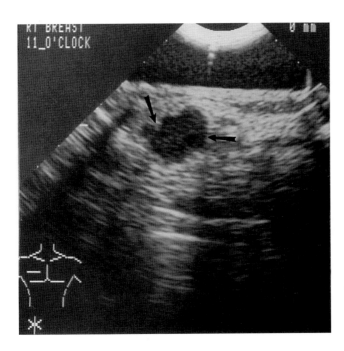

FIGURE 11-3. Breast cancer. Ultrasound image demonstrating a solid mass with irregular borders (arrows) consistent with cancer. *(Reproduced from Brunicardi FC, Andersen DK, Billiar TR, et al. Schwartz's Principles of Surgery. 9th ed. http://www. accessmedicine.com. Copyright © The McGraw-Hill Companies, Inc. All rights reserved.)*

BREAST CANCER

Most aggressive subtype of ductal carcinoma in situ (DCIS):
Comedo pattern

Risk of lymph node metastasis with DCIS:
<2%

Surgical treatment for a <1 cm low-grade DCIS?
Excision with 2- to 3-mm margins ± radiation

Surgical treatment for a >1 cm DCIS?
Lumpectomy and radiation with 2- to 3-mm margins or total mastectomy without axillary dissection

Indications to perform a simple mastectomy for DCIS:
Contraindications to radiation, high grade, and diffuse breast involvement

In which breast does invasive cancer arise in the setting of DCIS?
Usually the ipsilateral breast

What percentage of patients get cancer in the ipsilateral breast with unresected DCIS?
50% to 60%

What percentage of patients get cancer in the contralateral breast with unresected DCIS?
5% to 10%

What percentage of patients develop cancer in either breast with lobular carcinoma in situ (LCIS)?
40%

How much does atypical lobular hyperplasia increase the chance of developing breast cancer?
4-fold

How much does atypical lobular hyperplasia in the setting of a strong family history of breast cancer increase the chance of developing breast cancer?
9-fold

How much does LCIS increase the chance of developing breast cancer?
9-fold

In which breast does invasive cancer arise in the setting of LCIS?
Carcinoma can arise in either breast.

True or False: LCIS is a premalignant lesion:
False; considered a marker for the development of breast cancer but not premalignant

True or False: LCIS needs to be excised to negative margins:
False; negative margins are not required.

What is the most likely type of breast cancer to develop in a patient with LCIS?
Ductal carcinoma (70%)

What is the percentage of finding a synchronous breast cancer at the time of diagnosis of LCIS?
5%

Treatment for LCIS:
Close-interval follow-up, treatment with tamoxifen, or bilateral simple mastectomy

What is the incidence of breast cancer?
1 in 8 women; 12% lifetime risk

What is the breast cancer risk in a patient with no risk factors?
4% to 5%

What percentage of women with breast cancer have no known risk factors?
75%

Name factors that place a patient at greatly increased risk for breast cancer:
2 primary relatives with bilateral or premenopausal breast cancer
BRCA gene in a patient with family history of breast cancer
DCIS or LCIS
Fibrocystic disease with atypical hyperplasia

Name factors that place a patient at moderately increased risk for breast cancer:
Early menarche (<12 years)
Late menopause (>55)
Nulliparity (or first birth after age 30)
Environmental risk factor (high-fat diet/obesity)
Family history of breast cancer (excluding BRCA gene)
Two primary relative with bilateral or premenopausal breast cancer
Previous breast cancer
Radiation

What is the median survival for a patient with untreated breast cancer?
2 to 3 years

What is the most common site of breast cancer?
Upper outer quadrant (~50%)

What is the most important prognostic staging factor for breast cancer?
Nodal status

Approximate 5-year survival for a patient with breast cancer with:
0 positive nodes: 75%
1 to 3 positive nodes: 60%
4 to 10 positive nodes: 40%

According to AJCC cancer staging, what is a:
T1 breast lesion: ≤2 cm
T2 breast lesion: 2 to 5 cm
T3 breast lesion: >5 cm
T4 breast lesion: Skin/chest wall involvement (excluding pectoral muscles)
Peau d'orange: Inflammatory breast cancer

According to AJCC cancer staging, what are N1, N2, and N3 nodal status in breast cancer?
N1- Ipsilateral axillary nodes
N2- Fixed ipsilateral axillary nodes
N3- Ipsilateral internal mammary nodes

According to AJCC cancer staging, what is M1 disease in breast cancer?
Distant metastasis including ipsilateral supraclavicular nodes

AJCC cancer staging:
Stage 0 breast cancer?
  Tis, N0, M0
Stage I breast cancer?
  T1, N0, M0
Stage IIa breast cancer?
  T0-1, N1, M0 or T2, N0, M0
Stage IIb breast cancer?
  T2, N1, M0 or T3, N0, M0
Stage IIIa breast cancer?
  T0-3, N2, M0 or T3, N1-2, M0
Stage IIIb breast cancer?
  Any T4 or N3 tumors
Stage IV breast cancer?
  M1

Most common type of breast cancer:
Infiltrating ductal carcinoma

Name in dications for breast biopsy:
Blood in cyst aspirate, bloody nipple discharge
Dermatitis/ulceration of nipple
Patient concern of persistent breast abnormality
Persistent mass after aspiration
Solid mass
Suspicious lesion by imaging studies

What are central/subareolar tumors at an increased risk for?
These tumors are usually multicentric.

How long does it take for a single malignant cell to become a 1-cm tumor?
5 to 7 years

What are the sites of metastasis for breast cancer?
Lymph nodes (most common)
Brain
Bones
Liver
Lung/pleura

Estrogen receptor (ER)- and progesterone receptor (PR)-positive tumors are associated with?
Better overall prognosis and prognosis following surgery
Better response to chemotherapy and hormone manipulation
More well-differentiated tumor

Most common place for distant metastasis for breast cancer:
Bone

Name malignant tumors with a well-circumscribed, benign appearance:
Phyllodes tumor, medullary carcinoma, and adenoid cystic carcinoma

What percentage of phyllodes tumors are malignant?
10%

What is the treatment of a Pyllodes tumor?
Wide local excision with 1-cm margin without axillary dissection

Name benign conditions that can mimic breast cancer:
Fat necrosis, fibromatosis, granular cell tumor, radial scar

Incidence of male breast cancer:
<1% of all breast cancer cases

Risk factors for male breast cancer:
BRCA2 carrier, estrogen therapy, gynecomastia (from increased estrogen), increased estrogen, Klinefelter syndrome (XXY), radiation

The type of breast cancer that males develop:
Ductal carcinoma

True or False: The prognosis for breast cancer is poorer in men than in women, stage for stage?
False; prognosis is the same stage for stage (overall prognosis is poorer secondary to men presenting at a later stage).

Approximate risk of ovarian cancer with BRCA1 versus BRCA2 mutation:
40% versus 20%

Approximate percentage of males with BRCA2 mutations that develop breast cancer:
6%

How are BRCA1 and BRCA2 transmitted?
Autosomal dominant transmission

True or False: The germ-line mutations BRCA1 and BRCA2 are completely penetrant.
False; they are incompletely penetrant and some carriers may not develop cancer.

Population with the highest incidence of BRCA mutations:
Ashkenazi Jews (1%–3%)

What kind of protein does the human epidermal growth factor receptor-2 (HER-2) encode for?
Transmembrane tyrosine kinase receptor with potent growth-stimulating activity

Inherited breast cancer syndrome associated with an increased incidence of adrenocortical cancers, brain tumors, leukemias, soft tissue, and osteosarcomas in the same family:
Li-Fraumeni syndrome

Treatment for male breast cancer:
Modified radical mastectomy

Causes of male gynecomastia:
Medications (cimetidine, ketoconazole, spironolactone, TCAs), androgen insensitivity, gonadal failure, decreased testosterone, increased estrogen, illicit drugs (marijuana), liver failure

Treatment for male gynecomastia:
Stop/change medications, correct any hormonal imbalances/underlying cause; if refractory to time and conservative measures, perform a biopsy versus simple mastectomy

Define a simple/total mastectomy:
Excision of breast and nipple-areolar complex without removal of axillary nodes

What is removed with a modified radical mastectomy?
Breast, nipple-areolar complex, and axillary nodes (level I, II)

Potential complications after modified radical mastectomy:
Hematoma/seroma, infection, ipsilateral arm lymphedema, nerve injury, Phantom breast syndrome, skin flap necrosis

Considerations for prophylactic mastectomy:
Family history and BRCA+ or LCIS with one of the following:
High patient anxiety
Lesion difficult to follow on exam/mammography
Poor access for follow-up
Patient preference for mastectomy

What are indications for radiation after mastectomy?
Tumor >5 cm
4 or more positive lymph nodes
Extracapsular nodal invasion
Fixed axillary nodes (N2) or internal mammary nodes (N3)
Inflammatory cancer
Positive margins
Skin/chest wall involvement

List complications of breast irradiation:
Cardiac toxicity, contralateral breast cancer, edema, erythema, pneumonitis, rib fractures, sarcoma, ulceration

Absolute contraindications for breast-conserving therapy in invasive carcinoma:
An area with a history of prior therapeutic irradiation
Diffuse malignant-appearing microcalcifications
Persistent positive margins after surgery
Pregnancy (except in 3rd trimester, can give radiation after delivery)
Two or more primary tumors in separate quadrants of the breast

List relative contraindications for breast-conserving therapy in invasive carcinoma:
Extensive gross multifocal disease in the same quadrant
History of scleroderma or active systemic lupus erythematosus
Large tumor in a small breast if it would result in unacceptable cosmesis
Genetic predisposition to breast cancer

What breast cancers can be treated with lumpectomy and radiation?
Tumors <5 cm (stage I and II)

Chance of local recurrence after lumpectomy with radiation:
10%, usually within 2 years of the first operation

Treatment for local recurrence of breast cancer after lumpectomy, axillary dissection, and radiation:
Salvage mastectomy

Chance of local recurrence after mastectomy:
5% (4%–8%)

What is the false-negative rate for sentinel node biopsy?
4% to 12%

What are the usual chemotherapeutic regimens for breast cancer?
AC (adriamycin and cyclophosphamide) followed by pacitaxel, TAC (adriamycin, cyclophosphamide, and docetaxel), TC (docetaxel and cyclophosphamide), or CMF (cyclophosphamide, methotrexate, 5-fluorouracil)

Standard dosage of tamoxifen in regards to adjuvant treatment for breast cancer:
20 mg daily for 5 years

For which patient population is Arimidex/Femara (aromotase inhibitors) useful?
Postmenopausal women

Name alternative hormonal/chemotherapy options for breast cancer:
Aminoglutethimide, anastrozole/letrozole (aromatase inhibitors), androgenic steroid,
bilateral oophorectomy, megace

Risk of blood clots with the use of tamoxifen:
1%

Risk of endometrial cancer with the use of tamoxifen:
0.10%

What is the increased relative risk of breast cancer with 5 years of hormone
replacement therapy?
1.35 (26% increased risk)

Recommendation for adjuvant therapy for:
Node negative, low-risk breast cancer?
   No treatment or endocrine therapy if ER+
Node negative, higher risk ER+ breast cancer?
   Chemotherapy + endocrine therapy or endocrine therapy
Node negative, higher risk ER– breast cancer?
   Chemotherapy
Node positive, ER+ breast cancer in a premenopausal pt.?
   Chemotherapy + endocrine therapy
Node positive, ER+ breast cancer in a postmenopausal pt.?
   Chemotherapy + endocrine therapy or endocrine therapy alone
Node positive, ER– breast cancer?
   Chemotherapy

What is the treatment of HER-2–positive breast cancer?
Chemotherapy plus Trastuzumab (Herceptin)

Treatment for breast cancer in pregnancy:
1st trimester: modified radical mastectomy
2nd trimester: modified radical mastectomy
3rd trimester: If late, can perform lumpectomy with ALND and postpartum radiation;
otherwise modified radical mastectomy

Indications for neoadjuvant therapy:
Primary tumors >5 cm, fixed or matted axillary nodes, and inflammatory breast
carcinoma

Contraindications to radiation therapy:
Previous radiation therapy to breast or severe collagen vascular disease, pregnancy

What is the mechanism of action of tamoxifen versus aromatase inhibitors?
Tamoxifen is a selective estrogen receptor (ER) modulator and binds to and inhibits ER
signaling in the breast. It produces antiestrogen effects in the breast. In postmenopausal
women, the primary source of estrogen is from the conversion of androstenedione to

estrone and testosterone to estradiol in peripheral tissues such as breast, skin, and adipose tissue by aromatase. The aromatase inhibitors block this conversion, explaining why they are only effective in postmenopausal women.

What are the side effects to aromatase inhibitors?
Osteoporosis, joint disorders, hypercholesterolemia

What other cancers are associated with BRCA1 and BRCA2 mutations?
Prostate cancer is associated with both mutations. BRCA-1: ovarian and endometrial. Consider prophylactic TAH-BSO. BRCA-2: male breast cancer, colon, pancreatic, stomach, gallbladder, melanoma.

What type of breast cancer is associated with BRCA1 and BRCA2 mutations?
BRCA1: poorly differentiated, receptor-negative
BRCA2: well-differentiated, receptor-positive

What is Paget disease (of the breast)?
Dermatitis/scaling rash of the nipple caused by invasion of the skin by ductal carcinoma cells

If Paget disease is confined to the nipple, how can it be treated?
Excision with **sentinel lymph node** (SLN) biopsy and radiation.

MISCELLANEOUS

What is Stewart-Treves syndrome?
Lymphangiosarcoma secondary to chronic lymphedema following axillary dissection

Term for thrombophlebitis of superficial breast veins:
Mondor disease

How do you treat Mondor disease?
Nonsteroidal anti-inflammatory drugs (NSAIDs)

Term for a benign tumor of the breast found with collagen arranged in swirls and consisting of stromal overgrowth:
Fibroadenoma

Term for a cellulitis/superficial infection of the breast:
Mastitis

Most common bacteria to cause mastitis:
Staphylococcus aureus

Treatment for mastitis:
Antibiotics, continue breast-feeding, heating packs, utilization of breast pumps

Why should a patient with mastitis have close follow-up?
To rule out inflammatory breast cancer

Most common breast abnormality:
Accessory nipple

Name of the syndrome associated with absence of the pectoralis muscle, amastia, hypoplasia of the chest wall, and hypoplastic shoulder?
Poland syndrome

Condition in which the nipple is present, but the breast mound is absent:
Amastia

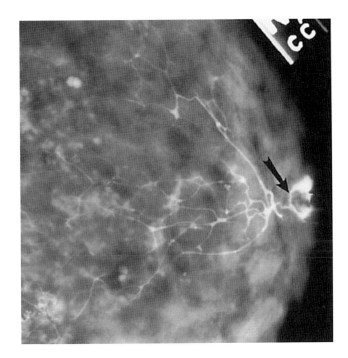

FIGURE 11-4. Ductogram. Craniocaudal mammographic view demonstrates a mass (arrow) posterior to the nipple and outlined by contrast, which also fills the proximal ductal structures. *(Courtesy of Dr. Barbara G. Steinbach.)*

Most common cause of bloody discharge from the nipple:
Intraductal papilloma

Treatment for an intraductal papilloma:
Resection (subareolar resection)

Most common cause of brown-, green-, or straw-colored nipple discharge:
Fibrocystic disease

Treatment for mastodynia:
Evening primrose oil, danazol, OCP

Dose of evening primrose oil to treat mastodynia:
3 to 4 g daily

Most common breast lesion in adolescents and young adults:
Fibroadenoma

MAKE THE DIAGNOSIS

Biopsy of a breast lesion shows prominent fibrous tissue compressing epithelial elements:
Fibroadenoma

Biopsy of a breast lesion shows nests of epithelial cells invading stroma in a random fashion with the suggestion of tubule formation:
Infiltrating ductal carcinoma

Biopsy of a breast lesion shows a uniform population of cells distorting, expanding, and filling the lobules:
LCIS

Biopsy of a breast lesion shows an ectatic duct with a single- or double-cell layer (epithelial or myoepithelial):
Fibrocystic disease

Fine-needle aspiration (FNA) of a breast lesion with the histologic appearance of poorly cohesive intact cells with variation in nuclear size with nuclear crowding, prominent nucleoli, clumping of chromatin, and radial dispersion in a highly cellular, monmorphic pattern:
Breast carcinoma

FNA of a breast lesion with the histologic appearance of broad sheets of cohesive cells with nuclei in uniform size and shape:
Fibroadenoma

MULTIPLE CHOICE QUESTIONS

1. A 65-year-old female presented with a 2.5-cm mass in her right breast that on core-needle biopsy had high-grade DCIS. She is taken to the operating room for lumpectomy and SLN biopsy. The patient was injected with both blue dye and radiotracer but no SLN could be identified. What will this patient's treatment include?

   A. Lumpectomy only
   B. Lumpectomy and radiation only
   C. Mastectomy and axillary lymph node dissection only
   D. Lumpectomy and radiation and axillary lymph node dissection
   E. Mastectomy and axillary lymph node dissection and radiation

2. A premenopausal 42-year-old female has been diagnosed with ER+/PR+ invasive ductal carcinoma. Her lesion is 2 cm in size and she has 2 positive lymph nodes. She had chosen to undergo breast-conserving therapy. What will her postsurgical treatment include?

   A. Chemotherapy only
   B. Radiation therapy only
   C. Anastrozole only
   D. Radiation therapy and tamoxifen
   E. Chemotherapy, radiation therapy, and tamoxifen

3. A 62-year-old female presents with scaly skin surrounding her nipple that has not resolved. A biopsy including skin was performed at this area. Pathology returns with large vacuolated cells in the epithelium and no other atypical cells or cancerous cells are present. Her treatment should be:

    A. Modified radical mastectomy
    B. Simple mastectomy
    C. Steroid cream
    D. Simple mastectomy with SLN
    E. Wide excision of the skin involved

4. A 36-year-old female who is 20 weeks' pregnant presents with a palpable mass. Ultrasound-guided core needle biopsy reveals a 3-cm invasive ductal carcinoma. She wishes to undergo breast-conserving therapy. What treatment is indicated for her?

    A. Perform the lumpectomy and wait until postpartum for radiation therapy.
    B. Give neoadjuvant therapy and wait until after delivery for breast-conserving surgery and radiation.
    C. The patient's condition is a contraindication to breast-conserving therapy and must undergo a modified radical mastectomy.
    D. Perform a lumpectomy, SLN biopsy, and radiation therapy after delivery.

5. A 47-year-old female presents with a palpable mass on physical exam. A mammogram was obtained and her lesion was characterized as a BIRADS3. Your next step is:

    A. An ultrasound
    B. Excision of mass
    C. Core needle biopsy
    D. Repeat mammogram in 6 months, since her mammogram result was a BIRADS3

6. A 70-year-old female presents with multiple nodules on her left arm that has been chronically swollen since her axillary lymph node dissection 7 years ago. How would you diagnose and treat this patient?

    A. Fine-needle biopsy and treat with radiation therapy
    B. Fine-needle biopsy with wide excision
    C. CT scan and chemotherapy
    D. Open biopsy and wide excision
    E. Open biopsy with radiation therapy

7. A 46-year-old female presents with a 4-cm palpable mass. Pathology and ultrasound-guided core needle biopsy reveal an invasive ductal carcinoma. The patient desires breast-conserving therapy. What treatment is indicated for her?

    A. Tell her that she is not a candidate for breast-conserving therapy and requires a modified radical mastectomy
    B. Neoadjuvant chemotherapy followed by breast-conserving therapy
    C. Tell her that she is not a candidate for breast-conserving therapy and requires a simple mastectomy with SLN biopsy
    D. Neoadjuvant chemotherapy followed by breast conservation and SLN biopsy if tumor has an appropriate response to chemotherapy

8. A 64-year-old female presents with spontaneous, unilateral, bloody nipple discharge. The rest of her exam is unremarkable, and mammogram and ultrasound do not reveal any abnormalities. What is the next step in management?

   A. Major duct excision
   B. Reassurance since nipple discharge is rarely associated with malignancy
   C. Ductography
   D. Repeat mammogram and ultrasound in 6 months

9. A 39-year-old female presents with a 2-cm palpable breast mass. On exam, she is also noted to have a warm, erythematous breast with peau d'orange changes. Biopsy of the mass reveals infiltrating ductal carcinoma. What is the next step in management?

   A. Breast-conserving surgery with SLN biopsy
   B. Modified radical mastectomy
   C. Breast-conserving surgery with SLN biopsy followed by chemotherapy
   D. Neoadjuvant chemotherapy followed by modified radical mastectomy
   E. Neoadjuvant chemotherapy followed by breast-conserving surgery

10. A 45-year-old female after a needle biopsy of a nonpalpable breast mass reveals LCIS. What is the next step in the management of this patient?

    A. Breast-conserving surgery with SLN biopsy
    B. Bilateral modified radical mastectomies
    C. Needle localized excisional biopsy of the lesion
    D. No further surgery is indicated
    E. Treat the patient with tamoxifen and close follow-up

ANSWERS

1. **Answer: D.** If no tracer or blue dye is taken up by the lymph nodes, then a lymph node dissection must be performed along with your breast-conserving therapy (ie, lumpectomy) and radiation.

2. **Answer: E.** Since the patient has positive nodal status, chemotherapy is necessary. Also undergoing breast-conserving therapy, the patient must receive radiation. Since she is premenopausal and her nodal status is positive, tamoxifen would also be given.

3. **Answer: B.** The patient has Paget disease that involves more than the nipple without evidence of malignancy; thus, the treatment is simple mastectomy.

4. **Answer: C.** Since the patient is in her second trimester, chemotherapy and radiation are contraindicated. She will need a modified radical mastectomy.

5. **Answer: C.** Even though her mammogram is BIRADS3, indicating a repeat mammogram in 6 months, the patient has a palpable mass. This alone necessitates immediate further work-up with core needle biopsy.

6. **Answer: D.** The patient has developed Stewart-Treves syndrome (lymphangiosarcoma). Her treatment would include an open biopsy to confirm diagnosis followed by wide excision.

7. **Answer: D.** Given the patient's wish for breast conservation, neoadjuvant chemotherapy can be given in an attempt to downsize the tumor. After neoadjuvant

chemotherapy if there is an appropriate response by the tumor, breast conservation can be undertaken. An SLN biopsy should also be performed to assess the lymph node status.

8. **Answer: A.** This patient has spontaneous, unilateral, bloody nipple discharge, which is suspicious for an underlying malignancy. The most common cause of bloody nipple discharge is a benign, intraductal papilloma. Major duct excision is warranted because of the risk of malignancy in this patient. Ductography has only a 60% sensitivity for malignancy, but could be a consideration in a patient who wishes to preserve breast-feeding.

9. **Answer: D.** This patient has inflammatory breast cancer and breast-conserving surgery is contraindicated. The management of inflammatory breast cancer is neoadjuvant chemotherapy followed by chemotherapy and radiation therapy.

10. **Answer: C.** In this patient with LCIS and an imaging abnormality she will need a wider biopsy to rule out an associated cancer. A negative margin is not required at the excisional biopsy, since LCIS can be extensive. The goal of the biopsy is to obtain a larger specimen. If a malignancy is found, then it should be appropriately treated.

CHAPTER 12
Endocrine

Danielle Press and Patty T. Liu

THYROID

EMBRYOLOGY, ANATOMY, AND PHYSIOLOGY

What embryologic structures does the thyroid originate from?
The medial thyroid comes from the first and second pharyngeal pouches
Lateral portions of the thyroid and parafollicular C cells arise from the fourth and fifth pharyngeal pouches

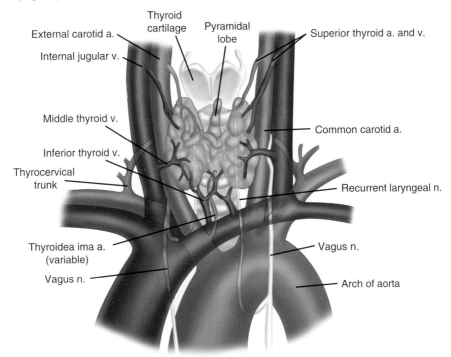

FIGURE 12-1. Anatomy of the thyroid gland and surrounding structures, viewed anteriorly. a., artery; n., nerve; v., vein. *(Reproduced from Brunicardi FC, Andersen DK, Billiar TR, et al. Schwartz's Principles of Surgery. 9th ed. http://www.accessmedicine.com. Copyright © The McGraw-Hill Companies, Inc. All rights reserved.)*

What is the arterial supply of the thyroid?
Superior thyroid artery (from external carotid artery)
Inferior thyroid artery (from thyrocervical trunk)

What is the venous drainage of the thyroid?
Superior and middle thyroid veins (drain into internal jugular vein)
Inferior thyroid veins (drain into innominate and brachiocephalic veins)

The recurrent laryngeal nerve innervates all of the muscles of the larynx except this muscle?
Cricothyroid muscle, which is innervated by the external branch of the superior laryngeal nerve

What structures do the recurrent laryngeal nerves wrap around?
Subclavian artery on the right
Arch of the aorta on the left

Injury to which nerve results in loss of projection and voice fatigability?
Superior laryngeal nerve

DRUGS

What is the mechanism of action of propylthiouracil (PTU) and methimazole?
Both drugs block peroxidase oxidation of iodide to iodine, thereby inhibiting incorporation of iodine into T4 and T3
PTU also inhibits peripheral conversion of T4 to T3

Which drug crosses the placenta: PTU or methimazole?
Methimazole
PTU is the safer choice in pregnancy

When steroids are given in severe or acute hyperthyroid conditions? How do they work?
Steroids inhibit peripheral conversion of T4 to T3 and lower serum TSH by suppressing the pituitary-thyroid axis

What is the Wolff-Chaikoff effect?
Large doses of iodine given after an antithyroid medication can inhibit thyroid hormone release by disrupting the coupling of iodide
This is a transient effect

HYPERTHYROIDISM/HYPOTHYROIDISM, AND GOITERS

What is the most common cause of hyperthyroidism?
Graves disease, also known as diffuse toxic goiter, is the cause of 60% to 80% of hyperthyroidism

What is the etiology of Graves disease?
Autoantibodies to TSH receptors (also called thyroid-stimulating antibodies or TSAb) bind and stimulate thyroid hormone production
This leads to thyrotoxicosis, diffuse goiter, pretibial myxedema, ophthalmopathy

What is the treatment for Graves disease?
Antithyroid medication
Thyroid ablation
With/without thyroidectomy

A 55-year-old woman presents with a 3-year history of fatigue and mild, diffuse, nontender thyroid enlargement and 15-lb weight loss. What is the most likely diagnosis?
Hashimoto thyroiditis

What is the most common cause of hypothyroidism in adults?
Hashimoto thyroiditis

What is the first-line treatment for Hashimoto thyroiditis?
Thyroid hormone replacement

What will pathology show in a patient with Hashimoto thyroiditis?
Lymphocytic infiltrate

A 35-year-old female presents with sudden onset of severe pain and associated swelling and tenderness of her thyroid with fever, chills, and dysphagia following an acute upper respiratory infection. What is the most likely diagnosis?
Acute suppurative thyroiditis

What is the treatment for acute suppurative thyroiditis?
Antibiotics
Occasionally, abscess drainage

A 35-year-old female presents with moderate swelling and tenderness of her thyroid with repeated exacerbations and remissions over several months following an acute upper respiratory infection. What is the most likely diagnosis?
Subacute (de Quervain) thyroiditis

What is the treatment for subacute (de Quervain) thyroiditis?
NSAIDs, steroids

A 40-year-old female presents with hypothyroidism and symptoms of tracheal and esophageal compression and is found to have dense fibrosis throughout her thyroid gland. What is the most likely diagnosis?
Riedel fibrous struma
Painless, progressive goiter
Usually euthyroid may become hypothyroid

What is the treatment for Riedel fibrous struma?
Thyroid hormone replacement and steroids
Surgery may be necessary to relieve obstructive symptoms

What is the treatment of thyroid storm?
PTU or methimazole q4 to 6 hours and inorganic iodide to block synthesis and release of thyroid hormones
Dexamethasone to inhibit peripheral conversion of T4 to T3
Propanolol
Fever reduction
General resuscitation

What is the most common cause of thyroid enlargement?
Multinodular goiter

What are indications for surgery with a multinodular goiter?
Inability to rule out cancer
Compressive symptoms
Cosmetic deformity

CANCER

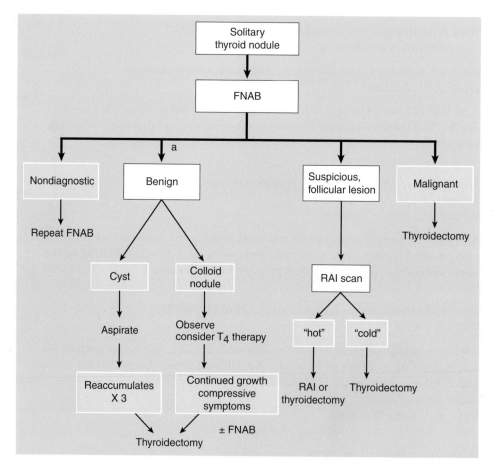

FIGURE 12-2. Management of a solitary thyroid nodule. a, except in patients with a history of external radiation exposure or a family history of thyroid cancer; FNAB, fine-needle aspiration biopsy; RAI, radioactive iodine; T4, thyroxine. (*Reproduced from Brunicardi FC, Andersen DK, Billiar TR, et al. Schwartz's Principles of Surgery. 9th ed. http://www.accessmedicine.com. Copyright © The McGraw-Hill Companies, Inc. All rights reserved.*)

What is the diagnostic test of choice for the evaluation of a thyroid nodule?
FNA
It has a sensitivity of 86% and specificity of 91%
Initial cytology is nondiagnostic in 20% to 25% of cases
However, a diagnosis of malignancy in FNA is highly accurate, approaching 100%

What is usually the first manifestation of multiple endocrine neoplasia (MEN) 2a and 2b?
Medullary thyroid carcinoma (MTC)

What are the cytologic features of MTC?
Amyloid among neoplastic cells
Immunohistochemistry positive for calcitonin
Positive staining for carcinoembryonic antigen (CEA) or calcitonin gene-related peptide
Heterogeneity with polygonal or spindle-shaped cells

What percentage of MTC is sporadic?
75% to 80%
Unable to differentiate familial versus sporadic at presentation—all should be tested
for rearranged during transfection (RET) mutation, pheochromocytoma, and
hyperparathyroidism

What operation should be done for MTC?
Total thyroidectomy
High incidence of multicentric disease

By what age should MEN 2a and MEN 2b patients undergo total thyroidectomy?
MEN 2a—age 6
MEN 2b—age 1 to 2

How can you follow patients after thyroidectomy for MTC?
Calcitonin levels
History and physical examination

What are the cytologic features indicative of anaplastic thyroid carcinoma?
Grossly firm and white
Marked heterogeneity with spindle, polygonal, or multinucleated cells

What is the prognosis for anaplastic thyroid carcinoma?
Poor—only few survive more than 6 months

Who typically gets anaplastic thyroid carcinoma?
Elderly patients with a long-standing goiter

What is the treatment for a small anaplastic thyroid carcinoma?
Total thyroidectomy with or without external beam radiation
Has small improvement in survival, especially for younger patients

What is the treatment for anaplastic thyroid carcinoma with compressive symptoms?
Debulking surgery with tracheostomy

Which patient has a higher likelihood of malignancy: the patient with a solid thyroid lesion versus cystic thyroid lesion?
Solid thyroid lesion

Which patient has a higher likelihood of malignancy: the patient with a solitary thyroid lesion versus multiple thyroid lesions?
Solitary thyroid lesion

Which patient has a higher likelihood of malignancy: the patient with a hot thyroid lesion versus cold thyroid lesion?
Cold thyroid lesion

Which type is the most common thyroid cancer and has the best prognosis?
Papillary thyroid cancer, about 70% to 80% of all thyroid cancers

Which subtypes carry a worse prognosis?
Insular
Columnar
Tall cell

What are the histologic findings for papillary thyroid carcinoma?
Psammoma bodies
Orphan Annie nuclei

What is the treatment for papillary thyroid carcinoma?
High-risk, large (>2 cm), or bilateral tumors—total thyroidectomy
Low-risk, small (<1 cm), or unilateral tumors—thyroid lobectomy and isthmusectomy

What laboratory test is followed after surgery to monitor recurrence?
Thyroglobulin

True or False: Positive cervical nodes affect the prognosis of papillary thyroid carcinoma?
False; positive cervical nodes do not affect the prognosis of papillary thyroid carcinoma as long as disease is resectable.

What are the histologic findings needed to define malignancy in follicular cancer?
Blood vessel, capsular invasion

What is the most common site of distant metastasis for follicular thyroid carcinoma?
Bone
Next most common is lung
Spread is hematogenous

Which has a worse prognosis: Hurthle cell carcinoma or Follicular carcinoma?
Hurthle cell carcinoma
Higher recurrence rate usually to regional lymph nodes

Name the 3 classifications systems specific to papillary thyroid cancer:
AGES (age, grade of tumor, extent of tumor, size)
AMES (age, metastasis, extent of tumor, size)
MACIS (metastasis, age, completeness of resection, local invasion, size)
High-risk patients by AGES or AMES criteria: >40 years old, male, capsular invasion or extrathyroidal extension, regional or distant metastases, size >4 cm, or poorly differentiated carcinoma

What is the (tumor, node, metastasis) (TNM) stage for a 57-year-old patient who underwent a total thyroidectomy for a 2.5-cm mass that was determined to be papillary thyroid carcinoma? All lymph nodes were free of disease and there was no extrathyroidal disease.
This patient has T2N0M0 disease
Because the patient is older than 45 years, this is stage II papillary thyroid cancer
See Table 12-1

Table 12-1	TNM Classification of Thyroid Tumors

TNM Staging of Thyroid Cancer (AJCC 7th Edition)	
TX–can not be assessed	NX–regional lymph nodes can not be assessed
T0–no evidence of primary tumor	N0–no regional lymph node metastasis
T1–2 cm or less, limited to thyroid T1a–1 cm or less, limited to thyroid T1b–1 to 2 cm, limited to thyroid	N1–regional lymph metastasis N1a–metastasis to level VI lymph nodes N1b–metastasis to ipsilateral, bilateral, or contralateral level I, II, III, IV, or V lymph nodes or level VII lymph nodes
T2–2 to 4 cm, limited to thyroid	
T3–more than 4 cm and limited to thyroid or any tumor with minimal extrathyroid extension	M0–no distant metastasis
T4a–moderately advanced disease; any size tumor extending beyond thyroid capsule to subcutaneous soft tissue, trachea, esophagus, larynx, or recurrent laryngeal nerve T4b–very advanced disease; invades prevertebral fascia or encases carotid artery or mediastinal vessel All anaplastic cancers are T4: T4a–intrathyroidal anaplastic carcinoma T4b–gross extrathyroid extension	M1–distant metastasis

T	N	M
Follicular and Papillary Carcinoma		
Under 45 Years		
Stage I	Any T	Any N	M0
Stage II	Any T	Any N	M1
45 Years and Older		
Stage I	T1	N0	M0
Stage II	T2	N0	M0
Stage III	T3	N0	M0
	T1	N1a	M0
	T2	N1a	M0
	T3	N1a	M0
Stage IVA	T4a	N0	M0
	T4a	N1a	M0
	T1	N1b	M0
	T2	N1b	M0
	T3	N1b	M0
	T4a	N1b	M0
Stage IVB	T4b	Any N	M0
Stage IVC	Any T	Any N	M1
Medullary Carcinoma		
Stage I	T1	N0	M0
Stage II	T2	N0	M0
	T3	N0	M0
Stage III	T1	N1a	M0
	T2	N1a	M0
	T3	N1a	M0

(continued)

Table 12-1	TNM Classification of Thyroid Tumors (*Continued*)		
	Medullary Carcinoma		
Stage IVA	T4a	N0	M0
	T4a	N1a	M0
	T1	N1b	M0
	T2	N1b	M0
	T3	N1b	M0
	T4a	N1b	M0
Stage IVB	T4b	Any N	M0
Stage IVC	Any T	Any N	M1
	Anaplastic Carcinoma		
Stage IVA	T4a	Any N	M0
Stage IVB	T4b	Any N	M0
Stage IVC	Any T	Any N	M1

Used with the permission of the American Joint Committee on Cancer (AJCC), Chicago, Ilinois. The original source for this material is the AJCC Cancer Staging Manual, Seventh Edition (2010) published by Springer Science and Business Media LLC, www.springerlink.com.

What are the indications for I-131 therapy?
All stage III or IV disease
All stage II disease younger than 45 years old
Most patients 45 years or older with stage II disease
Stage I disease who have aggressive histologies, nodal metastases, multifocal disease, and extrathyroid or vascular invasion

PARATHYROID GLAND

PARATHYROID EMBRYOLOGY, ANATOMY, AND PHYSIOLOGY

What structure are the superior parathyroid glands embryologically derived from?
Fourth branchial pouch

What structure are the inferior parathyroid glands embryologically derived from?
Third branchial pouch

What structure is the thymus embryologically derived from?
Third branchial pouch

What is the arterial blood supply to the superior parathyroid glands?
Inferior thyroid artery (occasionally by branches of the superior thyroid artery)

What is the arterial blood supply to the inferior parathyroid glands?
Inferior thyroid artery

What is the spatial relationship of the inferior parathyroid gland to the recurrent laryngeal nerve and inferior thyroid artery?
Inferior parathyroid glands are medial to the recurrent laryngeal nerves and located below the inferior thyroid artery

What is the spatial relationship of the superior parathyroid gland to the recurrent laryngeal nerve and inferior thyroid artery?
Superior parathyroid glands are lateral to the recurrent laryngeal nerves and located above the inferior thyroid artery

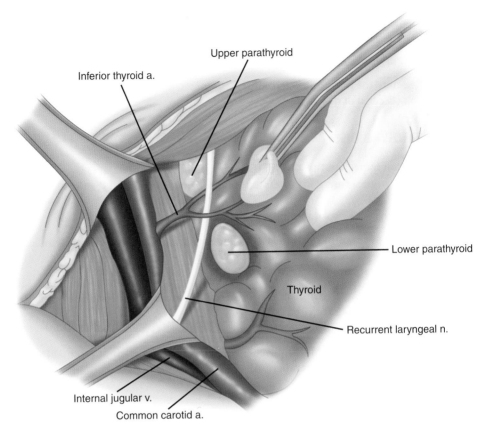

FIGURE 12-3. Relationship of the parathyroids to the recurrent laryngeal nerve. a., artery; v., vein. *(Reproduced from Brunicardi FC, Andersen DK, Billiar TR, et al. Schwartz's Principles of Surgery. 9th ed. http://www.accessmedicine.com. Copyright © The McGraw-Hill Companies, Inc. All rights reserved.)*

Describe the mechanisms by which PTH increases serum calcium concentration:
Bone—enhances resorption of bone matrix by osteoclasts
Kidney—increases tubular reabsorption of filtered calcium and decreases tubular reabsorption of filtered phosphate
Intestine—stimulates renal vitamin D complex synthesis, which increases intestinal absorption of calcium (indirect effect)

What laboratory test is the most sensitive and specific way to diagnose hyperparathyroidism?
Intact parathyroid hormone level (elevated in >95% of patients with primary hyperparathyroidism)

What is the half-life of parathyroid hormone?
2 to 4 minutes

What is the desired decline in the intraoperative parathyroid hormone assay that confirms that the suspected abnormal parathyroid tissue was resected?
50% decrease from baseline PTH or a drop of the PTH to the normal range

Describe the process of vitamin D formation and activation:
7-dehydrocholesterol undergoes ultraviolet activation to form vitamin D3 (cholecalciferol) → hydroxylated in the liver to form 25-hydroxycholecalciferol → undergoes a second hydroxylation in the kidneys to its most active form 1,25-dihydroxycholecalciferol

What cells secrete the hormone calcitonin?
Parafollicular (C cells) of the thyroid

HYPERPARATHYROIDISM

Which type(s) of hyperparathyroidism (primary, secondary, or tertiary) is associated with high serum PTH levels and high-normal to elevated serum calcium levels?
Primary and tertiary hyperparathyroidism

Which type of hyperparathyroidism is associated with high serum PTH levels and low-normal to low serum calcium levels?
Secondary hyperparathyroidism

Which type of hyperparathyroidism is considered a compensatory response of the parathyroid glands to hypocalcemia?
Secondary hyperparathyroidism

Which type of hyperparathyroidism occurs when long-standing stimulation of the parathyroid glands by hypocalcemia results in autonomous hyperfunctioning of the parathyroid glands?
Tertiary hyperparathyroidism

What acid-base disturbance can be seen with primary hyperparathyroidism?
Hyperchloremic metabolic acidosis

What chloride:phosphate ratio is highly suggestive of primary hyperparathyroidism?
Chloride:phosphate ratio >33 is highly suggestive of primary hyperparathyroidism

What is the most common cause of primary hyperparathyroidism? Second most common? Third most common?
Single adenoma (80%)
Diffuse hyperplasia (15%)
Multiple adenomas (4%)

What oncogene increases the risk for a parathyroid adenoma?
PRAD-1

What are the classic gross findings diagnostic of a parathyroid adenoma?
Single enlarged gland with 3 normal or small remaining glands associated with the histologic finding of hyperplastic tissue

Indications for initial parathyroidectomy for a patient with primary hyperparathyroidism:
Symptomatic:
Typical bone, renal, gastrointestinal, neuromuscular symptoms

Asymptomatic:
History of an episode of life-threatening hypercalcemia
Presence of kidney stones detected by abdominal imaging
Medical surveillance not desirable/possible
Serum calcium level >1 mg/dL above upper limit of normal
Age <50 years
Osteoporosis (bone density T-score <–2.5 at any site)
Creatinine clearance decreased by >30%
Elevated 24-hour urinary calcium excretion (>400 mg/d)

What is the difference between persistent and recurrent hyperparathyroidism?
Persistent refers to hypercalcemia that remains within 6 months of initial surgery
Recurrent refers to hypercalcemia that returns after 6 months of initial surgery

What is the most common cause of persistent hyperparathyroidism?
Missed adenoma

What are the causes for recurrent hyperparathyroidism?
New adenoma formation or recurrent parathyroid cancer

Indications for reoperative parathyroidectomy for persistent or recurrent disease:
Ongoing nephrolithiasis
Worsening renal function
Worsening bone disease as evidenced by bone mineral density scores
Associated neuromuscular symptoms
Associated psychiatric symptoms
Worrisome progressive hypercalcemia

Indications for parathyroidectomy in patients with secondary hyperparathyroidism:
Development of open ulcerative skin lesions from calcinosis or calciphylaxis
Persistent bone pain or pathologic fractures (renal osteodystrophy)
Ectopic calcifications
Intractable pruritus
Worsening disease with failure of medical management

General intraoperative algorithm for searching a "missing" parathyroid gland:
Open and inspect the thyroid capsule, palpate gland
Consider intraoperative US
Dissect superior thymic/paratracheal tissue and complete a cervical thymectomy for missing inferior parathyroid glands
Mobilize the pharynx and esophagus to look in the parapharyngeal/retropharyngeal/esophageal spaces for missing superior glands
Open the carotid sheath and expose the common carotid and inspect for potential parathyroid glands
Ligate the ipsilateral inferior thyroid artery and/or perform a thyroid lobectomy (record the location of all confirmed glands identified)
End the procedure and follow patient for any evidence of persistent hypercalcemia
Can reimage patient for evidence of ectopic parathyroid adenoma

What is the most common location for a "missing" parathyroid gland at reoperation?
Normal anatomic position

Generally what is the recommended period of time that cryopreserved parathyroid tissue should not be transplanted?
24 months after freezing

How is parathyroid tissue autotransplanted?
The resected parathyroid tissue is minced into 1-mm fragments. A pocket is then made in the desired muscle. Ten to 20 1-mm fragments of minced parathyroid tissue are inserted into the muscle pocket, which is closed and tagged with hemoclips/suture (for future identification)

Why is the forearm used preferentially over the sternocleidomastoid for autotransplantation of parathyroid tissue?
Easier to re-explore if patient develops persistent or recurrent disease from autotransplanted tissue
Easier to identify PTH gradients with peripheral blood draws in forearm versus neck (can place BP cuff)

Why do some patients experience postoperative hypocalcemia?
Bone hunger, hypomagnesemia, failure of parathyroid remnant or graft

What imaging study is used for preoperative localization for reoperative parathyroid surgery and for minimally invasive parathyroidectomy?
Technetium-sestamibi scan

In general, what is the most common cause of hypoparathyroidism?
Surgical trauma to parathyroid glands during thyroid or parathyroid exploration

What operation is performed for parathyroid carcinoma?
En bloc tumor resection that includes ipsilateral thyroid lobectomy, and resection of adjacent soft tissues

True or False: A frozen section biopsy for suspected parathyroid cancer should be performed before surgical excision?
False; capsular rupture may occur with the potential of spreading tumor cells in the neck.

What is the most common location for parathyroid cancer to metastasis?
Lung

What is the most common cause of hyperparathyroidism in MEN 1?
Parathyroid hyperplasia (90%)

Which of the following needs to be corrected first in MEN 1—hyperparathyroidism, gastrinoma, or prolactinoma?
Hyperparathyroidism; need to correct calcium first

Which of the following needs to be corrected first in MEN 2—hyperparathyroidism, pheochromocytoma, or MTC?
Pheochromocytoma

PITUITARY GLAND

ANATOMY AND PHYSIOLOGY

What hormones are released from the posterior pituitary?
ADH and oxytocin

What hormones are released from the anterior pituitary?
ACTH, FSH, LH, GH, TSH, and prolactin

What gonadotropic hormone promotes spermatogenesis or ovarian follicle maturation?
FSH

What gonadotropic hormone promotes testicular testosterone production?
LH

What drug may be given as primary therapy in patients who are not operative candidates with excessive production of GH by a pituitary adenoma?
Octreotide (decreases serum levels of GH and the downstream growth factor somatomedin C)

PROLACTINOMA AND OTHER PITUITARY LESIONS

What is the size cutoff to determine whether a pituitary lesion is a microadenoma versus macroadenoma?
Microadenoma <1 cm
Macroadenoma >1 cm

What imaging study is the gold standard for evaluating the pituitary?
MRI with gadolinium

What is the most common pituitary adenoma?
Prolactinoma

What is the treatment for prolactinoma?
Bromocriptine
Transsphenoidal resection for failure of medical management

OTHER PITUITARY PATHOPHYSIOLOGY

Name the syndrome

Meningococcal sepsis/infection results in adrenal gland hemorrhage leading to adrenal insufficiency:
Waterhouse-Friderichsen syndrome

Results from arachnoid herniation secondary to a congenital defect in the diaphragma sellae:
Empty sella syndrome (primary)

A 35-year-old female with 1-week postpartum history of placental hemorrhage who presents with trouble lactating and amenorrhea:
Sheehan syndrome

Hyperpigmentation and pituitary enlargement (resulting in amenorrhea and visual problems) after bilateral adrenalectomy:
Nelson syndrome

Calcified cyst that is remnant of Rathke pouch and can present with endocrine abnormalities, headache, hydrocephalus, and visual disturbances:
Craniopharyngioma

ADRENAL GLAND

ADRENAL ANATOMY AND PHYSIOLOGY

What are signs/symptoms of Cushing syndrome?
Acne, buffalo hump, depression, diabetes, easy bruising, hirsutism, hypertension, moon facies, myopathy, purple striae, truncal obesity, weakness

What enzyme is present almost exclusively in the adrenal medulla and organ of Zuckerkandl? What does it do?
Phenylethanolamine-*N*-methyltransferase (PNMT)
Converts norepinephrine to epinephrine via methylation

What enzyme is involved in the rate-limiting step of catecholamine synthesis?
Tyrosine hydroxylase (hydroxylates tyrosine to dihydroxyphenylalanine [DOPA])

What are the intermediate substrates involved in the synthesis of epinephrine from tyrosine?
Tyrosine→DOPA→Dopamine→Norepinephrine→Epinephrine

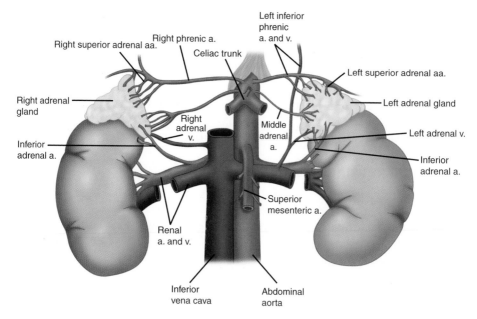

FIGURE 12-4. Anatomy of the adrenals and surrounding structures. a., artery; v., vein. *(Reproduced from Brunicardi FC, Andersen DK, Billiar TR, et al. Schwartz's Principles of Surgery. 9th ed. http://www.accessmedicine.com. Copyright © The McGraw-Hill Companies, Inc. All rights reserved.)*

Which artery does the superior adrenal artery originate from?
Inferior phrenic artery

Which artery does the middle adrenal artery originate from?
Aorta

Which artery does the inferior adrenal artery originate from?
Renal artery

The left adrenal vein empties into which vein?
Left renal vein

The right adrenal vein empties into which vein?
Inferior vena cava

What does the zona glomerulosa of the adrenal cortex produce?
Aldosterone

What does the zona fasciculata of the adrenal cortex produce?
Glucocorticoids

What does the zona reticularis of the adrenal cortex produce?
Androgens/estrogens

What is the most common deficiency seen with congenital adrenal hyperplasia?
21-hydroxylase deficiency (90%)

ADRENAL TUMORS

What are the indications for surgical resection of an adrenal mass?
More than 4 to 6 cm, enlarging (0.5 cm over 6 months), functioning, ominous characteristics (nonhomogenous) on imaging

What laboratory tests should be ordered in the workup of an adrenal mass?
Urine metanephrines/vanillylmandelic acid (VMA)/catecholamines, urine hydroxycorticosteroids, serum potassium
If decreased serum potassium or HTN, then obtain plasma renin and aldosterone

Primary hyperaldosteronism accounts for what percentage of all cases of HTN?
1%

Classic Conn syndrome is characterized by:
HTN, hypokalemia, polyuria

What test can differentiate primary hyperaldosteronism from secondary hyperaldosteronism?
Plasma renin level (suppressed with primary and not suppressed with secondary)

What is the #1 cause of primary hyperaldosteronism?
Adrenal adenoma

What is the aldosterone:renin ratio that is suggestive of an aldosteronoma?
20 is diagnostic for primary hyperaldosteronism

What is the aldosterone suppression test?
Give a saline infusion; if the urinary aldosterone level is elevated (>12 μg/d), the diagnosis of primary hyperaldosteronism is confirmed

What is the best imaging modality to distinguish aldosteronoma from bilateral hyperplasia?
CT scan of the abdomen with thin cuts (3–5 mm) through the adrenal glands

What acid-base disturbance will be seen with primary hyperaldosteronism?
Hypochloremic metabolic alkalosis

What test can be performed to lateralize an aldosterone producing hyperfunctioning adrenal gland in the setting of adrenal hypertrophy, bilateral nodules, or absence of lesions?
Selective venous catheterization for aldosterone sampling

What is the adrenal vein aldosterone-to-cortisol ratio required to lateralize an aldosteronoma/unilateral adrenal hyperplasia?
At least 5 times higher on the affected side; if ratios from both sides are similar, then suspect bilateral hyperplasia

If the captopril test is performed in a patient with an aldosterone-secreting tumor, what will happen to serum aldosterone levels?
No change
If the patient has bilateral adrenal hyperplasia, a captopril test will cause decreased aldosterone levels

What competitive inhibitor of aldosterone is usually given to control HTN and normalize potassium levels in a patient with an aldosteronoma/unilateral hyperplasia before surgery?
Spironolactone

What is the best treatment approach for an aldosteronoma or unilateral hyperplasia?
Laparoscopic adrenalectomy

What is the treatment for hyperaldosteronism from adrenal hyperplasia?
Medical therapy with calcium channel blockers, potassium, and spironolactone. If refractory hypokalemia, then bilateral adrenalectomy, steroids, and fludrocortisone

What is the most sensitive and specific test for making the diagnosis of Cushing syndrome?
24-hour urinary free cortisol

What is the most common site of ectopic ACTH-producing tumor? Second most common site?
#1 Small cell lung carcinoma
#2 Carcinoid

What ACTH level signifies an ACTH-independent cause of endogenous glucocorticoid hypersecretion?
<5 pg/mL (low)

What ACTH level signifies an ACTH-dependent cause of endogenous glucocorticoid hypersecretion?
15 pg/mL (high)

How is the low-dose overnight dexamethasone suppression test performed?
Administer dexamethasone 1 mg PO at 11 PM; check plasma cortisol at 8 AM the next day. Cortisol level will be markedly suppressed (<1.8 µg/dL) in normal individuals. If cortisol level is not suppressed, the patient has Cushing syndrome.

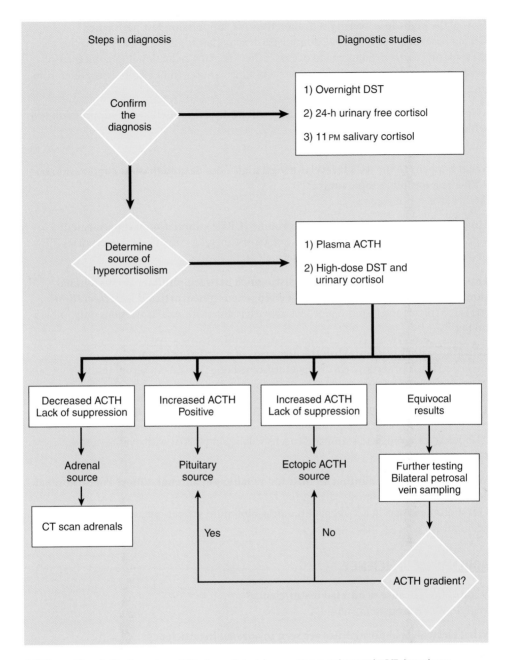

FIGURE 12-5. Diagnosis of Cushing syndrome. ACTH, adrenocorticotropic hormone; CT, computed tomography; DST, dexamethasone suppression test. *(Reproduced from Brunicardi FC, Andersen DK, Billiar TR, et al. Schwartz's Principles of Surgery. 9th ed. http://www. accessmedicine.com. Copyright © The McGraw-Hill Companies, Inc. All rights reserved.)*

How is the high-dose overnight dexamethasone suppression test performed?
Obtain baseline plasma cortisol; administer dexamethasone 8 mg PO at 11 PM; check 8 AM plasma cortisol. Suppression occurs if there is >50% reduction in plasma cortisol, which indicates Cushing syndrome from a pituitary source (if not suppressed, then from an adrenal or ectopic cause).

What happens to the ACTH level during a high-dose dexamethasone suppression test with a responsible pituitary tumor?
ACTH level is suppressed

What happens to the ACTH level during a high-dose dexamethasone suppression test with a responsible ectopic source?
ACTH level is not suppressed

How is the corticotropin-releasing hormone (CRH) stimulation test performed?
Check baseline serum ACTH and cortisol. Give 1 mcg/kg CRH IV. Draw serum ACTH and cortisol 15 minutes after administering CRH.

How does the CRH stimulation test distinguish between pituitary versus adrenal tumor versus ectopic ACTH causes of endogenous glucocorticoid hypersecretion?
ACTH increases at a minimum of 35% above baseline with pituitary lesions only (others do not)

What laboratory tests establish the diagnosis of a virilizing tumor?
Increased levels of serum dehydroepiandrostenedione (DHEA-S), serum testosterone, and 24-hour urine 7-hydroxysteroids and 17-ketosteroids

How does a dexamethasone suppression test differentiate between an adrenal versus ovarian cause for a virilizing tumor?
24-hour ketosteroids and serum androgens will be suppressed with ovarian tumors but not adrenal tumors

What happens to gadolinium on MRI for a malignant adrenal tumor? For an adrenal adenoma?
Gadolinium persists in a malignant tumor; gadolinium washes out rapidly from an adenoma

ADRENAL INSUFFICIENCY

What is the #1 cause of adrenal insufficiency?
Withdrawal of exogenous steroids

What electrolyte abnormalities are seen in adrenal insufficiency?
Hyponatremia, hyperkalemia

What test can be performed to diagnose adrenal insufficiency?
ACTH stimulation test

What is one of the first signs for the loss of hypothalamic regulation of cortisol secretion?
Loss of diurnal variation of cortisol levels

ADRENOCORTICAL CARCINOMA, PHEOCHROMOCYTOMA, AND MEN

What is the safest operation for patients with suspected adrenocortical carcinoma?
Open adrenalectomy

What medication is commonly used for adjuvant therapy with residual, recurrent, or metastatic adrenocortical carcinoma?
Mitotane, a synthetic derivative of the insecticide dichlorodiphenyltrichloroethane (DDT) that directly suppresses the adrenal cortex and modifies the peripheral metabolism of steroids

What follow-up is needed for a patient with adrenal tumor <4 cm or 4 to 6 cm treated nonoperatively?
Repeat abdominal imaging Q6 months to a year and annual screening for cortisol and catecholamines for 5 years

What is the treatment for a patient with adrenal mass >6 cm?
Adrenalectomy; most likely malignant

What disease process needs to be ruled out before performing a fine-needle aspiration of a solitary adrenal mass?
Pheochromocytoma; inadvertent biopsy can be potentially lethal

What laboratory test is the most sensitive for the detection of pheochromocytoma?
Plasma metanephrines (96%)

What is the rule of 10's for pheochromocytoma?
10% bilateral, 10% malignant, 10% extra-adrenal, 10% hereditary, 10% in children

What ectopic sites can a pheochromocytoma be found?
Organ of Zuckerkandl, thorax/mediastinum, bladder, scrotum

What familial syndromes are associated with pheochromocytoma?
MEN type 2, Sturge-Weber syndrome, tuberous sclerosis, von Hippel-Lindau disease, neurofibromatosis type I

What is usually seen with a hypertensive "spell," the hallmark clinical presentation of pheochromocytoma?
Diaphoresis, headache, palpitations, and paroxysmal HTN

True or False: Paragangliomas and pheochromocytomas located in the organ of Zuckerkandl can use PNMT to metabolize norepinephrine to epinephrine?
True; paragangliomas and pheochromocytomas in the organ of Zuckerkandl contain PNMT.

What medications should be given preoperatively for pheochromocytoma?
Phenoxybenzamine 10 mg BID and increase by 20 mg/d until BP and symptoms controlled; add β-blocker 3 days prior to surgery (inderal 10 mg TID); IVF hydration starting 2 days prior to surgery (typically patients are volume contracted)

What rapid-acting agents should be available in the operating room when operating on a pheochromocytoma?
Neosynephrine, nitroprusside, lidocaine, esmolol, phentolamine

What follow-up is recommended after adrenalectomy for pheochromocytoma?
Yearly 24-hour urinary metanephrines/catecholamines

What is the localizing test of choice for adrenal pheochromocytoma?
CT scan of the abdomen with thin cuts (3–5 mm) through the adrenal glands

What is the approximate percentage of MEN 2 patients with pheochromocytoma?
40%

What is the surgical treatment for pheochromocytoma in MEN 2?
Bilateral adrenalectomy; trend now is to remove the affected side and observe the contralateral side until there is radiographic/biochemical evidence of disease

What is the most common cancer to metastasize to the adrenal gland?
Breast cancer

MULTIPLE CHOICE QUESTIONS

1. **A 27-year-old woman presents to your office with a left-sided neck mass approximately 2.5 cm in size. FNA reveals papillary thyroid neoplasm. She has no palpable lymph nodes. What is the best management for this patient?**

   A. Left thyroid lobectomy with left modified radical neck dissection
   B. Total thyroidectomy with bilateral modified radical neck dissection
   C. Left thyroid lobectomy with postoperative I-131 therapy
   D. Total thyroidectomy with postoperative I-131 therapy
   E. Total thyroidectomy alone

2. **A 27-year-old woman presents to your office with a left-sided neck mass approximately 2.5 cm in size. FNA reveals papillary thyroid neoplasm. She has a 1-cm palpable left cervical lymph node. What is the best management for this patient?**

   A. Left thyroid lobectomy alone
   B. Left thyroid lobectomy with left modified radical neck dissection
   C. Total thyroidectomy with left modified radical neck dissection
   D. Total thyroidectomy with postoperative I-131 therapy
   E. Total thyroidectomy alone

3. **A 17-year-old male has a 2-cm right cervical nodule. An FNA is done and cells stain positive for calcitonin. Labs also reveal elevated calcium. What is the most likely diagnosis?**

   A. Familial MTC
   B. Follicular thyroid cancer
   C. MEN 1
   D. MEN 2a
   E. MEN 2b

4. **A 46-year-old woman presents to the emergency department with fever, tachycardia, diaphoresis, and tremors. She has a history of a goiter. Initial management should include all of the following except:**

   A. PTU
   B. Steroids
   C. β-blocker
   D. Oxygen
   E. I-131

5. **Which of the following is NOT commonly seen in patients with MEN 1 syndrome?**
   A. Gastrinoma
   B. Insulinoma
   C. Prolactinoma
   D. Parathyroid hyperplasia
   E. MTC

6. **What is the most common adrenal incidentaloma found on CT scan?**
   A. Adrenocortical carcinoma
   B. Cortical adenoma
   C. Pheochromocytoma
   D. Aldosteronoma
   E. Adrenal cyst

7. **Which of the following is an indication for surgery in a patient with asymptomatic primary hyperparathyroidism?**
   A. History of an episode of life-threatening hypercalcemia
   B. Medical surveillance not desirable/possible
   C. Age <50 years
   D. Osteoporosis (bone density T-score <−2.5 at any site)
   E. All of the above

8. **A 65-year-old male is found to have an incidental right adrenal mass on CT scan during workup for trauma. He does not have a history of hypertension or any malignancies. Physical examination is negative. Blood work demonstrates normal electrolytes and plasma metanephrines. Urinary free cortisol is normal and low-dose overnight dexamethasone suppression test shows a low cortisol level the following morning. The CT scan demonstrates a 6-cm irregularly shaped heterogenous mass. What is the next appropriate step in management?**
   A. Perform CT-guided needle biopsy of adrenal mass
   B. Repeat CT scan in 6 months
   C. Perform open adrenalectomy
   D. Give patient mitotane

9. **A 50-year-old woman presents with truncal obesity and hirsutism. A 24-hour urinary free cortisol is markedly elevated. Low-dose dexamethasone suppression test fails to suppress plasma cortisol levels. Plasma ACTH levels are also elevated. High-dose dexamethasone suppression test yields low plasma cortisol levels. Which imaging study would most likely demonstrate the cause of her symptoms?**
   A. CT of the chest
   B. CT of the abdomen
   C. MRI of the sella turcica
   D. Metaiodobenzylguanidine (MIBG) scan

10. **A 55-year-old male with newly diagnosed hypertension complains of muscle weakness. Laboratory data demonstrates hypokalemia and low plasma renin activity. CT scan shows bilaterally enlarged adrenal glands without a definite mass. What is the next best step in management?**

   A. Give spironolactone
   B. Perform selective venous catheterization
   C. Perform unilateral adrenalectomy
   D. Perform bilateral adrenalectomy

ANSWERS

1. **Answer: E.** For papillary thyroid cancers larger than 2 cm, total thyroidectomy is indicated. Postoperative I-131 therapy is given for tumors >4 cm or extrathyroidal disease. Neck dissection is unnecessary without evidence of nodal disease.

2. **Answer: C.** The size of the tumor necessitates a total thyroidectomy. This patient has a palpable cervical lymph node, and thus a unilateral modified radical neck dissection or excision of the enlarged lymph node should be done.

3. **Answer: D.** Calcitonin-positive cells indicate a diagnosis of MTC. Elevated calcium suggests hyperparathyroidism. Along with pheochromocytoma, these diagnoses make up MEN 2a. MEN 2b would include MTC, pheochromocytoma, and mucosal neuromas.

4. **Answer: E.** This patient has thyroid storm. β-blockers are used to control heart rate with reported inhibition of peripheral conversion of T4 to T3. Steroids and PTU work by decreasing production and release of thyroid hormones. IV fluids and oxygen are part of routine resuscitative care. I-131 has no role in the treatment of thyroid storm.

5. **Answer: E.** MTC is seen in patients with MEN 2a and 2b. Parathyroid hyperplasia is the earliest and most common manifestation of MEN 1. It develops in 80% to 100% of patients by age 40. Gastrinomas are the most common pancreatic islet cell tumor in MEN 1, which occurs in about 50% of patients, followed by insulinomas, which develop in 10% to 15% of cases. Prolactinomas are the most common pituitary lesion, which occurs in 10% to 50% of MEN 1 cases.

6. **Answer: B.** Nonfunctioning cortical adenomas comprise the majority of adrenal incidentalomas in patients without a history of cancer.

7. **Answer: E.** The 2002 NIH consensus conference guidelines for parathyroidectomy in patients with asymptomatic primary hyperparathyroidism are serum calcium >1 mg/dL above the upper limits of normal, life-threatening hypercalcemia episode, creatine clearance reduced by 30%, kidney stones on abdominal x-ray, markedly elevated 24-hour urinary calcium excretion >400 mg/dL, age <50 years, long-term medical surveillance not desired or possible, and substantially decreased bone mineral density at the lumbar spine, hip, or distal radius (T score <−2.5).

8. **Answer: C.** The patient is found to have an incidentaloma that is asymptomatic and nonfunctioning. However, given its size of 6 cm and CT findings that suggest malignancy, the patient should undergo adrenalectomy. Other CT scan features that suggest malignancy include evidence of necrosis, hemorrhage, local invasion, lymph node metastasis, and high attenuation. Needle biopsy of an adrenal mass should

only be performed in patients with a history of malignancy to rule out an adrenal metastasis after ruling out pheochromocytoma. Mitotane is an adrenal cytotoxic agent that is used as adjuvant therapy for adrenocortical carcinoma.

9. **Answer: C.** When Cushing syndrome is suspected, the first test should be a 24-hour urinary free cortisol. If it is elevated, a low-dose dexamethasone suppression test is performed. Failure to suppress cortisol levels indicates Cushing syndrome. ACTH levels are then measured. Low ACTH levels indicate a cortisol-secreting tumor such as a primary adrenal source. A CT scan of the abdomen would be helpful in this case. A high ACTH level suggests a pituitary or ectopic source of ACTH. A high-dose dexamethasone suppression test will differentiate this. The pituitary source will be suppressed; thus, pituitary MRI should be performed. Failure to suppress production suggests an ectopic ACTH tumor, which most commonly is small cell lung cancer or bronchial tumors. CT of the chest would be warranted in this case.

10. **Answer: B.** The patient is suspected to have primary hyperaldosteronism, which may be due to bilateral adrenal hyperplasia or an aldosteronoma. Selective venous catheterization for aldosterone sampling in adrenal veins can aid in localizing the aldosteronoma, thus determining if surgical intervention would be beneficial. If the aldosteronoma is localized to 1 adrenal gland, then the patient should undergo unilateral adrenalectomy. If bilateral adrenal glands are hyperfunctioning or if there is failure to localize the aldosteronoma, then medical management with spironolactone would be the mainstay therapy. There is increased morbidity with bilateral resection, which is reserved for refractory hypokalemia for cases of bilateral hyperplasia. NP-59 scintography can also be used to differentiate adenoma from hyperplasia.

CHAPTER 13
Abdominal Wall and Hernias

Dale A. Dangleben and James Lee

ANATOMY

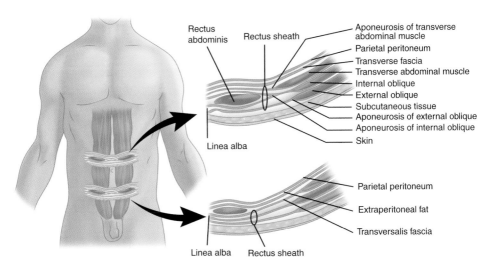

FIGURE 13-1. Cross-sectional anatomy of the abdominal wall above and below the arcuate line of Douglas. The lower right abdominal wall segment shows clearly the absence of an aponeurotic covering of the posterior aspect of the rectus abdominis muscle inferior to the arcuate line. Superior to the arcuate line, there are both internal oblique and transversus abdominis aponeurotic contributions to the posterior rectus sheath. *(Reproduced with permission from Moore KL, Dalley AF, eds. Clinically Oriented Anatomy. 4th ed. Philadelphia: Lippincott Williams & Wilkins; 1999:185.)*

What are the 9 layers of the abdominal wall?

Skin, subcutaneous tissue, superficial fascia, external oblique muscle, internal oblique muscle, transversus abdominis muscle, transversalis fascia, preperitoneal adipose and areolar tissue, and peritoneum

What is the portion of the external oblique aponeurosis that extends from the anterior superior iliac spine to the pubic tubercle called?
Inguinal (Poupart) ligament

What directions do the fibers of the external oblique course?
Superolateral to inferomedial

What directions do the fibers of the internal oblique course?
Inferolateral to superomedial

What directions do the fibers of the transversus abdominis course?
Transverse

Where does the aponeurosis, which is originally divided into anterior and posterior lamella that envelops the rectus abdominis muscle, begin to course anteriorly to the rectus abdominis muscle and become part of the anterior rectus sheath?
Semicircular line (of Douglas/arcuate line)

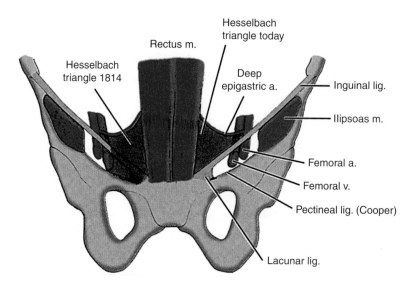

FIGURE 13-2. Hesselbach triangle as originally described (left) and as accepted today (right). Note that part of supravesical fossa lies within triangle. *(Modified from Skandalakis PN, Skandalakis LJ, Gray SW, Skandalakis JE. Supravesical hernia. In: Nyhus LM, Condon RE, eds. Hernia. 4th ed. Philadelphia: JB Lippincott; 1995:400–411, with permission.)*

What are the borders of Hesselbach triangle?
Inguinal ligament inferiorly, lateral margin of the rectus sheath medially, and inferior epigastric vessels laterally

What makes up the floor of Hesselbach triangle?
Transversalis fascia

What structures course through the preperitoneal space?
Inferior epigastric artery and vein; median umbilical ligament (urachus—remnant of fetal allantoic stalk); medial umbilical ligaments (vestiges of fetal umbilical arteries); falciform ligament

What are the 9 potential spaces of the abdomen?
Right subphrenic; left subphrenic; right paracolic gutter; left paracolic gutter; subhepatic; supramesenteric; inframesenteric; lesser space; pelvis

PHYSIOLOGY

What is the function of the peritoneum?
To promote sequestration and removal of bacteria from the peritoneal cavity, control the amount of fluid in the peritoneal cavity, and facilitate the migration of inflammatory cells from the microcirculation into the peritoneal cavity

What is the most reliable method to help determine the cause of ascites?
The serum-ascites albumin gradient (SAAG)

How do you calculate the SAAG?
Serum albumin concentration – ascites albumin concentration

What does a SAAG <1.1 g/dL signify?
Absence of portal hypertension (biliary ascites, nephrotic syndrome, pancreatic ascites, peritoneal carcinomatosis, post-op lymphatic leak, serositis with connective tissue disease, tuberculous peritonitis)

What does a SAAG >1.1 g/dL signify?
Presence of portal hypertension (alcoholic hepatitis, Budd-Chiari syndrome, cardiac ascites, cirrhosis, fulminant liver failure, massive liver mets, myxedema, portal vein thrombosis)

How much albumin should be given for every liter of ascites removed after large volume paracentesis (>5 L)?
6 to 8 g of albumin/L of ascites removed

Most common malignancy associated with chylous ascites:
Lymphoma

Term for bacterial infection of ascitic fluid in the absence of an intra-abdominal, surgically treatable source of infection:
Spontaneous bacterial peritonitis

What is the management of spontaneous bacterial peritonitis?
Third-generation cephalosporin (eg, ceftriaxone)

Treatment for tuberculous peritonitis:
Antituberculous drugs (isoniazid and rifampin daily for 9 months commonly used)

Initial treatment for peritoneal dialysis–associated peritonitis:
Intraperitoneal administration of antibiotics (usually first-generation cephalosporin)

Treatment for recurrent/persistent peritoneal dialysis-associated peritonitis:
Removal of the dialysis catheter and resumption of hemodialysis

What disease entails a mucous-secreting tumor coating the peritoneum and filling the peritoneal cavity with mucus and large loculated cystic masses?
Pseudomyxoma peritonei

Treatment for pseudomyxoma peritonei:
Drainage of mucus and intraperitoneal fluid
Peritonectomy and omentectomy with cytoreduction of primary and secondary tumor implants
Right colectomy for appendiceal adenocarcinoma or total abdominal hysterectomy and bilateral salpingo-oophorectomy for ovarian carcinoma
Post-op intraperitoneal chemo/mucolytics

Term for the dilated superficial paraumbilical veins in this seen with portal venous obstruction:
Caput medusae

What nodal system do the supraumbilical lymphatic vessels drain?
Axillary lymph nodes

What nodal system do the infraumbilical lymphatic vessels drain?
Superficial inguinal lymph nodes

Where does visceral pain from inflammation of the stomach, duodenum, or biliary tract (foregut) localize?
Epigastrium

Where does visceral pain from inflammation of the small intestine, appendix, or right colon (midgut) localize?
Periumbilical region

Where does visceral pain from inflammation of the left colon and rectum (hindgut) localize?
Hypogastrium

Why is visceral pain felt in the midline rather than lateralize?
Organs transmit sympathetic sensory afferents to both sides of the spinal cord.

Where would you expect referred pain with irritation of the diaphragm?
Shoulder pain

Where would you expect referred pain with acute biliary tract disease?
Scapular pain

Where would you expect referred pain with retroperitoneal inflammation?
Testicular or labial pain

DISEASES

Make the diagnosis: a newborn is noted to have passage of meconium and mucus from the umbilicus in the first few days of life:
Patent omphalomesenteric duct

What is the treatment for a patent omphalomesenteric duct?
Laparotomy with excision of the fistulous tract

How can an umbilical polyp (persistence of distal omphalomesenteric duct) be differentiated from an umbilical granuloma?
Umbilical polyp will not disappear after silver nitrate cauterization; umbilical granuloma will disappear after silver nitrate cauterization

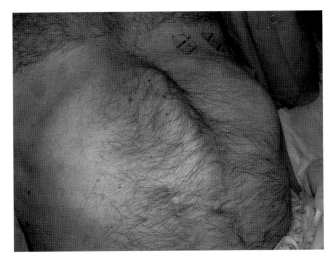

FIGURE 13-3. Diastasis recti visible in the midepigastrium with Valsalva maneuver. The edges of the rectus abdominis muscle, rigid with voluntary contraction, are palpable along the entire length of the bulging area. This should not be mistaken for a ventral hernia. *(Reproduced from Brunicardi FC, Andersen DK, Billiar TR, et al. Schwartz's Principles of Surgery. 9th ed. http://www.accessmedicine.com. Copyright © The McGraw-Hill Companies, Inc. All rights reserved.)*

What is the treatment for a vesicocutaneous fistula (patent urachus)?
Excision of the urachal remnant with closure of the bladder if needed

Term for a midline protrusion of the anterior abdominal wall secondary to thinning of the linea alba in the epigastrium with intact transversalis fascia:
Diastasis recti

Treatment for diastasis recti:
Reassurance

How is a rectus sheath hematoma usually managed?
Rest and analgesics, correction of coagulopathy, and blood transfusion if necessary

How do you manage a rectus sheath hematoma that progresses despite nonoperative measures?
Angiographic embolization of the bleeding vessel or operative evacuation of the hematoma and hemostasis (uncommon).

What is the treatment of an abdominal wall desmoid tumor?
Complete resection with a tumor-free margin with or without adjuvant radiation; if deemed unresectable, it can be treated with radiation therapy alone or with antiproliferative agents and cytotoxic chemotherapy.

What are the 2 most widely used groups of noncytotoxic drugs used for the palliation of abdominal wall desmoid tumors?
Antiestrogens (Tamoxifen) and nonsteroidal anti-inflammatory drugs (NSAIDs) (Sulindac)

What are clinical characteristics suggestive of an abdominal wall malignancy?
Fixation to the abdominal wall, fixation to abdominal organs, recent increase in size, size >5 cm, and nonreducible lesion arising from below the superficial fascia

How is the definitive diagnosis of an abdominal wall sarcoma made?
Core needle biopsy (choose this one on the test) or by incisional biopsy oriented in the same plane as the underlying muscle.

Treatment for an abdominal wall sarcoma:
Resection with tumor-free margins with reconstruction accomplished primarily, with myocutaneous flaps, or with prosthetic meshes.

Treatment for an omental cyst:
Local excision

Most common malignancy of the omentum:
Metastases

The greater omentum derives its arterial blood supply from which arteries:
Omental branches of the right and left gastroepiploic arteries

Make the diagnosis: a patient presents with acute right lower quadrant abdominal pain and is explored for suspected appendicitis and is subsequently found with enlarged mesenteric lymph nodes and a normal appendix:
Acute mesenteric lymphadenitis

Infection with what organism is associated with acute mesenteric lymphadenitis in children?
Yersinia enterocolitica

Term for a rare inflammatory disease of the mesentery characterized by fat necrosis, acute and chronic inflammation, and fibrosis:
Mesenteric panniculitis

Treatment of mesenteric panniculitis:
Usually resolves spontaneously; if it does not resolve, can try corticosteroids or other anti-inflammatory/immunosuppressive agents.

Term for a congenital hernia in which the small intestine herniates behind the mesocolon:
Mesocolic (paraduodenal) hernia

Operative management for a patient with a right mesocolic (paraduodenal) hernia:
Incise the lateral peritoneal reflections along the right colon with reflection of the right colon and cecum to the left without opening the hernia neck (could injure superior mesenteric vessels).

Operative management for a patient with a left mesocolic hernia:
Incise the peritoneal attachments and adhesions along the right side of the inferior mesenteric vein; reduce herniated small intestine from beneath the inferior mesenteric vein; return inferior mesenteric vein to the left side of the base of the small bowel mesentery; close the neck of the hernia by suturing the peritoneum adjacent to the vein to the retroperitoneum.

Most common location for a mesenteric hernia:
Near the ileocolic junction

Treatment for a mesenteric hernia:
Reduce the hernia and close the mesenteric defect

Most common primary malignancy of the mesentery:
Desmoid tumor

Treatment for desmoid tumor of the mesentery:
Surgical resection versus watchful waiting with sulindac and antiestrogen therapy versus imatinib mesylate (Gleevec)

Treatment for a retroperitoneal abscess:
Antibiotics and CT-guided drainage; if not amenable to percutaneous drainage or if fails to resolve with percutaneous drainage, then perform operative drainage through a retroperitoneal approach.

How do you make the diagnosis of retroperitoneal fibrosis?
Patient's history and IV urography demonstrating medial deviation of the ureters and hydronephrosis and hydroureter associated with delayed excretion

Treatment for primary, idiopathic retroperitoneal fibrosis:
Ureteral stenting and immunosuppression (methylprednisolone, azathioprine, penicillamine, tamoxifen)

Usual treatment for secondary cases of retroperitoneal fibrosis with compromised renal function:
Midline transperitoneal ureterolysis with wrapping of the ureter with an omental flap versus lateral retroperitoneal ureteral transposition

Most common malignant retroperitoneal tumor:
Lymphoma

Most common primary malignancy of the retroperitoneum:
Sarcoma (liposarcoma)

Prognostic factors for retroperitoneal sarcoma:
Histologic grade and tumor size

Treatment for retroperitoneal sarcoma:
Complete en bloc resection of the tumor with any involved adjacent organs (primary treatment); if invading inferior vena cava (IVC), the IVC can be excised and bypassed in the absence of sufficient collaterals. There used to be no role for radiation secondary to visceral toxicity, but with the advent of better radiation some institutions are giving radiation either pre- or postoperatively. If inoperable, symptomatic disease can consider chemotherapy with radiation.

HERNIAS

Type of hernia with an indirect and direct hernia component:
Pantaloon hernia

Most common hernia:
Indirect inguinal hernia

What is your differential diagnosis for a groin mass?
Abscess, epidermal inclusion cyst, femoral artery aneurysm, hernia, hydrocele, hematoma, seroma, lymphadenopathy, sarcoma, testicular torsion, and undescended testicle

On what side do inguinal hernias usually occur?
Right side (delay in atrophy of processus vaginalis after slower descent of right testis to scrotum during fetal development)

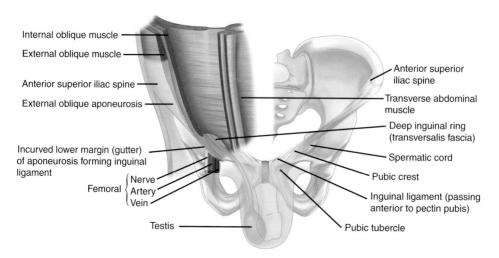

FIGURE 13-4. The 3 muscular layers of the abdominal wall lateral to the rectus abdominis are the external oblique, internal oblique, and transversus abdominis muscles, shown here on the low abdomen, where the lower margin of the external oblique reflects posteriorly as the inguinal ligament. (*Reproduced with permission from Moore KL, Dalley AF, eds. Clinically Oriented Anatomy. 4th ed. Philadelphia: Lippincott Williams & Wilkins; 1999:181.*)

On what side do femoral hernias usually occur?
Right side (possibly from tamponading effect of sigmoid colon on left femoral canal)

What type of hernia are most strangulated hernias?
Indirect inguinal hernia

What ligament is formed by the periosteum and fascia along the superior pubic ramus?
Cooper ligament

What attaches the testicle to the scrotum?
The gubernaculum

Name the contents of the spermatic cord:
Cremasteric muscle fibers, testicular artery, testicular pampiniform venous plexus, genital branch of the genitofemoral nerve, vas deferens, and processus vaginalis ± hernia sac

What are the boundaries of the inguinal canal?
Anterior—external oblique aponeurosis
Posterior—transversalis fascia and the aponeurosis of transversus abdominis
Superior—internal oblique and transversus abdominis musculoaponeurosis
Inferior—inguinal ligament and lacunar ligament

Where do direct inguinal hernias occur with regards to Hesselbach triangle?
Direct hernias occur within Hesselbach triangle

Where do indirect inguinal hernias occur with regards to Hesselbach triangle?
Indirect inguinal hernias occur lateral to Hesselbach triangle

What nerve runs anterior to the spermatic cord in the inguinal canal and branches at the superficial inguinal ring?
Ilioinguinal nerve

What nerve innervates the skin on the lateral side of the scrotum and labia and the cremaster muscle?
The genital branch of the genitofemoral nerve

Which nerves provide sensation to the base of the penis, skin of the groin, and ipsilateral upper medial thigh?
The iliohypogastric and ilioinguinal nerves

What are the boundaries of the femoral canal?
Superior—iliopubic tract
Inferior—Cooper ligament
Lateral—femoral vein
Medial—junction of iliopubic tract and Cooper ligament (lacunar ligament)

What kind of femoral hernias need to be repaired?
All femoral hernias need to be repaired (high incidence of strangulation)

What are the various methods through which a femoral hernia can be repaired?
Cooper ligament repair, via a preperitoneal approach, or a laparoscopic approach

What are the essential steps of femoral hernia repair?
Dissection and reduction of the hernia sac; obliteration of the femoral canal defect in the femoral canal by approximation of the iliopubic tract to Cooper ligament versus placement of prosthetic mesh.

What is the primary danger associated with a sliding hernia?
Failure to recognize the visceral component of the hernia sac before injury to bowel/bladder

Most common organ found in a sliding hernia in a female patient:
Ovaries/fallopian tubes

Most common organ found in a sliding hernia in a male patient:
Cecum/sigmoid colon

Next step if you cannot reduce an incarcerated femoral hernia:
Divide the inguinal or lacunar ligament

What should you do if during repair of an incarcerated inguinal hernia with a concern for strangulation you lose control of the hernia sac and the contents of the hernia drop back into the abdomen?
Explore through preperitoneal incision by opening the peritoneum versus laparoscopy

What procedure do you perform to repair an inguinal hernia in infants and children?
High ligation of the hernia sac

What is the percentage risk for hernia incarceration with watchful waiting?
0.03%

What does a cord lipoma represent?
Retroperitoneal fat that has herniated through the deep inguinal ring

How many cm of mobilization can be obtained when component separation is applied to both sides of the abdominal wall?
Up to 20 cm of mobilization

Term for the space that is first entered in an extraperitoneal hernia repair that lies between the posterior rectus sheath and pubic bone anteriorly and the vesicoumbilical fascia posteriorly:
The space of Retzius

Which types of patients may benefit from a laparoscopic hernia repair?
Patients with bilateral or recurrent inguinal hernias

What are relative contraindications to laparoscopic inguinal hernia repair?
Nonreducible, incarcerated inguinal hernia; prior laparoscopic herniorrhaphy; massive scrotal hernia; prior pelvic lymph node resection; prior groin irradiation

What are absolute contraindications to laparoscopic inguinal hernia repair?
Inability to tolerate general anesthesia

BORDERS OF THE TRIANGLE OF DOOM

What are the borders of the Triangle of Doom?
Vas deferens medially; spermatic vessels laterally; external iliac vessels inferiorly

What structures are contained within the Triangle of Doom?
External iliac vessels, deep circumflex iliac vein, genital branch of genitofemoral nerve, femoral nerve

TRIANGLE OF PAIN

What are the borders for the Triangle of Pain?
Spermatic vessels medially, iliopubic tract superolaterally

What structures are contained within the Triangle of Pain?
Lateral femoral cutaneous nerve and anterior femoral cutaneous nerve of the thigh

Why is the Triangle of Pain significant?
Placing tacks in this area may lead to chronic pain from injury to the lateral femoral cutaneous nerve/anterior femoral cutaneous nerve of the thigh.

What is the Circle of Death in regards to hernia repair?
Also known as the corona mortis, a vascular ring formed by the joining of an aberrant artery with the normal obturator artery arising from a branch of the internal iliac artery; during a laparoscopic hernia repair this vessel can be torn from both ends and bleed profusely

What must you remember to do before leaving the operating room after repairing an inguinal hernia in a male patient?
Pull the testicle back down into the scrotum

Most common early complication following hernia repair:
Urinary retention

Overall complication rate from hernia repair:
10%

Risk for surgical-site infection with open hernia repair:
Estimated to be 1% to 2%

Do you need to administer routine preoperative antibiotics to patients undergoing hernia repair?
No, consider a clean operation

Which patients undergoing hernia repair might you consider giving preoperative antibiotics?
Patients with significant underlying disease (ASA score >3)

If you have to give preoperative antibiotics before a hernia repair, what antibiotics do you give? How about a penicillin allergic patient?
Cefazolin, 1 to 2 g IV 30 to 60 minutes before incision; if penicillin allergic, give clindamycin 600 mg IV or vancomycin 1 g IV

What nerves are most commonly affected during open hernia repair?
Ilioinguinal, iliohypogastric, and genital branch of the genitofemoral nerve

What nerves are most commonly affected during laparoscopic hernia repair?
Lateral femoral cutaneous and genitofemoral nerves

What is the usual best treatment for patients who present with a nerve entrapment syndrome after open inguinal hernia repair?
Initial treatment should include a long trial of observation, NSAIDS, and possibly nerve blocks (exhaust every possible solution before taking the patient back; unless the patient is experiencing nerve entrapment immediately postoperatively in the PACU, in that case take them back). Repeat exploration with neurectomy and mesh removal as needed.

What is the pathogenesis of ischemic orchitis after inguinal hernia repair?
Thrombosis of the small veins of the pampiniform plexus within the spermatic cord resulting in venous congestion of the testis with resultant progressive pain and swelling usually resulting in testicular atrophy (the most common cause is extensive dissection of a scrotal hernia sac).

Where does recurrence of an inguinal hernia usually occur?
The floor of the inguinal canal near the pubic tubercle where the tension on the suture line is the greatest.

What is the rate of hernia recurrence?
1% to 3%

What is the time period that hernias usually recur?
Usually within the first 2 years after repair

How would you repair an incisional hernia with a small defect (<2 cm in diameter) with viable surrounding tissue?
Primary repair

When would you use a prosthetic mesh to repair an incisional hernia?
Incisional hernia with a large defect (>2–3 cm diameter)

What is the minimal desired overlap of mesh around the defect when performing a laparoscopic ventral hernia repair?
4 cm

What kind of hernia occurs at sites where vessels and nerves perforate the linea alba?
Epigastric hernia

What kind of hernia occurs between the rectus muscle medially and the semilunar line laterally?
Spigelian hernia

Why is it recommended that spigelian hernias be repaired?
The risk for incarceration associated with its relatively narrow neck.

What is Howship-Romberg sign?
Obturator hernia causing pain along the medial aspect of the proximal thigh from nerve compression.

What are the borders of the superior lumbar (Grynfeltt) triangle?
Medial—quadratus lumborum
Lateral—internal abdominal oblique
Superior—12th rib (floor—transversalis fascia; roof—external abdominal oblique)

What are the borders of the inferior lumbar (Petit) triangle?
Medial—latissimus dorsi
Lateral—external abdominal oblique
Inferior—iliac crest (floor—internal abdominal oblique)

Which lumbar hernia is more common? Grynfeltt hernia or Petit hernia?
Grynfeltt hernia

The most common symptom of a sciatic hernia:
Presence of an uncomfortable or slowly enlarging mass in the gluteal or intragluteal area

What options do you have after an inadvertent enterotomy during an elective hernia repair (after repair of the enterotomy)?
Abort the hernia repair; perform a primary tissue or biologic tissue repair; perform a delayed repair using prosthetic mesh in 3 to 4 days

What is an Amyand hernia?
Hernia sac containing a ruptured appendix

What is a Bochdalek hernia?
A posterior diaphragmatic hernia usually occurring on the left (Bochdalek = back and to the left)

What is a Morgagni hernia?
An anterior parasternal diaphragmatic hernia

What is a Cooper hernia?
A femoral hernia with 2 sacs that tracks into the scrotum or labia majorum through the femoral canal.

What is a Littre hernia?
Hernia containing a Meckel diverticulum

What is a Spigelian hernia?
Hernia through the linea semilunaris

What is a Hesselbach hernia?
A hernia that is lateral to the femoral vessels and under the inguinal ligament

What is a pantaloon hernia?
A hernia that straddles the inferior epigastric vessels representing both a direct hernia through the floor of the canal and an indirect hernia protruding through the internal ring

What is a Richter hernia?
Incarcerated/strangulated hernia involving only 1 sidewall of the bowel

What is an intraparietal hernia?
Hernia containing abdominal contents occurring between the layers of the abdominal wall

What is a Sports hernia?
Characterized by a dilated superficial ring of the inguinal canal and chronic groin pain in athletes (not a true hernia)

NAME THE HERNIA REPAIR

Name the repair: approximation of the transversus abdominis aponeurotic arch to the iliopubic tract with the use of interrupted sutures beginning at the pubic tubercle and extending laterally past the internal inguinal ring with or without the use of a relaxing incision.
The iliopubic tract

Name the repair: suturing the transversus abdominis and internal oblique musculoaponeurotic arches or conjoined tendon to the inguinal ligament.
The Bassini repair

Name the repair: a multilayer imbricated repair of the posterior wall of the inguinal canal with a continuous running suture technique by superimposing running suture lines progressing from deep to more superficial layers (initial suture line—transversus abdominis aponeurotic arch to iliopubic tract, next suture line—internal oblique and transversus abdominis muscles and aponeuroses to the inguinal ligament).
The Shouldice repair

Name the repair: the edge of the transversus abdominis aponeurosis is approximated to Cooper ligament with interrupted, nonabsorbable sutures; a transition suture is then placed to incorporate Cooper ligament and the iliopubic tract when the medial aspect of the femoral canal is reached; the transversus abdominis aponeurosis is then secured to the iliopubic tract lateral to the transition stitch; a relaxing incision is then made throughout the extent of the anterior sheath to near its lateral border.
McVay (Cooper ligament) repair

Name the tension-free inguinal hernia repair: prosthetic nonabsorbable mesh is sutured to the aponeurotic tissue overlying the pubic bone medially continuing along the transversus abdominis or conjoined tendon superiorly and the iliopubic tract or the shelving edge of the inguinal (Poupart) ligament inferolaterally using nonabsorbable monofilament suture in a continuous fashion.
Lichtenstein repair

Name the tension-free inguinal hernia repair: a cone-shaped plug of polypropylene is inserted into the internal inguinal ring and sewn to the surrounding tissues, occluding the hernia, and held in place by an overlying mesh patch (with or without sutures).
Plug and patch repair

Name the tension-free inguinal hernia repair: a repair that uses a bilayered device with 3 polypropylene components (underlay circular patch, connector, and onlay patch) covers the posterior inguinal floor.
Prolene hernia system (PHS) repair

Name the hernia repair: a hernia repair that utilizes an infraumbilical incision and blunt dissection to create a space beneath the rectus with placement of a dissecting balloon deep to the posterior rectus sheath and advanced to the pubic symphysis and inflated under direct laparoscopic vision.
Totally extraperitoneal (TEP) repair

Name the hernia repair: a hernia repair that utilizes an infraumbilical incision to gain access to the peritoneal cavity directly; placement of two 5-mm ports lateral to the inferior epigastric vessels at the level of the umbilicus; creation of a peritoneal flap.
Transabdominal preperitoneal (TAPP) repair

Name the hernia repair: a large piece of mesh is placed with an extensive fascial underlay in the retromuscular space on top of either the posterior rectus sheath or peritoneum.
Stoppa repair

Name the hernia repair: large subcutaneous flaps above the external oblique fascia are created; a relaxing incision is performed on the lateral external oblique aponeurosis from the costal margin to the pubis; the external oblique is then bluntly dissected from the internal oblique with the option of performing further relaxing incisions (aponeurotic layers of the internal oblique, transversus abdominis, or posterior rectus sheath); primary fascial closure at midline. These techniques, when applied to both sides of the abdominal wall, can yield up to 20 cm of mobilization.
Component separation technique

MULTIPLE CHOICE QUESTIONS

1. **Which of the following is the most common location for recurrence at reoperation following laparoscopic repair of an inguinal hernia?**
   A. Anterior
   B. Posterior
   C. Medial
   D. Lateral

2. **A 55-year-old female presents with a tender mass below the inguinal ligament. During repair of the femoral hernia through an inguinal approach you are unable to reduce the bowel. Which of the following is the next best step?**
   A. Push up on the bowel inferiorly while pulling up on the bowel superiorly
   B. Perform a small segmental bowel resection
   C. Divide the inguinal ligament
   D. Make a small contralateral inguinal incision to place a laparoscope

3. **Which of the following is the most common presentation of an obturator hernia?**

   A. Bowel obstruction
   B. Dysuria
   C. Testicular torsion
   D. Paresthesias of the lateral thigh

4. **In which of the following patients is laparoscopic hernia repair indicated?**

   A. 65-year-old male with bilateral inguinal hernias with a prior radical retropubic prostatectomy
   B. 37-year-old pregnant female in the second trimester with an incarcerated left inguinal hernia with a previous caesarean section
   C. 45-year-old female with bilateral recurrent inguinal hernias after laparoscopic repair who recently underwent pelvic radiation
   D. 27-year-old male with a history of laparoscopic cholecystectomy with bilateral inguinal hernias

5. **Which of the following is the most likely cause of ischemic orchitis following inguinal hernia repair?**

   A. Ligation of the testicular artery
   B. Complete excision of a large scrotal hernia sac
   C. Inadvertent torsion of the testicular cord during the repair
   D. Reconstruction of an internal ring that causes compression of the testicular cord

6. **A 52-year-old chronic alcoholic male, who has never been to a hospital, presents with slow oozing of clear fluid through thin skin at the apex of his large umbilical hernia. He has a shifting dullness on physical examination. Which of the following is the next best step in management?**

   A. Immediate umbilical hernia repair with mesh
   B. Perform paracentesis, primarily repair the skin defect, and place an abdominal binder
   C. Treat with salt and fluid restriction, oral antibiotics, and place a negative pressure wound dressing over the skin defect
   D. Aggressive diuresis, IV antibiotics, and bed rest followed by hernia repair during the same hospital admission

7. **Which of the following nerves is not at risk during a laparoscopic repair of an inguinal hernia?**

   A. Pudendal nerve
   B. Femoral branch of the genitofemoral nerve
   C. Lateral cutaneous nerve of the thigh
   D. Intermediate cutaneous branch of the anterior branch of the femoral nerve

8. **Which of the following statements regarding umbilical hernia is true?**

   A. Early repair of umbilical hernias in infants should be performed because of the risk of incarceration
   B. Umbilical hernias are more common in white infants than in African-American infants
   C. Repair of umbilical hernias in adults is usually indicated
   D. Umbilical hernias in infants usually require surgery

9. **Which of the following is the best choice for repairing a unilateral indirect inguinal hernia in a 5-month-old-male infant?**

   A. Open repair with PHS
   B. High ligation of the hernia sac
   C. Laparoscopic TEP hernia repair
   D. Cooper ligament (McVay) repair

10. **Which of the following statements is true regarding hernias?**

   A. Femoral hernias are more common in males than in females
   B. Inguinal hernias occur more frequently in females than in males
   C. Indirect inguinal hernias account for two-thirds of all inguinal hernias
   D. Indirect hernias are a rare occurrence in women

ANSWERS

1. **Answer: C.** The most common location for recurrence following laparoscopic hernia repair is the medial aspect of the mesh. This relates to failure to secure the mesh medially and using a piece of mesh that is too small. With a large direct defect, it is important to have adequate coverage anteriorly or the mesh can prolapse into the hernia defect.

2. **Answer: C.** If you are unable to reduce the bowel during a femoral hernia repair through an inguinal approach, the next best step is to incise the inguinal ligament. Make sure to control the neck of the hernia so that you can ensure viability of the bowel and then repair the hernia and inguinal ligament.

3. **Answer: A.** Obturator hernias are very rare but occur more frequently in multiparous elderly women. They can be associated with the Howship-Romberg sign, which is pain on internal rotation of the thigh. An obturator hernia occurs through a weakened obturator membrane. The defect is usually narrow in diameter, which predisposes to small bowel incarceration and strangulation.

4. **Answer: D.** Laparoscopic inguinal hernia repair has advantages in the setting of bilateral and/or recurrent hernias. Contraindications include patients who have had prior laparoscopic hernia repair, prior preperitoneal pelvic surgery or previous lower midline incision, prior pelvic radiation, or cannot tolerate general anesthesia.

5. **Answer: B.** Extensive dissection of the spermatic cord is the most common risk factor in the development of ischemic orchitis following inguinal hernia repair. Ischemic orchitis likely results from testicular venous congestion from thrombosis of the pampiniform venous plexus. To help prevent this, the spermatic cord should not be dissected past the pubic tubercle and the hernia sac can be ligated and divided leaving the distal sac in place. Ligation of the testicular artery is usually well tolerated, as evidenced by the 2-stage Fowler-Stevens orchiopexy for high undescended testis, because the testicle has a rich collateral blood supply from the cremasteric artery (branch of inferior epigastric artery) and the artery to the ductus deferens (branch of inferior vesical artery).

6. **Answer: D.** Umbilical hernia repair in cirrhotics with uncontrolled ascites has a high morbidity and mortality rate. Optimal therapy includes aggressive diuresis and sodium/fluid restriction to control ascites, IV antibiotics to combat possible bacterial peritonitis, bed rest to reduce stress on the hernia and leaking site, followed by repair of the hernia after the ascites is controlled.

7. **Answer: A.** The pudendal nerve is not at risk of injury during laparoscopic hernia repair. To help reduce the incidence of nerve injury during laparoscopic hernia repair, placing tacks lateral to the epigastric vessels is avoided.

8. **Answer: C.** Umbilical hernias in adults should usually be performed promptly because of the risk of incarceration. Umbilical hernias are rarely incarcerate and most surgeons will defer surgery until about 4 to 5 years of age because the majority of umbilical hernias in infants will close spontaneously by 2 years of age. Umbilical hernias are about 8 times more common in African-American children than in white children.

9. **Answer: B.** Inguinal hernia in infants results from a patent processus vaginalis and not from a weakness in the floor of the inguinal canal. High ligation of the hernia sac is usually all that is required except in the instance of a large defect, which may require tightening of the internal ring or reconstruction of the inguinal floor.

10. **Answer: C.** Indirect inguinal hernias account for two-thirds of inguinal hernias. Femoral hernias account for approximately 5% of abdominal wall hernias and occur more frequently in women. Inguinal hernias are approximately 25 times more common in men than in women. The most common hernia in both men and women is an indirect inguinal hernia.

CHAPTER 14
Stomach

Rona Altaras and Dale A. Dangleben

ANATOMY

Where does the lesser curvature abruptly angle to the right and the body of the stomach ends and the antrum begins?
Angularis incisura

Term for where the fundus forms with the left margin of the esophagus:
Angle of His

What is the arterial blood supply to the stomach?
4 main arteries: left gastric and right gastric arteries along lesser curvature and left and right gastroepiploic arteries along greater curvature; blood is also supplied to the proximal stomach by the inferior phrenic arteries and short gastric arteries

Approximate percentage that an aberrant left hepatic artery originates from the left gastric artery?
15% to 20%

What is the largest artery to the stomach?
Left gastric artery

In general, what is the maximal number of arteries that can be ligated, provided that the arcades along the greater and lesser curvatures are intact, that will still supply enough blood flow for the stomach to survive?
3 of 4 arteries can be ligated

Describe the venous drainage of the stomach:
Left gastric (coronary) and right gastric veins usually drain into the portal vein; left gastroepiploic vein drains into the splenic vein; right gastroepiploic vein drains into the superior mesenteric vein

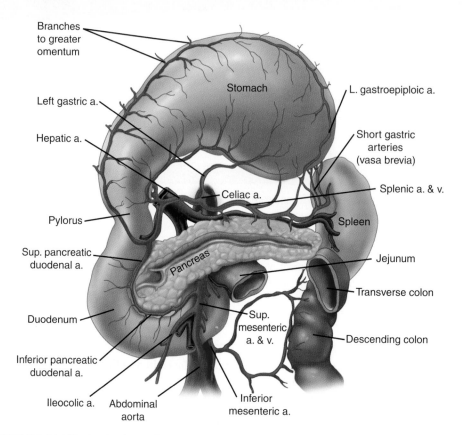

FIGURE 14-1. Arterial blood supply to the stomach. a., artery; v., vein. *(This article was published in Mercer DW, Liu TH, Castaneda A. Anatomy and physiology of the stomach. In: Zuidema GD, Yeo CJ, et al, eds. Shackelford's Surgery of the Alimentary Tract. 5th ed. Vol II. Philadelphia: Saunders; 2002:3, Copyright © Elsevier 2002.)*

What happens to the left vagus and right vagus at the gastroesophageal (GE) junction?
Left vagus becomes anterior and the right vagus becomes posterior (LARP mnemonic)

Where does the stomach receive its extrinsic parasympathetic and sympathetic innervation?
Parasympathetic via the vagus and sympathetic via the celiac plexus

Where does the sympathetic nerve supply to the stomach originate from?
From T5 to T10 (travels in splanchnic nerve to celiac ganglion)

Which vagus gives off a hepatic branch to the liver and continues along the lesser curvature as the anterior nerve of Latarjet?
The left vagus

Which nerve gives off a branch to the celiac plexus and continues posteriorly along the lesser curvature?
The right vagus

Which nerve is the first branch of the right or posterior vagus nerve and can lead to recurrent ulcers if left undivided?
The criminal nerve of Grassi

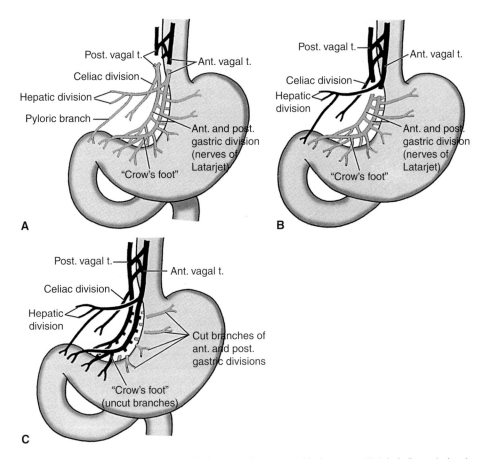

FIGURE 14-2. Vagotomy (nerves to be preserved are in black). (**A**) Truncal vagotomy. (**B**) Selective vagotomy. (**C**) Parietal cell or proximal gastric vagotomy. *(Modified from Skandalakis LJ, Gray SW, Skandalakis JE. The history and surgical anatomy of the vagus nerve. Surg Gynecol Obstet. 1986;162:75–85. Reprinted with permission from the Journal of the American College of Surgeons, formerly Surgery Gynecology & Obstetrics.)*

Where along the vagus is a truncal vagotomy performed?
Above the celiac and hepatic branches of the vagi

Where along the vagus nerve is a selective truncal vagotomy performed?
Below the celiac and hepatic branches of the vagi

Where along the vagus nerve is a highly selective vagotomy performed?
At the crow's feet to the proximal stomach while preserving the portion innervating the antrum and pylorus

The intrinsic or enteric nervous system of the stomach consists of which autonomic plexuses?
Auerbach and Meissner autonomic plexuses

What layer of the stomach lies between the mucosa and the muscularis propria that is the strongest layer of the gastric wall?
Submucosa

How many layers of smooth muscle make up the muscularis propria (muscularis externa) of the stomach?
3 layers of smooth muscle

Which layer of the muscularis propria (muscularis externa) is the only complete muscle layer of the stomach wall, is circular, and becomes progressively thicker and functions as a true anatomic sphincter at the pylorus?
The middle layer of smooth muscle

Gastric mucosa consists of what kind of epithelium?
Columnar glandular epithelium

PHYSIOLOGY

Where are parietal cells in the stomach mainly found? What do parietal cells secrete?
Body; secretion of intrinsic factor and acid

Where in the stomach will there be a complete absence of parietal cells?
The cardia and prepyloric antrum

Where are chief cells in the stomach mainly found? What do chief cells secrete?
Body; pepsinogen (converted to pepsin by gastric acid)

Where are G cells in the stomach mainly found? What do G cells secrete?
Antrum; gastrin

Where are D cells in the stomach mainly found? What do D cells secrete?
Body and antrum; somatostatin

Where are gastric mucosal interneurons mainly found? What peptide is released by gastric mucosal interneurons?
Body and antrum; gastrin-releasing peptide

Where are endocrine cells in the stomach mainly found? What hormone do endocrine cells in the stomach release?
Body; ghrelin

Process by which the proximal portion of the stomach relaxes in anticipation of food intake:
Receptive relaxation and gastric accommodation

Name ulcerogenic (excess acid secretion) causes of hypergastrinemia:
Antral G-cell hyperplasia or hyperfunction, gastric outlet obstruction, retained excluded antrum, short-gut syndrome, Zolinger-Ellison syndrome

Name nonulcerogenic (normal or low acid secretion) causes of hypergastrinemia:
Acid-reducing procedure (vagotomy), antisecretory agents (proton pump inhibitors [PPIs]), atrophic gastritis, chronic renal failure, *Helicobacter pylori* infection, pernicious anemia

What are the 3 local stimuli that regulate gastric acid secretion by the parietal cell?
Acetylcholine, gastrin, and histamine

The basal level of acid secretion accounts for roughly what percentage of maximal acid output?
~10%

What is the approximate rate of hydrochloric acid production during basal acid secretion?
1 to 5 mmol/h

What are the 3 phases of acid secretory response to a meal?
Cephalic, gastric, and intestinal

Histamine utilizes which second messenger to stimulate acid secretion by parietal cells?
Intracellular cyclic AMP

Acetylcholine and gastrin utilize which second messenger to stimulate acid secretion by parietal cells?
Calcium (phospholipase C converts membrane-bound phospholipids into inositol triphosphate (IP3), which mobilizes calcium from intracellular stores)

Mechanism by which PPIs inhibit acid secretion?
A covalent disulfate bond forms between the drug and the cysteine residues on the subunit of the H/K-ATPase leading to irreversible inhibition of the proton pump

Why do PPIs have a longer duration of action than their plasma half-life?
The drug is covalently bonded to the H/K-ATPase leading to irreversible inhibition, so new proton pumps need to be synthesized before the recovery of acid secretion occurs

What converts pepsinogen into pepsin?
Gastric acid

How is the maximal acid output (MAO) determined after gastric analysis?
By averaging the output of the last two 15-minute periods after secretogogue administration

What is the usual range for MAO?
10 to 15 mEq/h

How is the peak acid output obtained after gastric analysis?
It is the highest rate of secretion obtained during a 15-minute period following secretogogue administration

Gastric motility begins with the depolarization of which cells?
Gastric pacemaker cells of Cajal located in the midbody of the stomach along the greater curvature

How many phases are in the myoelectric migrating complex (MMC)?
4 phases

How long does each cycle of the MMC last?
90 to 120 minutes

What happens in phase I of the MMC?
Also known as the quiescent phase; slow waves are present without action potentials; increase in gastric tone but no gastric contraction

What happens in phase II of the MMC?
Motor spikes are associated with slow waves and occasional gastric contractions; gallbladder contraction

What happens in phase III of the MMC?
Motor spike activity is associated with each slow wave; forceful gastric contractions happen every 15 to 20 seconds; the stomach is cleared of large indigestible food substances

What happens in phase IV of the MMC?
A brief recovery period before the next MMC cycle

List protective factors to gastric barrier function:
Blood flow, bicarbonate secretion, cell renewal, endogenous prostaglandins, growth factors, mucus production

List damaging factors to gastric barrier function:
Duodenal reflux of bile, ethanol ingestion, *H pylori*, hydrochloric acid secretion, hypoxia, ischemia, nonsteroidal anti-inflammatory drugs (NSAIDs), pepsins, smoking

BENIGN CONDITIONS

Approximate percentage of gastric ulcers associated with *H pylori*:
75%

Approximate percentage of duodenal ulcers associated with *H pylori*:
90%

Most common cause of peptic ulcer disease:
H pylori infection

What is the second most common cause of peptic ulcer disease?
NSAID ingestion

Where do gastric ulcers usually occur?
On the lesser curve near the incisura (~60%; type I)

What is a type I gastric ulcer?
Gastric ulcer occurring on the lesser curvature near the incisura

What is a type II gastric ulcer?
Gastric ulcer located in the body of the stomach in combination with a duodenal ulcer

What is a type III gastric ulcer?
Prepyloric gastric ulcer

What is a type IV gastric ulcer?
Gastric ulcer that occurs high on the lesser curve near the GE junction

What is a type V gastric ulcer?
Drug-induced (NSAIDs) gastric ulcer that may occur anywhere in the stomach

Which types of gastric ulcer are not associated with excess acid secretion?
Type I and IV

Which types of gastric ulcer are associated with excess acid secretion?
Type II and III

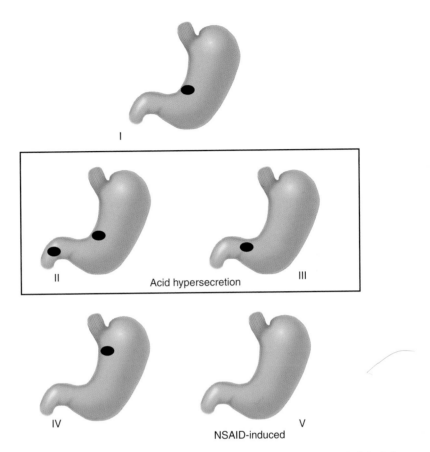

FIGURE 14-3. Modified Johnson classification for gastric ulcer. I, lesser curve, incisura; II, body of stomach, incisura + duodenal ulcer (active or healed); III, prepyloric; IV, high on lesser curve, near gastroesophageal junction; V, medication-induced (NSAID/acetylsalicylic acid), anywhere in stomach. NSAID, nonsteroidal anti-inflammatory drug. *(This article was published in Zinner MJ. Benign gastric ulcer. In: Cameron JL, ed. Current Surgical Therapy. 9th ed. Philadelphia: Mosby; 2007:81. Copyright © Elsevier 2007.)*

Name the ulcer: multiple, superficial erosions that begin in the proximal stomach and progress distally in a patient with central nervous system disease:
Cushing ulcer

Name the ulcer: multiple, superficial erosions that begin in the proximal stomach and progress distally in a patient with >30% body surface area burn:
Curling ulcer

Where in the stomach is stress gastritis usually seen?
Fundus

Initial management for a patient with stress gastritis with UGI bleeding:
A,B,Cs; fluid resuscitation with correction of any platelet/coagulation abnormalities; blood transfusion if needed; administration of broad-spectrum IV antibiotics in patients with sepsis, saline lavage of the stomach through a nasogastric (NG) tube; administration of antisecretory agents after the NGT aspirate runs clear

Dose of vasopressin for the control of acute GI bleeding?:
0.2 to 0.4 IU/min as a continuous infusion for a maximum of 48 to 72 hours

Indications for operation with stress gastritis:
Recurrent or persistent bleeding requiring >6 units of blood (3,000 mL)

After taking the patient to the operating room, how would you control the bleeding associated with stress gastritis in a hemodynamically stable patient?
Make a long anterior gastrotomy along the proximal stomach/fundus; clear the gastric lumen of blood; inspect the mucosal surface for bleeding points; oversew all bleeding areas with figure-of-eight stitches taken deep within the gastric wall; close the anterior gastrotomy; perform a truncal vagotomy and pyloroplasty (less commonly a partial gastrectomy with vagotomy can be performed)

After taking a patient with life-threatening hemorrhage refractory to other forms of therapy to the OR, what procedure would you perform to control the bleeding?
Gastric devascularization procedure (faster) versus total gastrectomy

Term for a disruption of the gastric mucosa (high on lesser curve at GE junction) that results from forceful vomiting, retching, coughing, or straining:
Mallory-Weiss tear

What percentage of acute UGI bleeds are accounted for by Mallory-Weiss tears?
15%

What is the overall mortality rate from a Mallory-Weiss tear?
3% to 4%

Treatment for active bleeding from a Mallory-Weiss tear that continues after initial resuscitation?
Esophagogastroduodenoscopy (EGD) (band ligation, epinephrine injection, hemoclipping, multipolar electric coagulation) versus angiographic intra-arterial infusion of vasopressin or transcatheter embolization (in patients with severe comorbidities)

Indications for surgery in a patient with an acute bleed from a Mallory-Weiss tear?
>6 U packed red blood cells (PRBC) transfused; failure of EGD to stop bleeding; failure of angiographic embolization (in patients with severe comorbidities)

If surgery for active bleeding from a Mallory-Weiss tear is indicated, what procedure would you perform?
Anterior gastrotomy and oversewing of the bleeding site with deep 2-0 silk ligatures with reapproximation of the gastric mucosa

If surgery for active bleeding from a Mallory-Weiss tear in the distal esophagus is indicated, how might your operative approach change?
Rather than laparotomy and anterior gastrotomy, you may need a left thoracotomy and esophagotomy followed by suture ligation

What disease process is characterized by erosion of the superficial mucosa overlying an abnormally large (1–3 mm) tortuous resulting in bleeding?
Dieulafoy lesion

Are Dieulafoy lesions more common in men or in women?
Men (M:F = 2:1)

Peak incidence for Dieulafoy lesion:
5th decade

Diagnostic modality of choice for Dieulafoy lesion:
EGD

Where do Dieulafoy lesions usually occur in the stomach?
6 to 10 cm from the GE junction generally in the fundus near the cardia

What is the classic presentation of a patient with a Dieulafoy lesion?
Sudden onset of massive, painless, recurrent hematemesis with hypotension

After resuscitation, what initial attempts should be made to stop acute bleeding from a Dieulafoy lesion?
Endoscopic modalities (band ligation, heater probe, hemoclipping, injection sclerotherapy, multipolar electrocoagulation, noncontact laser photocoagulation) or angiography if endoscopy cannot identify the bleeding source

Surgical management of a patient with Dieulafoy lesion:
Gastric wedge resection to include the offending vessel (laparotomy with gastrotomy vs laparoscopically with intra-op endoscopy)

What are the 2 ways that gastric varices can develop?
In conjunction with esophageal varices in the setting of portal hypertension (HTN); sinistral HTN from splenic vein thrombosis

Treatment for gastric varices in the setting of splenic vein thrombosis:
Splenectomy

Treatment for gastric varices in the setting of portal HTN:
Volume resuscitation and correction of any coagulopathy; temporary tamponade with Sengstaken-Blakemore tube; endoscopic banding or sclerotherapy; transjugular intrahepatic portosystemic shunt (with possible balloon-occluded retrograde transvenous obliteration of a gastrorenal shunt with ethanolamine oleate)

What study should be performed in patients with bleeding gastric varices prior to surgical intervention?
Abdominal ultrasound to document splenic vein thrombosis (portal HTN often accompanies gastric varices)

Term for when a gastric volvulus occurs along the stomach's longitudinal axis:
Organoaxial

Term for when a gastric volvulus occurs along the stomach's vertical axis:
Mesenteroaxial

Which type of gastric volvulus is more common: organoaxial or mesenteroaxial?
Organoaxial (two thirds of cases)

What is Borchardt triad?
Sudden onset of constant, severe upper abdominal pain; recurrent retching with inability to vomit; inability to pass an NG tube

Which type of gastric volvulus more often occurs acutely and is associated with a diaphragmatic defect?
Organoaxial gastric volvulus (mesenteroaxial volvulus usually recurrent and not associated with a diaphragmatic defect)

What might you see on plain film of the abdomen in a patient with gastric volvulus?
A gas-filled viscus in the chest or upper abdomen

Surgical treatment for a spontaneous gastric volvulus without an associated diaphragmatic defect:
Detorsion and fixation of the stomach by gastropexy or tube gastrostomy through a transabdominal approach

Surgical treatment for a gastric volvulus with an associated diaphragmatic defect:
Reduction and uncoiling of the stomach through a transabdominal approach; repair of the diaphragmatic defect; resection of compromised stomach if necessary; consideration to perform fundoplication; fixation of stomach with gastropexy versus tube gastrostomy

Term for a collection of nondigestible vegetable matter formed from within the GI tract:
Phytobezoar

Term for a collection of hair formed from within the GI tract?
Trichobezoar

What types of patients usually get phytobezoars?
Patients with impaired gastric emptying after gastric surgery; diabetics with autonomic neuropathy

What enzyme can be administered to attempt dissolution of a bezoar?
Papain

How is papain administered?
1 teaspoon of Papain (found in Adolph Meat Tenderizer) in 150 to 300 mL of water is given several times daily

Treatment for a phytobezoar?
Enzymatic débridement followed by endoscopic fragmentation versus aggressive Ewald tube lavage; surgical removal if these methods fail

Describe the typical patient who presents with a trichobezoar:
Long-haired females who often deny eating their own hair

Treatment for a trichobezoar:
Surgical removal; may attempt enzymatic therapy, endoscopic fragmentation, or vigorous lavage for small trichobezoars; psychiatric evaluation (recurrent bezoar formation common)

TUMORS

In what percentage of hyperplastic polyps in the stomach can adenocarcinoma be found?
2%

Treatment for a patient with a hyperplastic polyp in the stomach:
Endoscopic polypectomy for histologic examination

In what percentage of adenomatous polyps in the stomach can adenocarcinoma be found?
20%

Treatment for a patient with an adenomatous gastric polyp:
Endoscopic polypectomy as long as the entire polyp can be removed and no invasive cancer is in the specimen with close follow-up with serial endoscopies because of the increased risk for coincident gastric carcinoma

Name nutritional factors associated with an increased risk of developing gastric cancer:
Salted meat or fish, high complex-carbohydrate consumption, high nitrate consumption, low fat or protein consumption

Name medical factors associated with an increased risk of developing gastric cancer:
Adenomatous polyps, gastric atrophy and gastritis, *H pylori* infection, male gender, prior gastric surgery

Name environmental factors associated with an increased risk of developing gastric cancer:
Lack of refrigeration, low socioeconomic status, poor drinking water (well water), poor food preparation (salted, smoked), smoking

What percentage of all malignant gastric neoplasms are adenocarcinomas?
95%

Term for a diffusely infiltrating gastric carcinoma that involves the entire stomach:
Linitis plastica

According to the 6th edition of the AJCC Cancer Staging Manual, what is a T1 gastric cancer?
Tumor invades lamina propria or submucosa

According to the 6th edition of the AJCC Cancer Staging Manual, what is a T2 gastric cancer?
Tumor invades muscularis propria or subserosa

According to the 6th edition of the AJCC Cancer Staging Manual, what is a T2a gastric cancer?
Tumor invades muscularis propria

According to the 6th edition of the AJCC Cancer Staging Manual, what is a T2b gastric cancer?
Tumor invades subserosa

According to the 6th edition of the AJCC Cancer Staging Manual, what is a T3 gastric cancer?
Tumor penetrates serosa (visceral peritoneum) without invasion of adjacent structures

According to the 6th edition of the AJCC Cancer Staging Manual, what is a T4 gastric cancer?
Tumor invades adjacent structures

According to the 6th edition of the AJCC Cancer Staging Manual for gastric cancer, what is N1 nodal status?
Metastasis in 1 to 6 regional lymph nodes

According to the 6th edition of the AJCC Cancer Staging Manual for gastric cancer, what is N2 nodal status?
Metastasis in 7 to 15 regional lymph nodes

According to the 6th edition of the AJCC Cancer Staging Manual for gastric cancer, what is N3 nodal status?
Metastasis in more than 15 regional lymph nodes

Table 14-1	TNM Gastric Cancer Staging		
Stage	T	N	M
0	Tis	N0	M0
IA	T1	N0	M0
IB	T2	N0	M0
	T1	N1	M0
IIA	T3	N0	M0
	T2	N1	M0
	T1	N2	M0
IIB	T4a	N0	M0
	T3	N1	M0
	T2	N2	M0
	T1	N3	M0
IIIA	T4a	N1	M0
	T3	N2	M0
IIIB	T4b	N0	M0
	T4b	N1	M0
	T4a	N2	M0
	T3	N3	M0
IIIC	T4b	N2	M0
	T4b	N3	M0
	T4a	N3	M0
IV	Any T	Any N	M1

What is the minimum number of nodes that must be evaluated for accurate staging of gastric carcinoma?
15 nodes

In regards to gastric cancer, what is an R0 resection?
Microscopically margin-negative resection with no gross or microscopic tumor remaining in the tumor bed

In regards to gastric cancer, what is an R1 resection?
Removal of all macroscopic disease with positive microscopic margins for tumor

In regards to gastric cancer, what is an R2 resection?
Gross residual disease

In regards to gastric cancer, what is a D1 resection?
Removal of group 1 lymph nodes (right paracardial, left paracardial, lesser curvature, short gastric, right gastroepiploic, left gastroepiploic, suprapyloric, infrapyloric)

In regards to gastric cancer, what is a D2 resection?
Removal of group 1 and 2 lymph nodes (right paracardial, left paracardial, lesser curvature, short gastric, right gastroepiploic, left gastroepiploic, suprapyloric, infrapyloric + left gastric, anterior common hepatic, celiac artery, splenic hilum, proximal splenic, distal splenic, left hepatoduodenal, superior mesenteric vein)

In regards to gastric cancer, what is a D3 resection?
D2 resection with removal of paraaortic nodes

Diagnostic modality of choice for gastric cancer:
Flexible upper endoscopy

Desired margin of resection for gastric cancer:
5 to 6 cm

What procedure needs to be performed to completely remove station 10 nodes during a Japanese-style D2 resection?
Splenectomy (station 10 nodes are parasplenic)

What procedure needs to be performed to completely remove station 11 nodes during a Japanese-style D2 resection?
Partial pancreatectomy (station 11 nodes are parapancreatic)

Which patients should receive adjuvant chemoradiation following complete surgical resection for gastric cancer?
Patients with T3/T4 lesion, node-positive cancers, or microscopically positive resection margins

Usual time period for the recurrence of gastric cancer after gastrectomy for gastric cancer:
Within the first 3 years after gastrectomy

What are the most common sites of locoregional recurrence after gastrectomy for gastric cancer?
Gastric remnant at the anastomosis, gastric bed, regional nodes

Areas where gastric cancer hematogenously spreads:
Liver, lung, bone

How should patients treated with gastrectomy for gastric cancer be followed?
Complete history and physical examination every 3 to 4 months for 1 year
Every 6 months for 2 years
Yearly thereafter
Labs (CBC and LFTs) obtained as clinically indicated
CXR/CT A/P where indicated
If a subtotal gastrectomy was performed yearly endoscopy may be necessary.

Most common site of lymphoma in the GI tract:
Stomach

Most common gastric lymphoma:
Diffused large B-cell lymphoma (55%)

Second most common gastric lymphoma:
Extranodal marginal cell lymphoma (mucosa-associated lymphoid tissue [MALT])

Treatment for gastric lymphoma:
Chemoradiation (cyclophosphamide, hydroxydaunorubicin, oncovin, prednisone [CHOP] regimen usually employed) versus multimodal therapy (resection for gastric lymphoma controversial)

Treatment for early-stage gastric MALT lymphoma:
H pylori eradication alone with repeat endoscopy in 2 months to document clearance of infection and biannual endoscopy for 3 years to document regression

What characteristics of MALT lymphoma predict failure after *H pylori* eradication alone?
Nodal involvement, nuclear Bcl-10 expression, transformation into a large cell phenotype t(11;18), transmural tumor extension

Most common mesenchymal tumor of the GI tract?
GIST

What mutation is associated with GISTs?
c-kit

What is the goal of surgery when treating GISTs?
A margin-negative resection with en bloc resection of adjacent organs if involved by direct extension

What competitive tyrosine kinase inhibitor can be given to patients with unresectable and metastatic GISTs and as adjuvant therapy in clinical trials?
Imatinib mesylate (Gleevec)

What disease is otherwise known as a hypoproteinemic hypertrophic gastropathy and is characterized by gastric mucosa with a cobblestone/cerebriform appearance from massive gastric folds in the fundus and corpus of the stomach?
Ménétrier disease

What will be seen on histological examination with Ménétrier disease?
Expansion of surface mucous cells (foveolar hyperplasia); absent parietal cells

What is the treatment for a patient with Ménétrier disease who develops dysplasia/ carcinoma or continues to have massive protein loss despite optimal medical therapy?
Total gastrectomy

MULTIPLE CHOICE QUESTIONS

1. A 45-year-old male presents with sudden onset of severe abdominal pain and recurrent retching with inability to vomit. Attempts at placing an NG tube are not successful. What is the most likely diagnosis?
   A. Small bowel obstruction
   B. Gastritis
   C. Colonic obstruction
   D. Gastric volvulus

2. A 65-year-old male presents with prolonged vomiting. He undergoes an EGD and is diagnosed with a gastric outlet obstruction. Which of the following would correspond with the metabolic abnormality seen with this type of patients?

   A. Hypochloremic, hypokalemic metabolic alkalosis
   B. Hyperchloremic, hyperkalemic metabolic acidosis
   C. Hyponatremic, hypochloremic metabolic acidosis
   D. Hypernatremic, hypochloremic metabolic alkalosis

3. A 55-year-old critically ill intubated patient has large amount of bloody drainage from his NG tube. He is hemodynamically labile and received 8 U of PRBC and is not coagulopathic. What is the next step in treatment of this patient?

   A. EGD
   B. Observation with IV PPI
   C. Angiogram
   D. Operative intervention

4. A 35-year-old woman has underwent an EGD, which shows a prepyloric ulcer. What type of ulcer is this?

   A. Type I
   B. Type II
   C. Type III
   D. Type V

5. Where are the chief cells of stomach found?

   A. Fundus
   B. Body
   C. Antrum
   D. Pylorus

6. A 35-year-old burn patient with 40% TBSA burns is being treated in the intensive care unit (ICU). The patient undergoes an EGD after UGI bleeding and a stomach ulcer is seen during this procedure. What is the name of this type of ulcer?

   A. Marginal ulcer
   B. Cushing ulcer
   C. Curling ulcer
   D. Dieulafoy lesion

7. Which of these patients has to be on stress gastritis prophylaxis with H_2 blockers?

   A. Intubated patient (>48 hours) with an international normalized ratio of 3
   B. Stable trauma patient with an isolated pelvic fracture
   C. Long-term ICU patient tolerating tube feeds at goal for 2 weeks
   D. NPO patient with a postoperative ileus following elective colon resection

8. Where is the most common site for a lymphoma in the GI tract?

   A. Small bowel
   B. Duodenum
   C. Right colon
   D. Stomach

9. **What is the treatment for an early-stage gastric MALT lymphoma?**
   A. Gastrectomy
   B. Radiation treatment
   C. Chemotherapy
   D. *H pylori* eradication followed by regular EGD follow-up

10. **An aberrant left hepatic artery originates from:**
    A. Right gastric artery
    B. Left gastric artery
    C. Left gastroepiploic artery
    D. SMA

ANSWERS

1. **Answer: D.** This is a classic presentation of gastric volvulus with Borchardt triad. Two thirds of the gastric volvulus are organoaxial with the rest being mesenteroaxial.

2. **Answer: A.** With prolonged vomiting and loss of hydrochloric acid and potassium, a hypochloremic, hypokalemic metabolic alkalosis is encountered. Primary treatment is replacement of lost volume with normal saline.

3. **Answer: D.** The patient is hemodynamically labile and has already received 8 U of PRBC. He needs to go to the operating room for operative intervention, which would include exploratory laparotomy, gastrotomy, and oversewing of bleeding areas. If the patient is stable preoperatively, a highly selective vagotomy or a pyloroplasty and truncal vagotomy can be performed.

4. **Answer: C.** Type III ulcer is located in the prepyloric area. The management includes antrectomy with incorporation of the ulcer and vagotomy.

5. **Answer: B.** The chief cells are found in the body and secrete pepsinogen.

6. **Answer: C.** The Curling ulcer is typically seen in burn patients and is a type of stress ulcer. Prophylaxis is with H_2 blockers.

7. **Answer: A.** A coagulopathic state and intubation for more than 48 hours is the classic indication for stress ulcer prophylaxis.

8. **Answer: D.** Most common site to develop a lymphoma in the GI tract is the stomach.

9. **Answer: D.** The treatment of choice for early-stage gastric MALT lymphoma is eradication of *H pylori* and EGD follow-up in regular intervals.

10. **Answer: B.** An aberrant left hepatic artery originates from the left gastric artery, and an aberrant right hepatic artery originates from the SMA 15% of the time.

CHAPTER 15
Hepatobiliary

Firas Madbak

ANATOMY

List the ligaments of the liver:
The falciform ligament, coronary ligaments, and the right and left triangular ligaments.

What structures are contained within the hepatoduodenal ligament?
Porta hepatis: proper hepatic artery, portal vein, common bile duct (CBD)

What line divides the liver into left and right lobes?
Cantlie line (runs from the middle of the gallbladder fossa anteriorly to the inferior vena cava posteriorly)

How many Couinaud segments are in the liver?
8

Which segments are removed in a right hepatectomy?
Segments 5 to 8

Which segments are removed in a right trisegmentectomy?
Segments 4 to 8

Which segments removed are in a left hepatectomy?
Segments 2 to 4

Which segments are removed in a left lateral trisegmentectomy?
Segments 2 and 3

Which segments are removed in a left trisegmentectomy?
Segments 2, 3, 4, 5, 8

How much percentage of blood flow does the portal vein supply to the liver?
70%

What percentage of cardiac output accounts for hepatic blood flow?
25%

How much of the liver's oxygen supply is provided by the hepatic artery?
50%

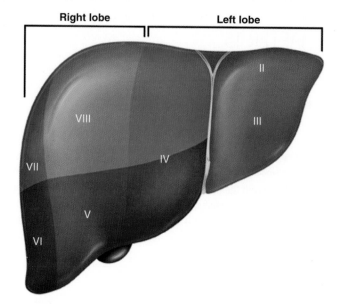

Right lobe   **Left lobe**

FIGURE 15-1. Couinaud's liver segments (I through VIII) numbered in a clockwise manner. The left lobe includes segments II to IV, the right lobe includes segments V to VIII, and the caudate lobe is segment I. *(Reproduced from Brunicardi FC, Andersen DK, Billiar TR, et al. Schwartz's Principles of Surgery. 9th ed. http://www.accessmedicine. com. Copyright © The McGraw-Hill Companies, Inc. All rights reserved.)*

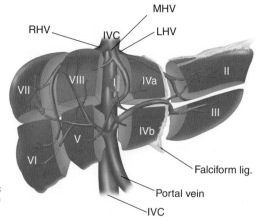

FIGURE 15-2. Hepatic resection nomenclature and anatomy. Hepatic segments removed in the formal major hepatic resections are indicated. The International Hepato-Pancreato-Biliary Association (IHPBA) Brisbane 2000 terminology also is presented. IVC, inferior vena cava; LHV, left hepatic vein; MHV, middle hepatic vein; RHV, right hepatic vein. *(Reproduced from Brunicardi FC, Andersen DK, Billiar TR, et al. Schwartz's Principles of Surgery. 9th ed. http://www.accessmedicine.com. Copyright © The McGraw-Hill Companies, Inc. All rights reserved.)*

How much does the portal vein contribute to total hepatic blood flow?
Two-thirds

How many hepatic veins are there?
Three (right, middle, and left)

What is the approximate length of the CBD?
Approximately 7 cm

What is normal CBD diameter?
0.5 to 1.5 cm

What is the arterial supply of the bile ducts?
Primarily the right hepatic artery

Where does the sympathetic innervation of the gallbladder originate?
Celiac axis

What is the parasympathetic innervation of gallbladder?
Vagus nerve

What are ducts of Luschka?
Accessory ducts directly from the liver bed into the gallbladder

PHYSIOLOGY

How much bilirubin is produced daily in normal adults?
About 250 to 350 mg

How much bilirubin is produced from turnover of senescent red blood cells?
Approximately 85%

What is the most common cause of hyperbilirubinemia in adults?
Cholelithiasis

What is the major metabolite of heme?
Bilirubin

What is the name of sinusoidal macrophages?
Kupffer cells

What is the half-life of albumin?
20 days

What is the half-life of transferrin?
6 days

Which major protein is produced by the liver?
Albumin

What are bile acids conjugated with to form bile salts?
Glycine and taurine

What is the major site of bile acid reabsorption?
Distal ileum

What autosomal recessive disorder causes an increase in conjugated bilirubin without elevation of liver function tests (LFTs)?
Dubin-Johnson syndrome

What percentage of the population has gallstones?
Approximately 10%

What group of Indians in southern Arizona are at high risk for gallstones?
Pima Indians

What population is at lowest risk for developing gallstones?
Sub-saharan Africans

How are gallstones classified?
Cholesterol, black pigment, or brown-pigment stones

What is the main composition of black pigmented stones?
Calcium bilirubinate

What is the main composition of brown pigmented stones?
Calcium salts of unconjugated bilirubin

What causes gallstone formation?
Cholesterol supersaturation, accelerated crystal nucleation, and gallbladder hypomotility

What are the 2 primary bile acids?
Cholate and chenodeoxycholate

What is the most common inherited cause of hyperbilirubinemia?
Gilbert syndrome (decreased activity of the enzyme glucuronyl transferase)

Which enzyme found in the cells of the bile duct rises with bile duct obstruction?
Alkaline phosphatase

The liver is the site of synthesis of all of the coagulation factors except:
von Willebrand factor

What is type I Crigler–Najjar syndrome?
Severe unconjugated hyperbilirubinemia, kernicterus, bilirubin deposits in the brain causing severe motor dysfunction and retardation.

What is type II Crigler–Najjar syndrome?
Less severe form, enzyme activity is 10% of normal

Which substance is metabolized by gut bacteria to lactic acid that converts ammonia to ammonium salt?
Lactulose

List the secondary bile salts:
Lithocholate, deoxycholate, and ursodeoxycholate

What hormone is a potent stimulator of gallbladder contraction?
Cholecystokinin

BENIGN BILIARY DISEASE

Is prophylactic cholecystectomy recommended in diabetics?
No

What is the incidence of endoscopic retrograde cholangiopancreatography (ERCP)-induced pancreatitis?
About 5%

Which is a rapid, noninvasive imaging study that provides detailed biliary tree and pancreatic duct images equal to those of ERCP?
Magnetic resonance cholangiopancreatography (MRCP)

What percentage of pigmented stones and cholesterol stones are seen on plain abdominal films?
50% and 20%, respectively

What is the principal imaging modality for the diagnosis of cholelithiasis?
Ultrasonography

What is the sensitivity of ultrasonography for stones greater than 2 mm?
>95%

What is the probability of complications requiring surgery in a patient with a history of biliary colic?
1% to 2% per year

What is the surgical management of uncomplicated biliary colic and documented gallstones?
Elective laparoscopic cholecystectomy

What percentage of patients with acute cholecystitis have positive enteric bacteria culture from the bile?
50%

What is hydrops of the gallbladder?
Chronic cystic duct obstruction and gallbladder distention with clear mucoid fluid.

What is Mirrizzi syndrome?
Impacted stone in the gallbladder neck causing extrinsic compression of the common (hepatic) duct

What is porcelain gallbladder?
Calcification of the gallbladder wall; cholecystectomy is indicated to prevent carcinoma

What is Murphy sign?
Inspiratory arrest upon right upper quadrant (RUQ) palpation

What percentage of patients with gallstones have CBD stones?
15% to 20%

What is the most common cause of cholangitis?
Stone impacted in the CBD (85% of the time)

Which organisms are most commonly cultured from bile?
Escherichia coli, *Klebsiella*, *Pseudomonas*, *Proteus*, enterococci

What is the constellation of RUQ pain, jaundice, and fever?
Charcot triad

What is Reynolds pentad?
Altered mental status and hypotension plus Charcot triad

Which autoimmune disease is associated with destruction of extrahepatic and intrahepatic bile ducts?
Primary sclerosing cholangitis

What is the type I choledochal cyst?
Saccular or fusiform dilatation of the common hepatic and CBDs

What is the type II choledochal cyst?
This choledochal cyst is characterized as a diverticulum protruding from the CBD

What is a type III choledochal cyst?
Choledochocele; found in the intraduodenal portion of the CBD

What is a type IV choledochal cyst?
Choledochal cyst that involves the extrahepatic bile duct and intrahepatic ducts

What is a type V choledochal cyst?
Caroli disease (multiple intrahepatic cysts)

List the areas where dilated collateral veins are seen in severe cirrhotics draining into the systemic circulation:
Hemorrhoidal, azygos, renal, and adrenal veins

What is the most common cause of hemobilia?
Iatrogenic trauma to the liver and biliary tree

What is the first test to rule out hemobilia?
Esophagogastroduodenoscopy

What is the first-line therapy for hemobilia?
Angiography (embolization)

BENIGN LIVER DISEASE

What is the treatment of pyogenic liver abscess?
Antibiotics and percutaneous drainage

What is the antibiotic course for pyogenic liver abscess?
Broad-spectrum intravenous antibiotics for 2 to 3 weeks followed by 4 to 6 weeks of oral antibiotics

What is the most common cause of hydatid disease?
Echinococcus granulosus

What cyst may rupture and result in anaphylactic shock?
Echinococcal cyst

What skin test is used in the diagnosis of hydatid disease?
Casoni test (intradermal injection of hydatid fluid)

What in the wall of a liver cyst is highly suggestive of hydatid disease?
Calcifications

What abnormality may be seen on complete blood count in about 25% of patients with echinococcal cyst?
Eosinophilia

What is the medical treatment of choice for *Echinococcus*?
Mebendazole/albendazole

What technique describes percutaneous management of hydatid cysts in patients who refuse or cannot undergo surgery?
PAIR—Percutaneous Aspiration, Injection, and Reaspiration

What is the most common scolicidal agent used in hydatid cyst injection?
20% sodium chloride solution

What are surgical options for hydatid cysts?
Partial cystectomy, pericystectomy, partial hepatectomy

What is the recurrence rate of postoperative hydatid cysts?
About 20%

What parasite causes amebiasis if transmitted through a fecal-oral route?
Entamoeba histolytica

What is the appropriate treatment of cyst rupture and bile duct obstruction?
ERCP with papillotomy

What liver abscess typically described as having anchovy paste appearance?
Amebic liver abscess

What is the treatment of amebic abscess?
750 mg of metronidazole 3 times a day for 10 days

What is the most common cause of intrahepatic presinusoidal hypertension worldwide?
Schistosomiasis

What is Budd-Chiari syndrome?
Hepatic venous outflow obstruction

What are some causes of Budd-Chiari syndrome?
Polycythemia vera, factor V Leiden mutation, thrombocytosis, Protein C and S, antithrombin III, antiphospholipid antibody syndrome.

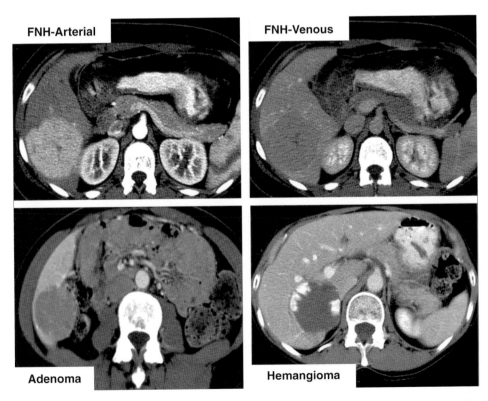

FIGURE 15-3. Computed tomographic scans showing classic appearance of benign liver lesions. Focal nodular hyperplasia (FNH) is hypervascular on arterial phase, isodense to liver on venous phase, and has a central scar (upper panels). Adenoma is hypovascular (lower left panel). Hemangioma shows asymmetrical peripheral enhancement (lower right panel). *(Reproduced from Brunicardi FC, Andersen DK, Billiar TR, et al. Schwartz's Principles of Surgery. 9th ed. http://www.accessmedicine.com. Copyright © The McGraw-Hill Companies, Inc. All rights reserved.)*

What are possible sequelae of hepatic adenomas?
Rupture or malignancy

What liver tumor is associated with oral contraceptive pill use?
Hepatic adenoma

How would you manage a patient with hepatic adenoma who wants to get pregnant?
Elective resection of hepatic adenoma

What liver mass is characterized by a central stellate scar seen on computed tomography (CT) imaging?
FNH

What is the indication for resection of FNH?
Symptomatic FNH or an enlarging lesion

What is Kasabach-Merritt syndrome?
Hepatic hemangioma, thrombocytopenia, and consumptive coagulopathy

What is the most common benign liver tumor?
Hemangioma

What are the 2 types of hepatic hemangioma?
Capillary hemangioma (clinically insignificant) and cavernous hemangioma

What diagnostic tests are indicated?
CT with IV contrast

Should biopsy be performed for a suspected hepatic hemangioma?
No (hemorrhage risk!)

Which hepatitis virus is transmitted by the fecal-oral route via contaminated food?
Hepatitis A

Which tests indicate acute hepatitis B virus (HBV) hepatitis?
IgM, anti-HBc, HBsAg

Which tests indicate chronic HBV hepatitis?
HBsAg, IgG anti-HBc, IgG anti-HB

What is caput medusae?
Dilation of paraumbilical veins arising from the left portal vein and extending to the umbilicus producing umbilical and abdominal wall varices

Where can collaterals form as a result of portal hypertension?
Esophagus, retroperitoneum, rectum, abdominal wall

What are the 3 categories of portosystemic shunts?
Nonselective, selective, partial shunts

What are 2 basic types of nonselective shunts?
End-to-side portacaval shunt, side-to-side portosystemic shunts

What procedure has all but supplanted nonselective shunts?
Transjugular intrahepatic portosystemic shunt (TIPS)

What is the only commonly applied partial portosystemic shunt?
Interposition portacaval shunt

MALIGNANT HEPATOBILIARY DISEASE

What is the surgical management of distal cholangiocarcinoma?
Pancreatoduodenectomy (Whipple)

What name is used to describe cholangiocarcinoma at the bifurcation of the common hepatic duct?
Klatskin tumor

What criteria for cholangiocarcinoma make it unresectable?
Bilateral hepatic artery involvement, encasement of the portal vein, bilateral hepatic duct involvement up to secondary radicals

What is the management of intrahepatic cholangiocarcinoma?
Hepatic resection

What is the management of perihilar cholangiocarcinoma?
Resection of the extrahepatic bile duct, cholecystectomy, and hepaticojejunostomy

Which potent hepatotoxin is produced by *Aspergillus* species?
Aflatoxin

What is the most common malignant hepatic tumor?
Metastases

What is the most common primary liver cancer worldwide?
Hepatocellular carcinoma (HCC)

What is the most common cause of HCC?
Hepatitis B and C

What distinct clinical variant of HCC is a well-circumscribed solitary lesion with a central scar?
Fibrolamellar carcinoma (better prognosis)

Which tumor marker may be helpful in the diagnosis of HCC?
α-Fetoprotein (AFP)

What are possible treatment options for HCC?
Partial hepatectomy, total hepatectomy with transplantation, ablation, embolization

This hepatic lesion does not produce AFP, but is associated with elevated neurotensin levels?
Fibrolamellar HCC

What is most common primary hepatic tumor of childhood?
Hepatoblastoma

What hepatic sarcoma is associated with vinyl chloride, thorotrast, and arsenic?
Angiosarcoma

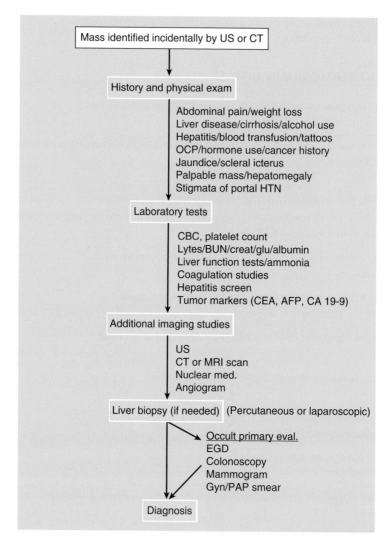

FIGURE 15-4. Algorithm for diagnostic workup of an incidental liver lesion. The evaluation includes history and physical examination, blood work, imaging studies, and liver biopsy (if needed). AFP, α-fetoprotein; BUN, blood urea nitrogen; CA 19-9, cancer antigen 19-9; CEA, carcinoembryonic antigen; creat, creatinine; CBC, complete blood count; CT, computed tomography; EGD, esophagogastroduodenoscopy; Gyn, gynecologic; HTN, hypertension; MRI, magnetic resonance imaging; OCP, oral contraceptive pill; PAP, papanicolaou; US, ultrasound. *(Reproduced from Brunicardi FC, Andersen DK, Billiar TR, et al. Schwartz's Principles of Surgery. 9th ed. http://www.accessmedicine.com. Copyright © The McGraw-Hill Companies, Inc. All rights reserved.)*

MULTIPLE CHOICE QUESTIONS

1. Which of the following lesions should be resected in the asymptomatic patient?

   A. 5-cm FNH
   B. 3-cm hepatic adenoma
   C. 4-cm hydatid cyst
   D. 6-cm hepatic hemangioma
   E. 2-cm hepatic hamartoma

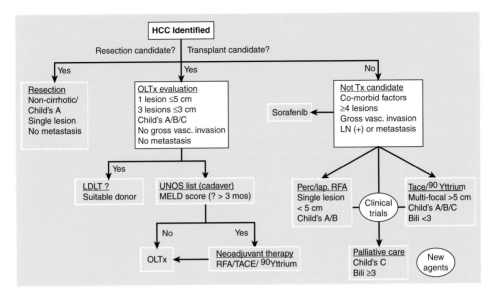

FIGURE 15-5. Algorithm for the management of hepatocellular carcinoma (HCC). The treatment algorithm for HCC begins with determining whether the patient is a resection candidate or liver transplant candidate. Bili, bilirubin level (in milligrams per deciliter); Child's, Child-Turcotte-Pugh class; lap, laparoscopic; LDLT, living-donor liver transplantation; LN, lymph node; MELD, model for end-stage liver disease; OLTx, orthotopic liver transplantation; Perc, percutaneous; RFA, radiofrequency ablation; TACE, transarterial chemoembolization; Tx, transplantation; UNOS, United Network for Organ Sharing; vasc., vascular. *(Reproduced from Brunicardi FC, Andersen DK, Billiar TR, et al. Schwartz's Principles of Surgery. 9th ed. http://www.accessmedicine.com. Copyright © The McGraw-Hill Companies, Inc. All rights reserved.)*

2. Which of the following is true regarding hemobilia?

   A. Cholelithiasis is the most important cause of hemobilia.
   B. Hepatoblastoma is the most commonly associated tumor.
   C. It always presents with acute upper or lower gastrointestinal bleeding.
   D. A tagged RBC scan is the diagnostic modality of choice.
   E. Angioembolization is initial definitive treatment of choice.

3. A 2-year-old boy is found to have fusiform dilation of the extrahepatic biliary duct. What is the best treatment option?

   A. Transduodenal cyst excision
   B. Excision with primary choledochorraphy
   C. Complete cyst excision with Roux-en-Y reconstruction
   D. Liver transplantation
   E. Observation

4. Regarding a 6-cm encapsulated cyst of the right lobe of the liver in a febrile patient, what is the best treatment?

   A. Right hepatectomy
   B. Percutaneous drainage
   C. Marsupialization
   D. Albendazole
   E. Metronidazole

5. Which of the following methods is the most accurate for detection of hepatic metastases?

   A. Intraoperative palpation
   B. CT
   C. Laparoscopy
   D. Transabdominal ultrasound
   E. Intraoperative ultrasound

6. A 55-year-old man presents undergoes a laparoscopic cholecystectomy for acute cholecystitis. The final pathology report indicates gallbladder carcinoma that invades the muscularis. Which of the following would be the most appropriate management?

   A. Radiation
   B. Chemotherapy
   C. Combined chemotherapy and radiation therapy
   D. Observation
   E. Reoperation with wedge resection of liver around the gallbladder fossa with regional lymph node dissection

7. A 25-year-old man presents with high fevers and RUQ pain. His WBC count is 19,000. An ultrasound shows a 6-cm fluid collection in the right lobe of the liver. On CT scan, the fluid collection shows a peripheral rim of edema. The cause of the fluid collection is most likely determined by:

   A. Blood and stool cultures
   B. Percutaneous aspiration of the liver lesion
   C. Serologic tests
   D. LFTs
   E. MRCP

8. A cirrhotic patient presents with a symptomatic umbilical hernia with overlying erythematous skin changes. What is the most appropriate management?

   A. Observation and delayed repair
   B. Repair with primary fascial closure
   C. Repair with synthetic permanent mesh
   D. Repair with biologic mesh
   E. Therapeutic paracentesis

9. A 38-year-old woman presents with RUQ. Imaging with CT shows a 3-cm mass in segment 7 of the liver that is well demarcated with a central fibrotic area. This central scar does not enhance in the arterial phase of the CT scan. Workup shows no evidence of cirrhosis, hepatitis and a normal AFP level, and slightly elevated neurotensin. What is the diagnosis?

   A. FNH
   B. Hepatic adenoma
   C. Fibrolamellar carcinoma
   D. Hepatoma
   E. Hemangioma

10. The model for end-stage liver disease (MELD) score is based on what 3 parameters?
    A. International normalized ratio (INR), creatinine, bilirubin
    B. Albumin, creatinine, alkaline phosphatase
    C. INR, bilirubin, AST
    D. Amylase, GGT, albumin
    E. AST, ALT, alkaline phosphatase

ANSWERS

1. **Answer: B.** Although regression of hepatic adenomas has been reported after discontinuation of oral contraceptives, the potential for bleeding and malignant transformation favors routine resection.

2. **Answer: E.** Hemobilia is bleeding within the biliary tract. Causes include trauma, surgery, malignancy, and infections. Angiography is the most accurate and helpful diagnostic and therapeutic modality.

3. **Answer: C.** Fusiform extrahepatic dilation is a type I choledochal cyst. Surgical resection is necessary to avoid recurrent episodes of infection from stasis of the bile within the cyst cavity as well as the risk of developing a cholangiocarcinoma. Type 3 cysts rarely progress to malignancy and usually do not require resection. However, types 1 and 2 do have a cancer risk. Therefore, the extrahepatic bile duct is resected and a Roux-en-Y choleenterostomy is performed.

4. **Answer: B.** Pyogenic liver abscesses are best treated with initial drainage and broad-spectrum antibiotics. Albendazole is reserved for hydatid/echinoccal cysts, while metronidazole is used for amebic cyts. Resection and marsupialization are not first-line treatments of benign liver cysts.

5. **Answer: E.** Performed with handheld or laparoscopic transducers, intraoperative ultrasound has been established as the most accurate method to detect hepatic metastases. It is a useful modality for identifying vascular structures and their relation to liver lesions, hence enabling an evaluation for resectability. CT scanning is accurate for larger lesions, usually measures more than 2 cm.

6. **Answer: E.** Gallbladder adenocarcinoma that is classified as carcinoma in situ or T1 (do not extend into perimuscular tissue) and have negative margins if discovered incidentally and removed can be managed by cholecystectomy alone.

   Lesions that are T1b (invades muscularis propria layer), T2 (invades the perimuscular connective tissue that is superficial to the muscularis propria) or greater are treated with a radical cholecystectomy, which consists of subsegmental resection of liver segments 4b and 5, in addition to a hepatoduodenal ligament lymphadenectomy. Remember that the gallbladder has no submucosa.

   Adjuvant chemotherapy and chemotherapy for unresectable disease can be considered.

7. **Answer: C.** Amebic liver abscesses are caused by *E histolytica*. Diagnosis is made by clinical presentation, ultrasound, and most notably and distinctly by CT or serologic testing. The classic finding on CT is a single fluid collection in the right lobe with a rim of peripheral edema, which distinguishes this entity from pyogenic and echinococcal cysts.

8. **Answer: C.** A recent Dutch study suggested that after excluding patients with an intact umbilical vein, umbilical hernia repair can be performed safely in patients with liver cirrhosis. The authors pointed out that the ideal time to repair such hernias would be at the time of transplantation. However, for many patients, the waiting time prior to transplantation can be prolonged, increasing the likelihood of an incarcerated hernia developing. Thus, it may be prudent to perform herniorrhaphy on some of these patients while they are awaiting liver transplantation.

    Moreover, permanent mesh can be used in complicated hernias in cirrhotic patients with minimal wound-related morbidity and a significantly lower rate of recurrence.

9. **Answer: C.** The fibrolamellar variant of HCC (or hepatoma) is now sometimes considered as a distinct pathologic entity. It occurs in younger patients. Unlike HCC, most patients are not cirrhotic, not hepatitis B positive, and have normal AFP levels and may have elevated neurotensin levels. They tend to have a better prognosis than HCC.

    The tumor is well demarcated and generally has a central fibrotic area. As opposed to the central scar seen in FNH, this is not a vascular lesion and therefore will not enhance in the arterial phase of the CT, nor with gadolinium-enhanced MRI, whereas FNH will.

10. **Answer: A.** The MELD is a scoring system for assessing the severity of chronic liver disease. It was initially developed to predict death within 3 months of surgery in patients who had undergone TIPS procedure, and was subsequently found to be useful in determining prognosis and prioritizing for receipt of a liver transplant. This score is now used by the United Network for Organ Sharing and Eurotransplant for prioritizing allocation of liver transplants instead of the older Child-Pugh score.

    It is based on the INR, creatinine, and bilirubin, thereby avoiding the inclusion of subjective parameters that are incorporated in the previously used Child score.

CHAPTER 16
Pancreas

Firas Madbak

ANATOMY/PHYSIOLOGY

What is the duct of Wirsung?
Major pancreatic duct that forms in the pancreatic head and descends inferiorly and joins the intrapancreatic portion of the common bile duct to form the common pancreaticobiliary channel proximal to the ampulla of Vater.

What is the duct of Santorini?
Accessory pancreatic duct that drains the anterior portion of the pancreatic head

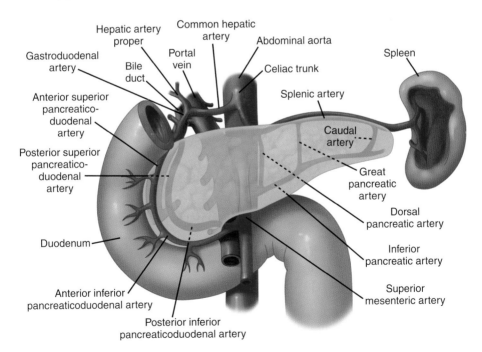

FIGURE 16-1. Arterial supply to the pancreas. Multiple arcades in the head and body of the pancreas provide a rich blood supply. The head of the pancreas cannot be resected without devascularizing the duodenum unless a rim of pancreas containing the pancreaticoduodenal arcade is preserved. (*Reproduced from Brunicardi FC, Andersen DK, Billiar TR, et al. Schwartz's Principles of Surgery. 9th ed. http://www.accessmedicine.com. Copyright © The McGraw-Hill Companies, Inc. All rights reserved.*)

What is the blood supply to the head of the pancreas?
Anterior and posterosuperior pancreaticoduodenal arteries from the gastroduodenal artery that form collaterals with branches of the superior mesenteric artery (SMA) (inferoanterior and posterior pancreaticoduodenal arteries)

What is the venous drainage?
It parallels the arterial supply; drains into the portal system via the superior mesenteric and splenic veins.

Which enzyme is responsible for pancreatic necrosis in presence of bile?
Phospholipase A

What defines a high-output pancreatic fistula?
Output in excess of 200 mL/d

BENIGN PANCREATIC DISEASES

What are the etiologies of acute pancreatitis?
Gallstones and alcohol account for >90% of cases. Other causes include hyperlipidemia, hypercalcemia, trauma, pancreatic duct obstruction, ischemia, drugs, familial, and idiopathic.

What are some common medications implicated as possible etiologies of pancreatitis?
Azathioprine, furosemide, thiazides, sulfonamide, tetracycline, steroids, estrogens, ethacrynic acid, and H_2 blockers

What metabolic conditions could cause pancreatitis?
Hyperlipidemia (types I, IV, and V have been implicated); hypercalcemia, which is most commonly found with hyperparathyroidism that could lead to intraductal precipitation of calcium

How is acute pancreatitis diagnosed?
The diagnosis of pancreatitis requires 2 of the following 3 features: abdominal pain characteristic of acute pancreatitis, a serum amylase or lipase level at least 3 times the upper limit of normal, and characteristic findings of acute pancreatitis on computed tomography (CT).

Which enzyme is implicated in etiology of pancreatitis?
Trypsin

Which serum enzyme rises within 2 hours of the onset of pancreatitis and peaks within 48 hours?
Amylase

What antibiotics are indicated for patients with mild pancreatitis?
None! Antibiotics neither improve the course nor prevent septic complications.

What CT scan findings are suggestive of chronic pancreatitis?
Dilated pancreatic duct, calcifications, and parenchymal atrophy

What are the early Ranson criteria (on admission)?
Glucose >200 mg/dL, Age >55, LDH >350 IU/L, AST >250 IU/L, WBC >16k

What are the late Ranson criteria (48 hours)?
Calcium <8.0 mg/dL, HCT drop >10%, PaO2 <60 mm Hg, BUN increase by 5 or more mg/dL, base deficit >4 mEq/L, fluid sequestration >6 L

How do Ranson criteria predict mortality?
0 to 2 signs, 2%
3 to 4 signs, 15%
5 to 6 signs, 40%
7 to 8 signs, ~100%

What are the indications for surgery in chronic pancreatitis?
Intractable abdominal pain, common bile duct obstruction, duodenal obstruction, persistent pseudocysts, pancreatic fistula or ascites, variceal hemorrhage secondary to splenic vein obstruction (treated by splenectomy), to rule out pancreatic malignancy, colonic obstruction

What are possible complications of pancreatitis?
Pancreatic necrosis, pseudocyst, pancreatic fistulas, hemorrhage, pancreatic ascites, abscess/sepsis

How does chronic pancreatitis present?
Abdominal pain, diabetes, steatorrhea, and pancreatic calcification. Amylase is not typically elevated in chronic pancreatitis

Initial management of pancreatic duct stricture from chronic pancreatitis:
Pancreatic duct stenting

What are some surgical procedures used in chronic pancreatitis?
Duval procedure (distal pancreatectomy with end-to-end pancreaticojejunostomy)
Puestow procedure (lateral side-to-side pancreaticojejunostomy), which is most widely used and preferred; pancreatic resection, pancreatic denervation, islet cell transplantation (for type I diabetes mellitus)
Frey procedure (coring out of diseased portion of pancreatic head and then lateral pancreaticojejunostomy for chronic pancreatitis)
Beger procedure (duodenum-preserving pancreatic head resection)

When is a follow-up CT scan for pancreatitis indicated?
Clinical deterioration (pseudocyst, abscess, or necrosis)

Why does shock occur in severe pancreatitis?
Hypotension and subsequent shock are related to hemodynamic changes resembling sepsis rather than hypovolemia. Cardiac output is generally increased with decreased peripheral vascular resistance

What percentage of pseudocysts spontaneously resolve within 4 to 6 weeks?
50%

How are pseudocysts managed?
Expectant, supportive management for 4 to 6 weeks
If no resolution occurs, wait until a thick, fibrous wall has formed and perform internal cyst drainage via a cystgastrostomy, cystjejunostomy, or cystduodenostomy.
A biopsy should always be performed to rule out malignancy
External drainage may be pursued for infected pseudocysts or ones with immature walls

How long does it take a pseudocyst to mature?
4 to 6 weeks

Indication for surgical intervention for pancreatic pseudocysts:
Pseudocyst has not resolved by 6 weeks and also persistently greater than 6 cm

List the enteric methods of pseudocyst drainage:
Cystogastrostomy, cystoduodenostomy, and Roux-en-y cystojejunostomy, lateral pancreaticojejunostomy

Most common cause of pancreatic abscess:
Infection of pseudocyst

What is the usual time frame for development of pancreatic abscesses associated with acute pancreatitis?
2 to 4 weeks

What CT scan criteria are used for diagnosis of pancreatic necrosis?
Well-demarcated areas of nonenhancing pancreatic tissue >3 cm or occupying more than 30% of the gland

How is infected pancreatic necrosis diagnosed?
CT-guided percutaneous fine-needle aspiration

What antibiotics are indicated in pancreatic necrosis involving >30% of the gland?
Imipenem or meropenem

Aspiration of the necrotic pancreas is negative, now what?
Continue nonoperative management

How are pancreatic fistulas managed?
NPO, parenteral nutrition. Somatostatin has been showed to accelerate closure rate. If no resolution, an endoscopic retrograde cholangiopancreatography (ERCP) to evaluate anatomy and ultimate surgical internal drainage or distal resection.

How does hemorrhage manifest in the setting of pancreatitis?
It usually is due to erosion of an arterial pseudoaneurysm secondary to pseudocyst, abscess, or necrotizing pancreatitis. Diagnosis is by angiography. Immediate surgery is indicated should the patient become unstable. Selective embolization may be possible in stable patients.

Which congential anomaly results from failure of fusion of the dorsal and ventral pancreatic ducts?
Pancreas divisum

BENIGN PANCREATIC TUMORS

What is the most common benign neoplasm in the pancreas?
Serous cystadenoma. These tumors have a low rate of malignant transformation.

What is the treatment for serous cystadenoma?
Resection generally recommended but this lesion can be closely followed in high-operative-risk patients.

What tumor exhibits sunburst central calcification on CT scan?
Serous cystadenoma

MALIGNANT PANCREATIC TUMORS

Overall 5-year survival rate for pancreatic cancer:
<5% in general. Recent reports have cited a 5-year survival of 20% to 25%.

Median survival time of pancreatic cancer patients:
4 to 6 months

What is the most significant modifiable risk factor for pancreatic cancer?
Cigarette smoking

What are the presenting signs of pancreatic cancer?
Abdominal pain, jaundice (could be painless jaundice but this is actually more commonly associated with ampullary and duodenal neoplasms), and weight loss

What imaging studies are needed for diagnosis?
Ultrasound to evaluate biliary anatomy, CT scan

What are some inherited disorders that increase the risk of pancreatic cancer?
MEN, hereditary pancreatitis, familial adenomatous polyposis, hereditary nonpolyposis colorectal cancer, Von Hippel-Lindau, Gardner syndrome

What serologic tumor markers are measured?
CA 19-9 (sensitivity 83%, specificity 82%), CEA (sensitivity 56%, specificity 75%)

What imaging modality is beneficial in assessing the T stage of the tumor in pancreatic cancer?
Endoscopic ultrasonography

Which chemotherapeutic agents are commonly used in adjuvant therapy?
The 2 most active agents are 5-fluorouracil and gemcitabine. Mitomycin C, streptozocin, doxorubicin, and lomustine have also been used. 5-FU potentiates radiation therapy.

FDA approved for combination with gemcitabine for first-line treatment of locally advanced, unresectable, or metastatic pancreatic cancer:
Erlotinib (Tarceva)

What percentage of patients with pancreatic cancer will have had a new diagnosis of diabetes?
20%

T1 pancreatic cancer:
Tumor limited to the pancreas, <2 cm

T2 pancreatic cancer:
Tumor limited to the pancreas, >2 cm

T3 pancreatic cancer:
Tumor extends beyond the pancreas but without involvement of the celiac axis or the SMA

T4 pancreatic cancer:
Tumor involves the celiac axis or the SMA

Choledochojejunostomy

Pancreaticojejunostomy

Gastrojejunostomy

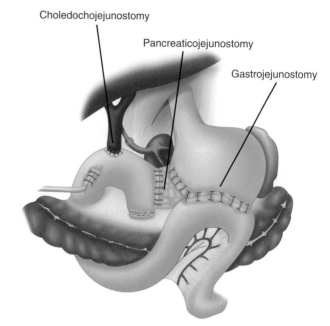

FIGURE 16-2. The pancreaticoduodenectomy (Whipple procedure) can be performed either with the standard technique, which includes distal gastrectomy (**A**) or with preservation of the pylorus (**B**). The pylorus-sparing version of the procedure is used most commonly. *(Reproduced from Gaw JU, Andersen DK. Pancreatic surgery. In: Wu GY, Aziz K, Whalen GF, eds. An Internist's Illustrated Guide to Gastrointestinal Surgery. Totowa, NJ: Humana Press; 2003:229. With kind permission of Springer Science+Business Media.)*

What T stage denotes unresectable disease?
T4, by definition

What reconstruction is performed during after standard pancreaticoduodenectomy (Whipple procedure)?
End-to-side pancreaticojejunostomy, hepaticojejunostomy, gastrojejunostomy

What percentage of pancreatic neoplasms are mucinous cystic neoplasms?
2%

What distinguishes mucinous cystic neoplasm from intraductal papillary mucinous neoplasm?
Mucinous cystic neoplasm rarely communicates with the main pancreatic duct.

Should mucinous cystic neoplasm be resected?
Yes, because of malignant potential.

What rash is seen with glucagonoma?
Necrolytic migratory erythema

From which islet cells do glucagonoma arise?
α-cells

What laboratory test confirms the diagnosis of glucagonoma?
Elevated plasma glucagon >150 pg/mL (many will have levels in excess of 500 pg/mL)

Which test is used for localization of glucagonoma?
CT or MRI

What is another name for VIPoma?
Verner Morrison syndrome

What triad is associated with VIPoma?
Watery diarrhea, hypokalemia, and achlorhydria

What tests are used for localization of VIPoma?
Ultrasound, CT (often tumor is 3 cm or larger), angiography, and transhepatic venous sampling may be used as second-line in difficult cases

What is the appropriate treatment of VIPoma?
Enucleation or surgical resection, depending on location

Where are 85% of all gastrinomas located?
In the gastrinoma triangle, the borders are the pancreatic neck/body junction, confluence of cystic and common hepatic ducts and the junction of second/third portions of duodenum

What percentage of islet cell tumors do insulinomas comprise?
25%

How can this condition be distinguished from factitious hyperinsulinemia?
C-peptide: insulin ratio is 1:1 in insulinoma

What percentage of insulinomas are malignant?
10%

What triad is suggestive of the diagnosis of insulinoma?
Whipple: symptoms of hypoglycemia with fasting, blood glucose <50 mg/dL, relief with glucose intake

What test is diagnostic for insulinoma?
72-hour fast. Insulin and glucose are measured every 6 hours. Symptoms of hypoglycemia develop in 12 hours. Insulin: glucose ratio >0.3 or serum insulin >6 µU/mL is diagnostic.

What is the surgical procedure of choice for insulinoma?
Enucleation

What are the 4Ds of glucagonoma
Diabetes, dermatitis, deep venous thrombosis, depression

What percentage of patients with glucagonoma have diabetes?
>75%

What does VIP in VIPoma stand for?
Vasoactive intestinal peptide

The diagnosis of VIPoma is supported by what serum VIP level:
>200 pg/mL

Management of the diarrhea of VIPoma:
Octreotide

What is the rarest pancreatic islet cell tumor?
Somatostatinoma

What somatostatin level confirms the diagnosis of somatostatinoma?
>10 ng/mL

What study should be used to define the extent of pancreatic islet cell tumors?
Octreotide scan

What is the most malignant pancreatic endocrine tumor?
Gastrinoma

What is the most benign pancreatic endocrine tumor?
Insulinoma

What is the surgical management of endocrine tumors in tail of the pancreas?
Distal pancreatectomy

What is the surgical management of endocrine tumors in head of the pancreas?
Whipple procedure

This receptor is found on many pancreatic islet cell tumors:
Somatostatin receptor

MULTIPLE CHOICE QUESTIONS

1. **Regarding pancreatic anatomy, which of the following is correct?**
   A. The uncinate process is located anterior to the superior mesenteric artery
   B. The blood supply of the pancreas is partly derived from the inferior mesenteric artery
   C. The body of the pancreas lies to the right of the SMA
   D. In 60% of cases, the ducts of Wirsung and Santorini empty into the duodenum independently
   E. The splenic artery usually runs posterior to the pancreatic body

2. **Regarding insulinomas, which of the following is correct?**
   A. Usually occur in the head of the pancreas, measure >4 cm, malignant, and single
   B. Usually occur in the tail of the pancreas, measure >4 cm, malignant, and single
   C. Usually occur in the body of the pancreas, measure <2 cm, benign, and multiple
   D. Uniformly distributed throughout the pancreas (head, body, and tail), measure <2 cm, benign, and single
   E. Usually occur in the body of the pancreas, measure <2 cm, malignant, and multiple

3. **A-33-year-old female is involved in a motor vehicle collision and found to have a complete transaction of the pancreas at the level of the pancreatic neck:**
   A. Oversewing of the proximal segment and distal pancreatectomy
   B. Drainage of the proximal and distal segments
   C. Drainage of the proximal segment and oversewing of the distal segment
   D. Oversewing of the proximal segment and drainage of the distal segment
   E. Roux-en-Y pancreaticojejunostomy of the proximal pancreas and distal pancreatectomy

4. **Which pancreatic head adenocarcinoma is considered resectable?**

    A. Tumor involves the celiac axis or the SMA
    B. T4 tumor
    C. Tumor extends beyond the pancreas but without involvement of the celiac axis or the SMA
    D. A 4-cm tumor limited to the pancreas with 1 peritoneal metastasis
    E. Periaortic lymph node involvement

5. **Which tumor suppressor gene is implicated in MEN I?**

    A. p53
    B. c-kit
    C. menin
    D. RET
    E. PRAD

6. **The earliest manifestation of pancreas transplant graft thrombosis is:**

    A. Fever
    B. Sepsis
    C. Hyperglycemia
    D. Elevated urinary amylase
    E. Altered mental status

7. **The most common pancreatic tumor in MEN I is:**

    A. Insulinoma
    B. Glucagonoma
    C. VIPoma
    D. Gastrinoma
    E. Somatostatinoma

8. **A patient with acute pancreatitis deteriorates clinically and is reimaged. CT scan shows findings of a fluid collection consistent with infected pancreatic necrosis that is adherent to the posterior gastric wall and close to the pancreatic head. What is the best management?**

    A. Endoscopic drainage
    B. Cystogastrostomy
    C. Roux-en-Y cystojejunostomy
    D. Percutaneous drainage
    E. ERCP

9. **Options for palliative chemotherapy for unresectable adenocarcinoma of the pancreas include which agent?**

    A. Doxorubicin
    B. Leucovorin
    C. Gemcitabine
    D. Vincristine
    E. Methotrexate

10. **The preferred treatment for annular pancreas is:**
    A. Lateral pancreaticojejunostomy (Puestow procedure)
    B. Sphincterotomy
    C. Gastrojejunostomy
    D. Pylorus preserving pancreaticoduodenectomy
    E. Duodenoduodenostomy or duodenojejunostomy

ANSWERS

1. **Answer: D.** The uncinate process is posterior to the superior mesenteric vessels. The pancreas is part of the midgut, which is supplied by the SMA and its branches. The SMA/SMV delineates the separation of the head and neck of the pancreas from the pancreatic body, which lay to the left of these blood vessels. The splenic vein is posterior to the body of the pancreas, while the artery usually runs along the superior edge.

2. **Answer: D.** Insulinoma are usually benign tumors, measuring less than 2 cm, and uniformly distributed in pancreatic tissue.

3. **Answer: A.** The best approach for repair in this case is distal pancreatectomy and oversewing of the proximal pancreatic remnant. Pancreatic duct injury can usually be assessed by inspection of the injury.

   In the absence of duct injury, only drainage is required. Pancreatography may be considered to evaluate the duct, although it is not essential if there is a low index of suspicion.

   Less favorable, such as distal cannulation of the pancreatic duct and transduodenal pancreaticography, should be avoided.

4. **Answer: C.** Extrapancreatic metastases preclude resection. Celiac axis or SMA involvement is the description of T4. A T4 tumor is unresectable, by definition.

5. **Answer: C.** PRAD is implicated in parathyroid tumors. RET is associated with MEN II. C-kit is seen with gastrointestinal stromal tumors. Mutations in p53 tumor suppressor gene occur in various malignancies: breast, colorectal, liver, lung, and ovarian cancer to name a few.

6. **Answer: C.** The most immediate and frequent complication is pancreatic graft thrombosis. Unexplained early hyperglycemia is usually the first manifestation.

7. **Answer: D.** About 33% of gastrinomas are associated with the MEN-I syndrome. The other tumors occur with far less frequency.

8. **Answer: D.** Infected pseudocysts are essentially pancreatic abscesses. Along with necrotizing pancreatic collections, these are treated with external drainage. Internal drainage is reserved for sterile collections such as uncomplicated large, refractory pseudocysts and encompasses surgical enteric drainage or endoscopic drainage. External drainage is usually inappropriate as this may seed and cause contamination.

9. **Answer: C.** Chemotherapy significantly reduced the 1-year mortality when compared to best supportive care in patients with inoperable pancreatic cancer as outlined in a 2006 Cochrane Review. Also, chemoradiation improved 1 year when compared to best supportive care. There was no significant difference in 1-year mortality for 5-FU alone versus 5-FU combinations (odds ratio [OR] 0.90, 95% confidence interval [CI] 0.62–1.30); single-agent chemotherapy versus gemcitabine

(OR 1.34, 95% CI 0.88–2.02, $P = 0.17$); or gemcitabine alone versus gemcitabine combinations (OR 0.88, 95% CI 0.74–1.05). However, subgroup analysis showed that platinum-gemcitabine combinations reduced 6-month mortality compared to gemcitabine alone (OR 0.59, 95% CI 0.43–0.81, P value 0.001). A qualitative overview suggested that chemoradiation produced better survivals than either best supportive care or radiotherapy. Chemoradiation treatment was associated with more toxicity.

The authors concluded that chemotherapy appears to prolong survival in people with advanced pancreatic cancer and can confer clinical benefits and improve quality of life. Combination chemotherapy did not improve overall survival compared to single-agent chemotherapy. Gemcitabine is an acceptable control arm for future trials investigating scheduling and combinations with novel agents. There is insufficient evidence to recommend chemoradiation in patients with locally advanced inoperable pancreatic cancer as a superior alternative to chemotherapy alone.

10. **Answer: E.** Annular pancreas is a congenital anomaly, which consists of a ring of pancreatic tissue partially or completely encircling the descending portion of the duodenum. It was first described by Tiedemann in 1818 and named "annular pancreas" by Ecker in 1862. The first surgical treatment of obstructive annular pancreas was performed on a neonate by Vidal et al in 1905. In the past, the diagnosis of this anomaly was usually made by surgery or autopsy. With the widespread use of ERCP and magnetic resonance cholangiopancreatography, more cases are diagnosed preoperatively. The surgical treatment is bypassing the obstructed duodenal segment, with either a duodenoduodenostomy or duodenojejunostomy.

CHAPTER 17
Spleen

Ryan Lawless

Test Taking Tips

1. Be wary about idiopathic thrombocytopenic purpura (ITP) questions. Pay close attention to the preoperative details regarding platelet count, patient status, and timing of platelet transfusion.
2. Treatment of gastric varices (sinistral hypertension) with splenectomy is frequently covered.
3. Don't forget about an accessory spleen in a refractory ITP patient.

ANATOMY

What is the arterial blood supply to the spleen?
Splenic artery from the celiac plexus; short gastric arteries (vasa brevia) from the gastroepiploic artery

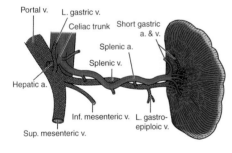

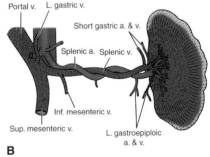

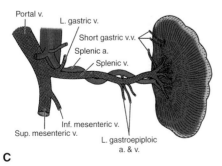

FIGURE 17-1. Relation of splenic artery and splenic vein. (A) Vein posterior to artery (this is the usual pattern); (B) vein both anterior and posterior to artery; (C) vein anterior to artery (this is the least common configuration). *(Modified from Skandalakis' Surgical Anatomy: The Embryologic Basis of Modern Surgery. Paschalidis Medical Publications; 2004, with permission.)*

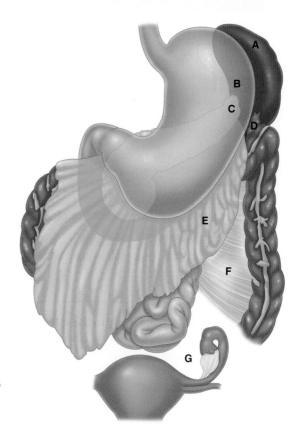

FIGURE 17-2. Sites where accessory spleens are found in order of importance. (A) Hilar region, 54%; (B) pedicle, 25%; (C) tail of pancreas, 6%; (D) splenocolic ligament, 2%; (E) greater omentum, 12%; (F) mesentery, 0.5%; (G) left ovary, 0.5%.

What is the relationship between the splenic artery and the splenic vein?
The splenic artery is anterior and superior to the splenic vein

What percentage of patients have an accessory spleen?
~20%

Where is an accessory spleen most commonly found?
The accessory spleen is found in the region of the splenic hilum and vascular pedicle in 80% of cases

What ligaments suspend the spleen?
Splenocolic, gastrosplenic, phrenosplenic, and splenorenal ligaments

PHYSIOLOGY

What is the function of the spleen?
Hematologic: removal of cytoplasmic inclusions in the erythrocytes (pitting); destruction of senescent erythrocytes (culling); hematopoiesis in the fetus or in patients with bone marrow destruction; reservoir for platelets and granulocytes

Immunologic: production of the opsonins tuftsin and properdin; antibody production in germinal follicles; filtration and trapping of circulatory antigens; lymphocyte stimulation and proliferation

What is the largest producer of IgM in the body?
The spleen

What 2 opsonins are produced by the spleen?
Tuftsin and properdin

NONTRAUMATIC DISEASES

What is idiopathic thrombocytopenic purpura (ITP)?
A condition in which circulating IgG antiplatelet antibodies destroy platelets

In which patient population does ITP usually resolve spontaneously?
Children (rarely requires surgery)

What is the first-line therapy for ITP?
Corticosteroids (*Note:* plasmapheresis and γ globulin can be used as adjuncts)

What time period should elapse prior to performing splenectomy in an ITP patient being treated with steroids?
6 weeks

When should platelets be administered during splenectomy for ITP?
Once the splenic hilum is ligated

What is the most common nontraumatic condition requiring splenectomy?
ITP

What is the most common cause of failure to correct thrombocytopenia after splenectomy for ITP?
Unidentified accessory spleen

What pentad of clinical findings can be seen with thrombotic thrombocytopenic purpura (TTP)?
Thrombocytopenic purpura, fever, renal failure, hemolytic anemia, and neurologic manifestations

What is the treatment of choice for TTP?
Daily plasmapheresis and fresh frozen plasma administration

True or False: G6PD deficiency is an indication for splenectomy?
False: G6PD deficiency is not an indication for splenectomy

What is the most common congenital hemolytic anemia not involving a membrane protein that requires splenectomy?
Pyruvate kinase deficiency

What is the most common congenital hemolytic anemia requiring splenectomy?
Spherocytosis

What is the definition of hypersplenism?
A decrease in the circulating cell count of any combination of leukocytes/erythrocytes/platelets with a normal compensatory hematopoietic response from bone marrow with correction of cytopenia by splenectomy with/without splenomegaly

What is Felty syndrome?
Splenomegaly, rheumatoid arthritis, and neutropenia (perform splenectomy for symptomatic patient with IgG present on the surface of neutrophils)

What is the #1 splenic tumor overall?
Hemangioma

What is the #1 benign splenic tumor?
Hemangioma

What is the most common primary splenic neoplasm?
Non-Hodgkins lymphoma

What is the first-line therapy for hairy cell leukemia?
Cladribine and Pentostatin (purine nucleoside analogs)

What are indications for surgery for a splenic cyst?
If >5 cm or symptomatic

POSTSPLENECTOMY MANAGEMENT

When is the optimal time to administer vaccines to prevent overwhelming postsplenectomy sepsis (OPSI) after splenectomy?
If possible 10 to 14 days before splenectomy; if emergent wait at least 14 days postprocedure to vaccinate (often given postoperative day 5 in trauma patients secondary to poor follow-up)

What is the optimal time period to wait before performing a splenectomy in a child?
Until age 5 (allows antibody formation and full immunization)

When do most cases of overwhelming OPSI occur?
Within 2 years of splenectomy

What are the most common bacteria involved in overwhelming OPSI?
Streptococcus pneumoniae

What measures are taken to help prevent overwhelming OPSI?
Vaccinate against *Streptococcus pneumoniae, Haemophilus influenzae, and Neisseria meningitidis*; antibiotic prophylaxis for children <5 years of age; prophylactic penicillin for all minor illnesses/infections; immediate medical evaluation for febrile illness; MedicAlert bracelet

What is the most consistent finding in the blood in all patients following splenectomy?
Howell-Jolly bodies

What will you find on a peripheral blood smear in a patient following splenectomy?
Howell-Jolly bodies; Heinz bodies; Pappenheimer bodies; target cells; polychromatophilia (reticulocytosis)

What are Howell-Jolly bodies?
Basophilic nuclear remnants (clusters of DNA)

What are Heinz bodies?
Formations of damaged hemoglobin component molecules (usually through oxidation)

What are Pappenheimer bodies?
Abnormal granules of iron formed by phagosomes that have engulfed excessive amounts of iron

SPLENIC TRAUMA

What is the most common intra-abdominal organ injured with blunt trauma?
The spleen

What is a grade III splenic injury?
Hematoma: subcapsular, >50% surface area or expanding, ruptured subcapsular or parenchymal hematoma; intraparenchymal hematoma, 5 cm or expanding
Laceration: >3 cm in parenchymal depth or involving the trabecular vessels

Table 17-1	The Splenic Organ Injury Scaling System of the American Association for the Surgery of Trauma, 1994 Revision	
Grade*		Injury Description
I	Hematoma	Subcapsular, <10% surface area
	Laceration	Capsular tear, <1 cm parenchymal depth
II	Hematoma	Subcapsular, 10%–50% surface area, <5 cm in diameter
	Laceration	1–3 cm parenchymal depth that does not involve a trabecular vessel
III	Hematoma	Subcapsular, >50% surface area or expanding; ruptured subcapsular or parenchymal hematoma intraparenchymal hematoma >5 cm or expanding
	Laceration	>3 cm parenchymal depth or involving trabecular vessels
IV	Laceration	Laceration involving segmental or hilar vessels producing major devascularization (>25% of spleen)
V	Laceration	Completely shattered spleen
	Vascular	Hilar vascular injury, which devascularizes spleen

*Advance one grade for multiple injuries up to grade III.
Feliciano DV, Mattox KL, Moore EE. *Trauma.* 6th ed. http://www.accesssurgery.com Copyright © The McGraw-Hill Companies, Inc. All rights reserved.

How would you manage a hemodynamically stable patient with a splenic injury and contrast extravasation on the arterial phase of abdominal CT scan?
Controversial: operative intervention versus angiographic embolization

How would you manage a hemodynamically stable patient with a splenic injury without contrast extravasation on abdominal CT scan?
Admission to ICU; serial hematocrit, vital signs, serial abdominal examinations; bed rest; NPO; if stable at 48 to 72 hours transfer to step-down unit, activity as tolerated, and advance diet

What classic criteria are used for the nonoperative management of splenic injury?
Absence of contrast extravasation on CT; absence of other associated injuries requiring surgical intervention; absence of health conditions with an increased risk for bleeding (coagulopathy, hepatic failure, anticoagulants, specific coagulation factor deficiency); hemodynamic stability; negative abdominal examination; splenic injury grade I to III

What are the indications for splenectomy in a patient with splenic injury?
Patients with multiple associated injuries (neuro injuries), unstable, or in DIC

After performing an exploratory laparotomy for trauma, you incidentally discover a capsular tear of the spleen; how should you control the bleeding?
With compression or with topical hemostatic agents

How should you manage a patient with an injury to the central portion of the spleen extending into the hilum?
Splenectomy

Table 17-2 Indications for and Expected Response to Splenectomy in Various Diseases and Conditions		
Disease/Condition	Indications for Splenectomy	Response to Splenectomy
Hereditary spherocytosis	Hemolytic anemia, recurrent transfusions, intractable leg ulcers	Improves or eliminates anemia
Hereditary elliptocytosis	Limited role for splenectomy	–
Pyruvate kinase deficiency	Only in severe cases, recurrent transfusions	Decreased transfusion requirement, palliative only
Glucose-6-phosphate dehydrogenase deficiency	None	–
Warm-antibody autoimmune hemolytic anemia	Failure of medical (steroid) therapy	60%–80% response rate, recurrences common
Sickle cell disease	History of acute sequestration crisis, splenic symptoms, or infarction (consider concomitant cholecystectomy)	Palliative, variable response
Thalassemia	Excessive transfusion requirements, symptomatic splenomegaly, or infarction	Diminished transfusion requirements, relief of symptoms
Acute myeloid leukemia (AML)	Intolerable symptomatic splenomegaly	Relief of abdominal pain and early satiety
Chronic myeloid leukemia	Symptomatic splenomegaly	Relief of abdominal pain and early satiety
Chronic myelomonocytic leukemia	Symptomatic splenomegaly	Relief of abdominal pain and early satiety
Essential thrombocythemia	Only for advanced disease (ie, transformation to myeloid metaplasia or AML) with severe symptomatic splenomegaly	Relief of abdominal pain and early satiety
Polycythemia vera	Only for advanced disease (ie, transformation to myeloid metaplasia or AML) with severe symptomatic splenomegaly	Relief of abdominal pain and early satiety
Myelofibrosis (agnogenic myeloid metaplasia)	Severe symptomatic splenomegaly	76% clinical response at 1 year, high risk of hemorrhagic, thrombotic, and infectious complications (26%)
Chronic lymphocytic leukemia	Cytopenias and anemia	75% response rate
Hairy cell leukemia	Cytopenias and symptomatic splenomegaly	40%–70% response rate

(continued)

Table 17-2	Indications for and Expected Response to Splenectomy in Various Diseases and Conditions (Continued)	
Disease/Condition	Indications for Splenectomy	Response to Splenectomy
Hodgkin's disease	Surgical staging in select cases	–
Non-Hodgkin's lymphoma	Cytopenias, symptomatic splenomegaly	Improved complete blood count values, relief of symptoms
ITP	Failure of medical therapy, recurrent disease	75%–85% rate of long-term response
TTP	Excessive plasma exchange requirement	Typically curative
Abscesses of the spleen	Therapy of choice	Curative
Symptomatic parasitic cysts	Therapy of choice	Curative; exercise caution not to spill cyst contents
Symptomatic nonparasitic cysts	Partial splenectomy for small cysts; unroofing for large cysts	Curative
Gaucher disease	Hypersplenism	Improves cytopenias; does not correct underlying disease
Niemann-Pick disease	Symptomatic splenomegaly	Improves symptoms; does not correct underlying disease
Amyloidosis	Symptomatic splenomegaly	Improves symptoms; does not correct underlying disease
Sarcoidosis	Hypersplenism or symptomatic splenomegaly	Improves symptoms and cytopenias; does not correct underlying disease
Felty's syndrome	Neutropenia	80% durable response rate
Splenic artery aneurysm	Splenectomy best for distal lesions near splenic hilum	Curative
Portal hypertension	Portal or sinistral hypertension due to splenic vein thrombosis	Palliative

MULTIPLE CHOICE QUESTIONS

1. **Splenectomy results in the loss of what immunologic protein?**

   A. Tuftsin
   B. Immunoglobulin A
   C. Membrane attack complex
   D. C3 convertase

2. **What is the most common cause of splenic artery/vein thrombosis?**

   A. Portal hypertension
   B. Pancreatitis
   C. Pancreatic cancer
   D. Factor V Leiden
   E. Antiphospholipid syndrome

3. **What ligament contains the vascular supply to the spleen?**

   A. Splenocolic ligament
   B. Gastrosplenic ligament
   C. Phrenosplenic ligament
   D. Splenorenal ligament

4. **What is the treatment for bleeding gastric varices in the setting of sinistral hypertension?**

   A. Gastrectomy
   B. Transjugular intrahepatic portosystemic shunt
   C. Mesocaval shunt
   D. Splenectomy
   E. Sclerotherapy

5. **Which of the following is not an indication to repair a splenic artery aneurysm?**

   A. Asymptomatic and size >2 cm
   B. Pregnancy
   C. Symptomatic and size = 1.5 cm
   D. Presence of collagen vascular disease

6. **When should a patient be vaccinated prior to elective splenectomy?**

   A. The day of surgery
   B. 7 days
   C. 14 days
   D. 21 days

7. **What is the embryologic origin of the spleen?**

   A. Endoderm
   B. Mesoderm
   C. Ectoderm
   D. Neural crest cells

8. **What is the optimal timing of platelet transfusion in a patient with ITP?**

   A. Preoperatively
   B. After ligation of the splenic vein
   C. After ligation of the splenic artery
   D. Postoperatively

9. **Which of the following conditions is an indication for splenectomy?**

   A. Sickle cell anemia
   B. Myelofibrosis
   C. TTP
   D. Asymptomatic 1.5 cm midsplenic artery aneurysm

10. **What type of bacteria does the spleen opsonize better than the liver?**

    A. Encapsulated organisms
    B. Yeast
    C. Parasites
    D. Gram positives

ANSWERS

1. **Answer: A.** Tuftsin and properdin are immunologic proteins produced by the spleen. After splenectomy these 2 immunologic proteins are absent, increasing the susceptibility to encapsulated organisms.

2. **Answer: B.** Pancreatitis is the most common cause of splenic artery/vein thrombosis.

3. **Answer: B.** The gastrosplenic ligament contains the splenic artery/vein and short gastric arteries. In the setting of portal hypertension, the splenorenal ligament may contain vascular supply.

4. **Answer: D.** Splenectomy is the treatment for isolated gastric varices in the setting of sinistral hypertension.

5. **Answer: D.** Resection, with or without splenectomy, or embolization of a splenic artery aneurysm should be performed in pregnant patients, asymptomatic aneurysms >2 cm, and any symptomatic aneurysm.

6. **Answer: C.** Patients should be vaccinated preoperatively if possible prior to a splenectomy. Two weeks prior to surgery is the preferred time frame for an adequate immune response to occur. Emergent splenectomy patients should be vaccinated prior to discharge. In the trauma population, recidivism is low, and therefore vaccination prior to discharge may help vaccinate patients who will not come back for vaccination 2 weeks post-op.

7. **Answer: B.** The spleen arises from the primitive mesoderm and is evident by the 5th week of gestation.

8. **Answer: C.** The optimal time to give a platelet transfusion to a patient undergoing splenectomy for ITP is after ligation of the splenic artery. Be aware that a question like this on the ABSITE will describe a patient with low platelets and not bleeding preoperatively, making it very tempting to transfuse prior to operation. If the patient is actively bleeding preoperatively, then a transfusion is required prior to surgery.

9. **Answer: B.** Myelofibrosis leads to extramedullary hematopoiesis and can be alleviated by splenectomy.

10. **Answer: A.** Encapsulated organisms are opsonized by the reticuloendothelial system, namely the spleen.

CHAPTER 18
Esophagus

Timothy Misselbeck and James Lee

ANATOMY

Name the layers of the esophagus:
Mucosa and muscularis propria (esophagus has no serosa)

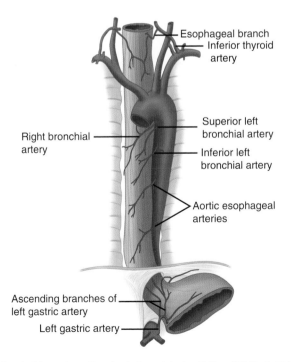

FIGURE 18-1. Arterial blood supply of the esophagus. *(Reproduced with permission from Rothberg M, DeMeester TR. Surgical anatomy of the esophagus. In: Shields TW, ed. General Thoracic Surgery. 3rd ed. Philadelphia: Lea & Febiger; 1989:84.)*

What is the arterial blood supply to the cervical esophagus?
Inferior thyroid arteries (branch of thyrocervical trunk on left and subclavian artery on right)

What is the arterial supply to the thoracic esophagus?
Direct blood supply from 4 to 6 esophageal arteries off of the aorta; esophageal branches off of right (R) and left (L) bronchial arteries; supplemented by descending branches off the inferior thyroid arteries, intercostal arteries, and ascending branches of the paired inferior phrenic arteries

What is the arterial blood supply to the abdominal esophagus?
Left gastric artery and the paired inferior phrenic arteries

Describe the venous drainage for the cervical esophagus:
The submucosal venous plexus drains into the inferior thyroid veins (tributaries of L subclavian vein and R brachiocephalic vein)

Describe the venous drainage for the thoracic esophagus:
The submucosal venous plexus of the thoracic esophagus joins with the more superficial esophageal venous plexus and the venae comitantes that surround the esophagus at this level. This plexus then drains into the azygos veins on the right and the hemiazygous veins on the left.

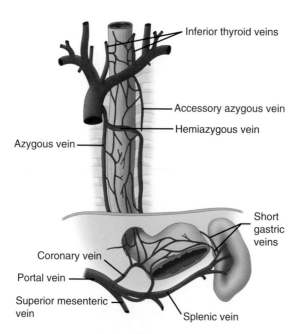

FIGURE 18-2. Venous drainage of the esophagus. *(Reproduced with permission from Rothberg M, DeMeester TR. Surgical anatomy of the esophagus. In: Shields TW, ed. General Thoracic Surgery. 3rd ed. Philadelphia: Lea & Febiger; 1989:85.)*

Describe the venous drainage of the abdominal esophagus?
Drains into both the systemic and portal venous systems through the L and R phrenic veins, and the L gastric (coronary) vein and short gastrics

In what direction is the lymphatic flow in the upper two-thirds of the esophagus?
Cephalad

In what direction is the lymphatic flow in the distal third of the esophagus?
Caudad

Describe the sympathetic innervation of the esophagus:
Cervical esophagus receives branches from the cervical sympathetic trunk (from superior ganglion in neck); the thoracic esophagus receives branches from the thoracic sympathetic trunk (from stellate ganglion), which form an esophageal plexus that envelops the thoracic esophagus anteriorly and posteriorly; the distal thoracic esophagus receives innervation from the greater and lesser splanchnic nerves.

The parasympathetic fibers to the esophagus arise from which cranial nerve?
Vagus nerve

The esophagus is composed of which 2 concentric muscle bundles?
Inner circular and outer longitudinal

What kind of muscle composes the upper one-third of the esophagus?
Striated muscle

What kind of muscle composes the lower two-thirds of the esophagus?
Smooth muscle

At what vertebral level does the esophagus enter the diaphragm through the esophageal hiatus?
T11

What are the areas of anatomical narrowing of the esophagus?
Cricopharyngeus muscle; compression by the left mainstem bronchus and aortic arch; diaphragm

What is the Z line?
The transition of the distal 1 to 2 cm of esophageal mucosa to cardiac mucosa/junctional columnar epithelium

Identification of gastroesophageal junction (external):
The collar of Helvetius (loop of Willis) and the gastroesophageal fat pad

Identification of gastroesophageal junction (internal):
The squamocolumnar epithelial junction (Z-line), provided the patient does not have Barrett.
The transition from the smooth esophageal lining to the rugal folds of the stomach.

PHYSIOLOGY

What are the 6 events that occur during the oropharyngeal phase of swallowing?
Elevation of the tongue, posterior movement of the tongue, elevation of the soft palate, elevation of the hyoid, elevation of the larynx, tilting of the epiglottis

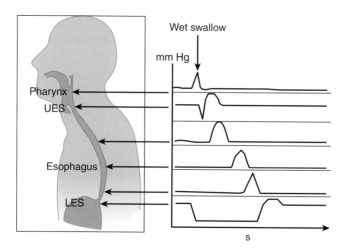

FIGURE 18-3. Swallowing process. Upper esophageal sphincter (UES), esophageal peristalsis, and lower esophageal sphincter (LES) in response to swallowing. *(Reproduced from Doherty GM. Current Diagnosis and Treatment: Surgery. 9th ed. http://www.accessmedicine.com. Copyright © The McGraw-Hill Companies, Inc. All rights reserved.)*

What are primary peristaltic contractions of the esophagus?
Progressive contractions (2 to 4 cm/s) that move down the esophagus and reach the LES after the initiation of swallowing (~9 seconds)

What are secondary peristaltic contractions of the esophagus?
Progressive contractions generated from distention/irritation of the esophagus or from an independent local reflex to clear the esophagus of material that was left behind after a primary peristaltic wave rather than voluntary swallowing

What are tertiary contractions of the esophagus?
Uncoordinated contractions of smooth muscle that are nonprogressive, nonperistaltic, monophasic, or multiphasic simultaneous waves that can occur either after voluntary swallowing or spontaneously between swallows

Normal upper esophageal sphincter pressure at rest:
50 to 70 mm Hg

Normal upper esophageal sphincter pressure with food bolus:
12 to 14 mm Hg

DIVERTICULUM

Give examples of pulsion (false; mucosa and submucosa herniate through esophageal musculature) diverticula in the esophagus:
Zenker diverticulum and epiphrenic diverticulum

What esophageal diverticulum is a traction (true) diverticulum that results from external inflammatory mediastinal lymph nodes adhering to the esophagus that heal and contract and pull the esophagus resulting in the diverticulum?
Parabronchial (midesophageal) diverticulum

What side are midesophageal diverticula usually found?
Typically present on the right secondary to the overabundance of structures in the midthoracic region of the left chest.

Treatment for a midesophageal diverticula:
If asymptomatic patient with inflamed mediastinal lymph nodes from tuberculosis or histoplasmosis, treat medically with antituberculin or antifungal agents; if diverticulum <2 cm, observe; if patient symptomatic or diverticulum >2 cm, perform diverticulopexy (suspend from thoracic vertebral fascia) and a long esophagomyotomy is indicated in patients with severe chest pain or dysphagia and a documented motor abnormality.

Treatment for epiphrenic diverticulum:
If diverticula <2 cm, perform diverticulopexy; in patients with severe chest pain, dysphagia, or a documented motor abnormality, perform long esophagomyotomy: if diverticulopexy, begin long esophagomyotomy at the neck of diverticulum and extend onto LES), and if diverticulectomy, perform esophagomyotomy on opposite esophageal wall, extending from the level of the diverticulum onto the LES; if large associated hiatal hernia, perform diverticulectomy, long esophagomyotomy, and repair of hiatal hernia

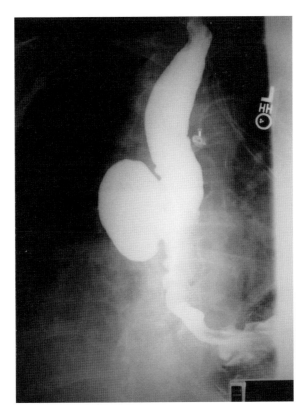

FIGURE 18-4. Epiphrenic diverticulum. *(Reproduced from Doherty GM. Current Diagnosis and Treatment: Surgery. 9th ed. http://www.accessmedicine.com. Copyright © The McGraw-Hill Companies, Inc. All rights reserved.)*

Killian triangle (site of a Zenker diverticulum):
Point of potential weakness at the transition between the oblique fibers of the thyropharyngeus muscle and the horizontal fibers of the cricopharyngeus muscle

The surgical treatment of a Zenker diverticulum:
If diverticulum >3 cm—cricopharyngeal myotomy with diverticulectomy with TA stapler versus invert and perform diverticulopexy to precervical fascia
If <2 cm—leave alone

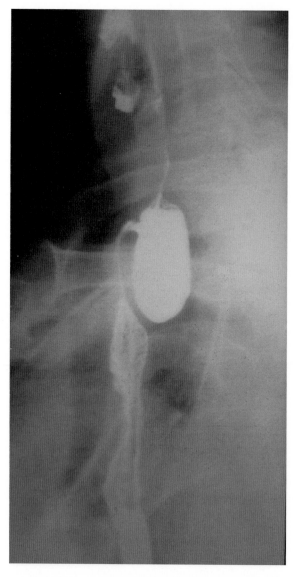

FIGURE 18-5. Pharyngoesophageal diverticulum (Zenker diverticulum). *(Reproduced from Doherty GM. Current Diagnosis and Treatment: Surgery. 9th ed. http://www.accessmedicine.com. Copyright © The McGraw-Hill Companies, Inc. All rights reserved.)*

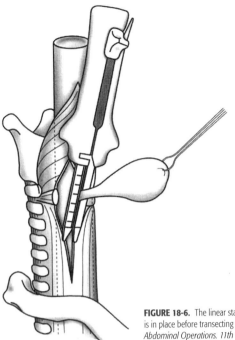

FIGURE 18-6. The linear stapler is placed across the neck of the diverticulum. Note that the bougie is in place before transecting the diverticulum. *(Reproduced from Zinner MJ, Ashley SW. Maningot's Abdominal Operations. 11th ed. http://www.accesssurgery.com. Copyright © The McGraw-Hill Companies, Inc. All rights reserved.)*

BENIGN DISEASE

Most common site of esophageal perforation:
Cricopharyngeus muscle

Recommended first test in any patient presenting with dysphagia:
Video-esophagram

Indications for a video-esophagram:
Regurgitation, globus sensation, dysphagia, GERD, noncardiac chest pain, esophageal neoplasm

What characteristics of the esophagus help determine if a lower esophageal sphincter is mechanically defective?
Pressure <6 mm Hg, total length <2 cm, abdominal length <1 cm

What is the definition of a hypertensive lower esophageal sphincter?
LES with a sphincter pressure above the 95th percentile of normal

What are the manometric characteristics of achalasia?
Hypertensive LES resting pressure, incomplete or nonrelaxing LES, aperistalsis of the esophageal body, esophageal pressurization, and elevated lower esophageal baseline pressure

What is the gold standard for the diagnosis of achalasia?
Esophageal manometry

Term for a patient with achalasia with preserved muscle function as demonstrated by simultaneous contraction waves of the esophagus with various amplitudes:
Vigorous achalasia

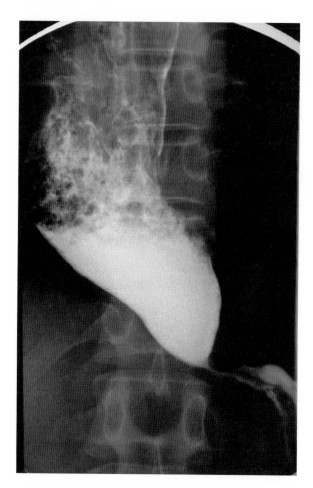

FIGURE 18-7. Esophageal achalasia. Note dilation of the esophageal body, retained barium, and distal esophageal narrowing (bird's beak). *(Reproduced from Doherty GM. Current Diagnosis and Treatment: Surgery. 9th ed. http://www.accessmedicine.com. Copyright © The McGraw-Hill Companies, Inc. All rights reserved.)*

What is presumed pathogenesis of achalasia?
Primary destruction of nerves to the LES with secondary degeneration of the neuromuscular function of the body of the esophagus from idiopathic or infectious neurogenic degeneration

What is the classic triad of presenting symptoms for achalasia?
Dysphagia, regurgitation, weight loss

What is the most common esophageal carcinoma identified with achalasia?
Squamous cell carcinoma

Standard surgical treatment for achalasia:
Heller myotomy

What are the classic manometry findings with diffuse esophageal spasm?
Simultaneous, multipeaked contractions of high amplitude (>120 mm Hg) or long duration (>2.5 seconds)

What is the mainstay of treatment for diffuse esophageal spasm?
Medical treatment or endoscopic intervention (nonsurgical)

Indications for surgery in a patient with diffuse esophageal spasm:
Incapacitating chest pain or dysphagia after failure of medical and endoscopic therapy or presence of a pulsion diverticulum of the thoracic esophagus

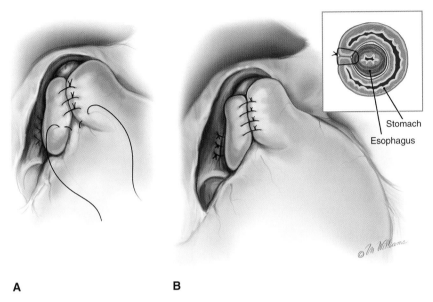

A   **B**

FIGURE 18-8. Nissen Fundoplication. **(A)** A 2 to 2.5 cm 360 degree fundoplication is created around the GE junction. **(B)** Completed Nissen fundoplication with sutures placed to reapproximate the diaphragmatic hiatus. *(Reproduced from Sugarbaker DJ, Bueno R, Krasna MJ, Mentzer SJ, Zellos L. Adult Chest Surgery. http://www.accesssurgery.com. Copyright © The McGraw-Hill Companies, Inc. All rights reserved.)*

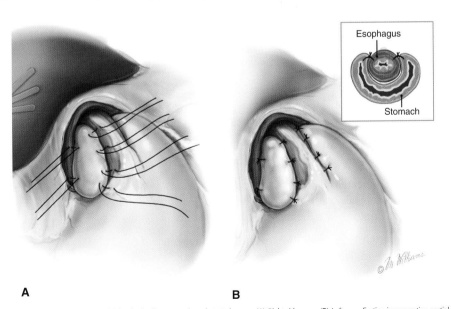

A   **B**

FIGURE 18-9. Toupet posterior partial fundoplication, approximately 270 degrees. **(A)** Right side wrap. **(B)** Left wrap fixation incorporating partial thickness bites of the esophagus and stomach. *(Reproduced from Sugarbaker DJ, Bueno R, Krasna MJ, Mentzer SJ, Zellos L. Adult Chest Surgery. http://www.accesssurgery.com. Copyright © The McGraw-Hill Companies, Inc. All rights reserved.)*

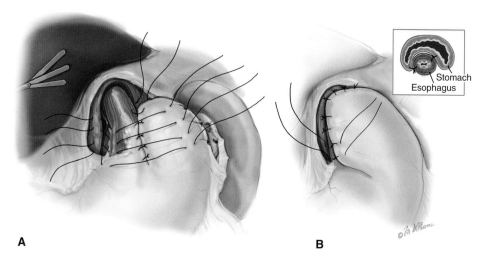

A **B**

FIGURE 18-10. Dor anterior partial fundoplication. (**A**) Left sided bites affix the gastric fundus to the esophagus with additional lateral fixation of the fundus incorporating the esophagus and fixation to the right crus of the diaphragm. (**B**) Completed repair. *(Reproduced from Sugarbaker DJ, Bueno R, Krasna MJ, Mentzer SJ, Zellos L. Adult Chest Surgery. http://www.accesssurgery.com. Copyright © The McGraw-Hill Companies, Inc. All rights reserved.)*

If indicated, what surgical procedure should be performed in patients with diffuse esophageal spasm?

Long esophagomyotomy with the proximal extent high enough to include the entire length of the abnormal motility as determined by manometric measurements and the distal extent of the myotomy down onto the LES with or without extension onto the stomach through a left thoracotomy or a left video-assisted technique; Dor fundoplication can be performed to provide protection from reflux and prevent healing of the myotomy site.

What is the gold standard for the diagnosis of nutcracker esophagus?

Subjective complaint of chest pain with simultaneous objective evidence of peristaltic esophageal contractions 2 standard deviations above the normal values on manometric tracings (amplitudes >400 mm Hg)

Treatment of nutcracker esophagus:

Medical (calcium channel blockers, nitrates, and antispasmodics) for temporary relief during acute spasms; avoidance of caffeine, cold, and hot foods

Manometric findings with hypertensive LES:

Elevated LES pressure (>26 mm Hg) and normal relaxation of the LES

Treatment of hypertensive LES:

Initially endoscopically with Botox injections and hydrostatic balloon dilation; surgery indicated in symptomatic patients who fail interventional treatments

If indicated, what is the operation of choice for hypertensive LES?

Laparoscopic modified Heller esophagomyotomy with a partial antireflux procedure (Dor, Toupet) in patients with normal esophageal motility

What is the manometric definition of ineffective esophageal motility?

The sum total of the number of low-amplitude contractions (<30 mm Hg) and nontransmitted contractions exceeds 30% of wet swallows

Best treatment for ineffective esophageal motility:
Prevention with effective treatment of GERD; altered motility is irreversible.

Treatment for a patient with Barrett esophagus with no dysplasia?
Acid suppression medication and yearly surveillance endoscopy with surveillance extended to every 2 to 3 years if there is no evidence of dysplasia on 3 consecutive yearly endoscopic exams

Treatment for a patient with Barrett esophagus with low-grade dysplasia:
Acid suppression medication and surveillance endoscopy performed at 6-month intervals for the first year and then yearly thereafter if there has been no change

Recommended treatment for a patient with Barrett esophagus with high-grade dysplasia:
Esophageal resection (near-total esophagectomy through a transhiatal approach); additional treatment options include ablative therapy or endoscopic mucosal resection in patients who are not acceptable surgical candidates

What is the most common aortic arch anomaly that creates an incomplete vascular ring around the esophagus?
Right subclavian artery arising from the descending aorta and traveling behind esophagus in its course to the right upper extremity

What is a pulmonary artery sling?
An anomaly of the pulmonary arterial trunk where the left pulmonary artery arises from the right pulmonary artery (instead of main pulmonary artery trunk) and courses between the trachea and the esophagus with resultant significant anterior compression of the esophagus

What can develop with a long-standing untreated pulmonary artery sling?
Tracheal stenosis and left pulmonary artery narrowing

Treatment of a pulmonary artery sling:
Open sternotomy with cardiopulmonary bypass and anatomic repositioning of the great vessels

What are the theories regarding the etiology of a Schatzki ring?
A result of reflux esophagitis versus overcontractility of the circular esophageal musculature of the inferior esophageal sphincter combined with the sliding gastric mucosa of a hiatal hernia results in persistent apposition of the 2 mucosal layers and fibrosis of the submucosal layer below

How is the diagnosis of a Schatzki ring made?
Barium esophagram

Treatment for an asymptomatic patient incidentally found to have a Schatzki ring:
No treatment

Treatment for a patient with a Schatzki ring who presents with acute obstruction:
Administration of oral papain (2.5% solution) in 5-mL aliquots every 30 minutes for a total of 4 doses for proteolytic digestion of impacted protein food; intravenous (IV) meperidine (25–50 mg) to encourage spontaneous dislodgment of the impacted food bolus; esophagoscopy with the use of an overtube (rigid or flexible) for extraction

Treatment for a patient with a Schatzki ring who presents with dysphagia:
Disruption of the ring by oral dilation (50-French tapered Maloney bougie) with sequential bougienage dilation as symptoms recur

Indications for surgery in a patient with a Schatzki ring:
Patients who fail bougienage or have intractable reflux intraoperative bougienage followed by a Nissen fundoplication is recommended, but excision of the ring is not indicated.

If indicated, what surgical procedure is performed in a patient with a Schatzki ring?
Intraoperative bougienage followed by Nissen fundoplication without excision of the ring

How is an esophageal web distinguished from a Schatzki ring based on epithelium?
Esophageal web has squamous cell epithelium above and below the web. Schatzki ring is composed of esophageal epithelium above and gastric epithelium below the ring.

What is the treatment for a thin esophageal web?
Membranous disruption through an endoscope or bougie versus piecemeal excision with biopsy forceps versus laser lysis versus balloon dilation

What is the treatment for a thick esophageal web refractory to bougienage?
Surgical mucosal resection via a transcervical or transthoracic approach, longitudinal myotomy created and circumferential excision of the web performed, mucosa is circumferentially reapproximated with interrupted absorbable sutures, and muscle is closed longitudinally

What is the characteristic appearance that a leiomyoma has on barium esophagram?
A smooth, well-defined, noncircumferential mass with distinct borders

What is the treatment for a leiomyoma?
Surgical enucleation; observation acceptable in patients with significant comorbidities or with small (<2 cm) asymptomatic tumors

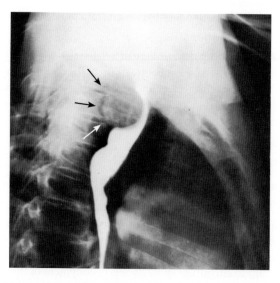

FIGURE 18-11. Leiomyoma of esophagus. Note smooth, rounded density causing extrinsic compression of esophageal lumen. Arrows are pointing at Leiomyoma of the esophagus. *(Reproduced from Doherty GM. Current Diagnosis and Treatment: Surgery. 9th ed. http://www.accessmedicine. com. Copyright © The McGraw-Hill Companies, Inc. All rights reserved.)*

What is a type I hiatal hernia?
Sliding hiatal hernia; simple herniation of GE junction into chest

What is a type II hiatal hernia?
GE junction remains at esophageal hiatus and gastric fundus herniates alongside the esophagus into the chest

What is a type III hiatal hernia?
Combination of type I and type II hiatal hernia; GE junction and gastric fundus/body in chest

What is a type IV hiatal hernia?
Advanced stage of hiatal hernia with entire stomach and other intraabdominal content is herniated into the chest

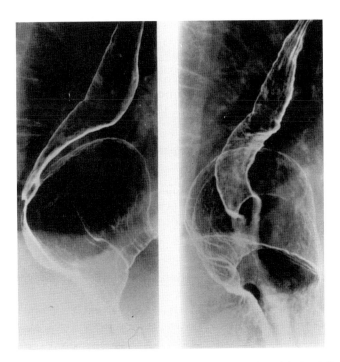

FIGURE 18-12. Radiogram of a type III (combined sliding-rolling or mixed) hernia. *(Reproduced with permission from DeMeester TR, Bonavina L. Paraesophageal hiatal hernia. In: Nyhus LM, Condon RE, eds. Hernia. 3rd ed. Philadelphia: Lippincott; 1989:684.)*

ACID/ALKALI INJURIES

What kind of necrosis occurs with a caustic esophageal injury from alkali?
Liquefaction necrosis

What kind of necrosis occurs with a caustic esophageal injury from acid?
Coagulation necrosis

What are the 3 phases of tissue injury from alkali ingestion?
Acute necrosis, ulceration and granulation, cicatrization and scarring

What is a grade I caustic injury to the esophagus and the associated endoscopic findings?
Superficial mucosal burn, mucosal edema, and hyperemia

What is a grade IIA caustic injury to the esophagus and the associated endoscopic findings?
Transmucosal injury, patchy ulcerations, exudates, sloughing mucosa

What is a grade IIB caustic injury to the esophagus and the associated endoscopic findings?
Transmucosal injury, circumferential injury

What is a grade III caustic injury to the esophagus and the associated endoscopic findings?
Transmural injury with periesophageal/perigastric extension; deep ulcerations; black/gray discoloration; full-thickness necrosis

Which grade or grades of caustic injury will progress to stricture?
Grade IIB and III

Treatment for a patient who presents within the first hour following alkali ingestion:
Neutralization with half-strength vinegar or citrus juice

Treatment for a patient who presents within the first hour following acid ingestion:
Neutralization with milk, egg whites, or antacids

Management for a patient with no evidence of burn on endoscopy or physical exam following corrosive ingestion in the acute phase:
Observation and oral nutrition when the patient can painlessly swallow saliva

Management for a patient with an endoscopically identified first-degree burn following corrosive ingestion in the acute phase:
48 hours of observation and oral nutrition when the patient can painlessly swallow saliva; repeat endoscopy and barium esophagram are performed in follow-up at intervals of 1, 2, and 8 months

Management for a patient with an endoscopically identified second- or third-degree burn following corrosive ingestion in the acute phase:
Monitor in the ICU and keep NPO with IV fluids; start IV antibiotics and a proton pump inhibitor; If evidence of acute airway involvement, airway obstruction can be relieved with aerosolized steroids with the possible need for fiberoptic intubation

How can the diagnosis of corrosive injury to the esophagus/stomach be made if not originally secured with endoscopy?
Exploratory laparoscopy in stable patients or laparotomy in unstable patients

After performing an exploratory laparotomy/laparoscopy after corrosive injury, a viable stomach and esophagus are encountered; what should be performed?
The viable stomach and esophagus are left in situ and a feeding jejunostomy tube is placed with endoscopic placement of an esophageal stent

After performing an exploratory laparotomy/laparoscopy after corrosive injury, a questionable esophagus and stomach are encountered; what should be performed?
The questionable esophagus and stomach are left in situ with a second-look operation performed in 36 hours with further management based on the findings.

After performing an exploratory laparotomy/laparoscopy after corrosive injury, full-thickness necrosis, or perforation of the esophagus/stomach is found; what should be performed?

Resection of the esophagus, stomach, and all affected surrounding organs and tissues; creation of an end-cervical esophagostomy; and placement of a feeding jejunostomy

How is a patient who develops an esophageal stricture secondary to corrosive injury managed?

After re-epithelialization, aggressive treatment with bougie dilation regardless of symptoms; dilations performed daily for 2 to 3 weeks, then every other day for 2 to 3 weeks, then weekly for months and lengthening the interval as time passes

Name some types of conduits that can be used for esophageal reconstruction:

Gastric pull-up, jejunal interposition, colon interposition

MALIGNANT DISEASE

How much does the presence of Barrett esophagus increase the risk of developing adenocarcinoma?

50×

What is the most common esophageal cancer?

Adenocarcinoma

Where does adenocarcinoma of the esophagus usually occur?

Lower one-third of the esophagus

Where does squamous cell carcinoma of the esophagus usually occur?

Upper two-thirds of the esophagus

Most common presentation of esophageal cancer:

Dysphagia

Complications of esophagectomy:

Bleeding, airway injury, insufficient conduit length, thoracic duct injury, respiratory (pneumonia), esophageal conduit necrosis, anastomotic leak, anastomotic stricture, hoarseness, chylothorax, transhiatal herniation of abdominal contents

What are the characteristic findings of a chylous effusion?

Turbid, milky white fluid, specific gravity 1.020 to 1.030, protein content 3 to 4 g/100 mL, fat content 1 to 4 g/100 mL, triglyceride content >110 mg/dL

What is the reported incidence of chylothorax as a complication of esophageal surgery?

~4%

Management for a chylous effusion with <500 cc/24 h chest tube output:

Nonoperative management (should stop spontaneously)

Management for a chylous effusion with (>500 cc but <1000 cc)/24 h chest tube output:

Initially, nonoperative management; if not resolved or significantly improved in 5 to 7 days, perform operative duct ligation

Management for a chylous effusion with >1000 cc/24 h chest tube output:

Early duct ligation

MULTIPLE CHOICE QUESTIONS

1. The most common cause of chylothorax is:

   A. Trauma to the spine and chest wall
   B. Lymphatic obstruction from mediastinal lymphoma
   C. Lymphatic leakage after mediastinal lymph node dissection
   D. Thoracic duct injury during esophagectomy

2. A 34-year-old male patient has been experiencing gastric reflux symptoms and recently underwent a workup, which included a upper endoscopy. The upper endoscopy revealed Barrett esophagus. The most appropriate therapy for this patient is:

   A. Esophagectomy
   B. Repeat endoscopy in 6 months
   C. Medical therapy with acid suppression
   D. Medical therapy with acid suppression and referral for fundoplication

3. What is the histologic subtype of Barrett tissue?

   A. Junctional epithelium
   B. Specialized columnar epithelium
   C. Gastric fundus epithelium
   D. Specialized squamous epithelium

4. After a 3-hole esophagectomy with a cervical anastomosis, the patient begins to develop leukocytosis, fever, and erythema of the wound. A barium swallow is performed and there is an anastomotic leak noted. What is the most appropriate management of this patient?

   A. Open the wound and redo the anastomosis
   B. Open the wound and widely drain the anastomosis
   C. Endoluminal stent
   D. IV antibiotics and NPO

5. Boerhaave esophageal rupture normally occurs at:

   A. Cervical esophagus
   B. Proximal thoracic esophagus
   C. Middle thoracic esophagus
   D. Distal thoracic esophagus

6. An elderly man was experiencing progressive dysphagia with regurgitation of undigested food. A thorough workup revealed he had a cervical Zenker diverticulum. What is the treatment of choice for this condition?

   A. Observation
   B. Ligation
   C. Diverticulectomy
   D. Diverticulectomy with cricopharyngeal myotomy
   E. Esophagectomy

7. A 32-year-old man is brought to the emergency room after ingesting some drain cleaner in a suicide attempt. He is hemodynamically stable and a referral is placed for surgical evaluation. A CT scan has already been performed and there is no evidence of perforation. What is the next step in management?

   A. Observation
   B. EGD
   C. Barium upper GI swallow
   D. Immediate laparotomy for exploration
   E. Immediate thoracotomy for exploration

8. A 48-year-old woman who is morbidly obese is referred to your office with an incidental CT finding of an aberrant right subclavian artery running in a retroesophageal path. What is the management strategy of choice?

   A. Reimplantation or bypass of the subclavian artery
   B. Upper GI swallow study
   C. EGD
   D. Observation
   E. Gastric bypass

9. A 50-year-old man comes in complaining of progressive dysphagia. CT scan shows no evidence of tumor. An upper GI study shows no tumor or functional obstruction. An EGD is performed and a small tear is iatrogenically created with the EGD scope. The patient has some mild chest pain and is started on antibiotics. A stat CT scan shows a small, contained perforation just above the GE junction. What is the treatment of choice?

   A. Immediate laparotomy and primary repair
   B. NPO, antibiotics, and observation
   C. Esophageal stenting
   D. Endoluminal repair with clips

10. A patient recently underwent an Ivor-lewis esophagectomy for cancer. The initial operation was straight-forward and the operation took 4 hours. On postoperative day 7, the patient began to develop fevers, tachycardia, and shortness of breath. He developed hypotension and was refractory to IV fluid boluses and is now on vasopressors to maintain an adequate perfusion pressure. A CT demonstrated a large right-sided pleural effusion and extravasation of the oral contrast material. The patient was brought back for re-exploration and the anastomosis was disrupted. In addition, the gastric conduit was dusky and there was concern about its viability. What is the best treatment option at this point?

    A. Staple off the necrotic stomach; perform a diverting esophagostomy
    B. Resect the necrotic stomach and redo the anastomosis
    C. Place an endoluminal stent across the anastomosis and allow it to granulate
    D. Resect the gastric conduit and perform jejunal interposition bypass
    E. Wide drainage with chest tubes and long-term antibiotics with total parenteral nutrition support

ANSWERS

1. **Answer: D.** The thoracic duct ascends in the mediastinum parallel to the esophagus and can easily be injured during mobilization for esophagectomy. Lymphatic leaks from lymph node dissections are often trivial and will usually seal on their own with no intervention.

2. **Answer: D.** In a patient with reflux symptoms and Barrett epithelium, this is an indication for antireflux surgery, that is, Nissen fundoplication.

3. **Answer: B.** Barrett is an acquired condition thought to be caused by chronic reflux. It is associated with ulceration and stricture and has a higher rate of malignant degeneration than normal esophageal endothelium.

4. **Answer: B.** Patients with anastomotic leaks at the cervical area need to be made NPO, given antibiotics, and have the neck wound explored, debrided, and drained. Revising the anastomosis is unlikely to be successful due to inadequate length and friability of the tissues. In cases of catastrophic conduit necrosis, the esophagus can be diverted proximally and reconstruction performed in a delayed fashion with alternative conduits (jejunum, colon).

5. **Answer: D.** Boerhaave ruptures normally occur in this area after periods of coughing or retching. The patient will normally present with severe chest pain, fever, and subcutaneous emphysema.

6. **Answer: D.** Symptoms may vary but this is largely a progressive disease. Smaller diverticuli may be left in situ; however, the key aspect to the procedure is to release the cricopharyngeal muscle by performing an adequate myotomy. The patient is at a higher risk for recurrence if an appropriate myotomy is not made.

7. **Answer: B.** Caustic injuries can cause catastrophic damage to the esophagus; aggressive management is necessary. An EGD should be the first invasive test to assess the degree of damage to the esophageal mucosa and needs to be serially repeated throughout the healing process. There is no role for exploratory surgery in the absence of perforation or sepsis.

8. **Answer: D.** An aberrant right subclavian artery is a common anomaly. Normally, it doesn't cause any symptoms and the patient can be reassured. In a patient with no symptoms of dysphagia and concomitant morbid obesity, there is little doubt that food intake is a problem and no specific treatment is necessary. In patients who present with dysphagia and weight loss, this can be termed "dysphagia lusoria" and consideration is made for reimplantation or bypass of the subclavian artery to provide relief of the esophageal obstruction.

9. **Answer: B.** A patient with a contained esophageal perforation may be treated conservatively provided there are no systemic signs of sepsis or peritonitis. These patients often heal within 2 weeks. Surgery should be reserved for patients who develop peritoneal signs, a leucocytosis, or an uncontained perforation. Esophageal stenting is a novel approach but would be difficult to place at the GE junction to create a good seal without creating significant reflux. The role of endoluminal repair is evolving and is not currently a standard approach.

10. **Answer: A.** In a septic patient with conduit necrosis, the best choice is a damage control type procedure: resect the obviously necrotic gastric conduit and perform an esophageal diversion (Spit fistula). Presumably, the patient already has a j tube for enteral feeds from the first operation. This will allow for resuscitation and stabilization, and delayed reconstruction can be considered with alternative conduits. There is no role for a complex operation in a septic patient with a failed bypass.

CHAPTER 19
Small Intestine

James Lee and Dale A. Dangleben

EMBRYOLOGY

What does the cranial limb of the midgut loop develop into?
Distal duodenum, jejunum, and proximal ilium

What does the caudal limb of the midgut loop develop into?
Distal ilium and proximal two-thirds of the transverse colon

What structure joins the yolk sac to the juncture of the cranial and caudal limbs of the midgut loop?
The vitelline duct

What is a persistent vitelline duct otherwise known as?
Meckel diverticulum

How much does midgut loop rotate during normal physiologic herniation of bowel?
270° counterclockwise rotation

ANATOMY

How long is the entire small intestine, from the pylorus to the cecum?
~6 m (20 ft)

How long is the duodenum?
26 cm (9.8 in.)

How long is the jejunum?
2.5 m (8.2 ft)

How long is the ileum?
3.5 m (11.5 ft)

What peritoneal fold supports the duodenojejunal angle, which marks where the duodenum ends and the jejunum begin?
Ligament of Treitz

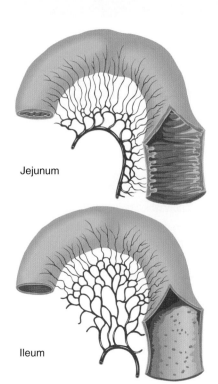

Jejunum

Ileum

FIGURE 19-1. Blood supply and luminal surface of the small bowel. The arterial arcades of the small intestine increase in number from 1 or 2 in the proximal jejunum to 4 or 5 in the distal ileum, a finding that helps to distinguish proximal from distal bowel at operation. Plicae circulares are more prominent in the jejunum. *(Reproduced with permission from Gerard M Doherty. CURRENT Diagnosis & Treatment: Surgery. 13th ed. http://www.accessmedicine.com. Copyright © The McGraw-Hill Companies, Inc. All rights reserved.)*

What are plicae circulares?
Circular folds of mucosa in the small bowel lumen (also known as valvulae conniventes)

Excluding the proximal duodenum, what artery supplies the entire blood supply of the small bowel?
Except for the proximal duodenum that is supplied by branches of the celiac axis, the supply comes entirely from the superior mesenteric artery (SMA).

Where is the parasympathetic innervation of the small bowel derived from?
Parasympathetic fibers are derived from the vagus, which traverse the celiac ganglion to supply the small bowel.

Where is the sympathetic innervation of the small bowel derived from?
Sympathetic fibers originate from 3 sets of splanchnic nerves; ganglion cells found in a plexus around base of SMA.

Describe the lymphatic drainage of the small intestine:
From mucosa through wall of the bowel
Mesenteric lymph nodes adjacent to the bowel
Regional nodes adjacent to the mesenteric arterial arcades
Group of lymph nodes at the base of the superior mesentery vessels
Cisterna chyli
Thoracic ducts
Return to venous system

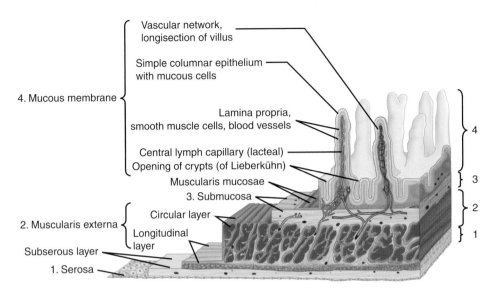

FIGURE 19-2. Layers of wall of the small intestine. The individual layers and their prominent features are represented schematically. *(Reproduced from Brunicardi FC, Anderson DK, Billiar TR, et al. Schwartz's Principles of Surgery. 9th ed. http://www.accessmedicine.com. Copyright © The McGraw-Hill Companies, Inc. All rights reserved.)*

What are the 4 layers of the small bowel? From out to in:
Serosa
Muscularis propria
Submucosa
Mucosa

The muscularis propria comprises what 2 muscle layers?
Thin outer longitudinal layer; thicker inner circular layer (with myenteric [Auerbach] plexus between the muscle layers)

The strongest layer of the small bowel:
Submucosa

What extensive plexus of nerve fibers and ganglion cells are found in the submucosa of the small bowel?
Meissner plexus

What 3 layers comprise the mucosa of the small bowel?
Muscularis mucosae (thin layer of muscle that separates mucosa from submucosa)
Lamina propria (connective tissue layer between epithelial cells and muscularis mucosae)
Epithelial layer (continual sheet of epithelial cells covering villi and lining crypts)

Which layer of small bowel mucosa is responsible for combating microorganisms that penetrate the overlying small bowel epithelium?
Lamina propria (contains a rich supply of immune cells)

What are the 4 main cell types found in the small bowel mucosal layer?
Absorptive enterocytes
Goblet cells (secretes mucus)
Paneth cells (secrete lysozyme, tumor necrosis factor)
Enteroendocrine cells (produce gastrointestinal hormones)

Term for the fuzzy coat of glycoprotein that covers the microvilli to further increase absorption:
Glycocalyx

The portions of the duodenum that are retroperitoneal:
Second portion (descending), third portion (transverse)

The vascular supply of the duodenum is:
Anterosuperior pancreaticoduodenal and posterosuperior pancreaticoduodenal arteries (from gastroduodenal artery) and anteroinferior pancreaticoduodenal and posteroinferior pancreaticoduodenal arteries (from SMA)

What is the first branch off of the SMA?
Anteroinferior pancreaticoduodenal and posteroinferior pancreaticoduodenal arteries

PHYSIOLOGY

What is the primary responsibility of the small bowel?
The absorption of carbohydrates, proteins, fats, ions, vitamins, and water

What does the terminal ileum absorb?
Fatty acids; bile salts; vitamin B_{12}

What enzymes involved in carbohydrate digestion are contained in the brush border of the small intestine?
Lactase; maltase; sucrase-isomaltase; trehalase

Name the substrate and the product for lactase, located in the brush border of the small intestine:
Substrate: lactose
Product: glucose, galactose

What brush border enzyme in the duodenum activates pancreatic trypsinogen that is secreted into the intestine?
Enterokinase

What 3 principal pancreatic proteases comprise the endopeptidases?
Trypsin
Chymotrypsin
Elastase

What 2 principal pancreatic proteases comprise the exopeptidases?
Carboxypeptidase A
Carboxypeptidase B

What is the primary action of trypsin?
Forms products with basic amino acids at carboxyl-terminal end by attacking peptide bonds involving basic amino acids.

What is the primary action of chymotrypsin?
Forms peptide products with aromatic amino acids, leucine, glutamine, and methionine at carboxyl-terminal ends by attacking peptide bonds involving aromatic amino acids, leucine, glutamine, and methionine.

What is the primary action of elastase?
Forms products with neutral amino acids at carboxyl-terminal end by attacking peptide bonds involving neutral aliphatic amino acids.

What is the primary action of carboxypeptidase A?
Attacks peptides with aromatic and neutral aliphatic amino acids at carboxyl-terminal end

What is the primary action of carboxypeptidase B?
Attacks peptides with basic amino acids at carboxyl-terminal end

Normally, what percentage of digestion and absorption of protein is completed in the jejunum?
80% to 90%

Describe the process of the fat digestion in the small bowel:
Fat globules from the diet are emulsified with the help of bile
Pancreatic lipase splits triglycerides into free fatty acids and 2-monoglycerides
Bile salts form micelles with the monoglycerides and free fatty acids (dissolved in central hydrophobic portion of micelles) formed from lipolysis
Micelles carry the products of fat hydrolysis to brush border where absorption occurs

What is a micelle?
A small spherical globule with a lipophilic sterol nucleus and a polar hydrophilic group that projects outward and is composed of 20 to 40 molecules of bile salts

What kind of fatty acids are absorbed directly into the portal blood?
Short- and medium-chain fatty acids

What kind of fatty acid is absorbed via chylomicrons passing from the epithelial cells into lacteals, which pass through the lymphatics into the venous system?
Long-chain fatty acids

What is the composition of a chylomicron?
~90% triacylglycerol; ~10% phospholipid; cholesterol; protein

What percentage of fat absorption occurs by way of the thoracic lymphatics?
80% to 90%

What percentage of bile salts are reabsorbed?
95%

How are unconjugated bile acids absorbed into the jejunum?
Passive diffusion

Only location of the small bowel where conjugated bile is absorbed:
Terminal ileum

What is bile conjugated to?
Glycine and taurine

What are the primary bile acids?
Chenodeoxycholic; cholic

What are the secondary bile acids?
Dexoycholic; lithocholic

How much is the total bile salt pool in humans?
2 to 3 g

Approximately how much bile is lost in the stool in 1 day?
0.5 g

Number of times the bile recirculates in 24 hours (enterohepatic circulation):
~6 times

In the ileal enterocyte, what binds and transports free vitamin B_{12} into the portal circulation?
Transcobalamin II

What are the 3 areas of the small bowel where gut-associated lymphoid tissue can be found?
Intraepithelial; lamina propria; Peyer patches

What cells contained within the follicle-associated epithelium of the small bowel serve as a site for the selective sampling of intraluminal antigens?
M cells (microfold cells)

What is the most important hormone in the migrating motor complex?
Motilin

During which phase of the migrating motor complex is motilin found at its peak plasma levels?
Phase III

What happens during Phase I of the migrating motor complex?
Rest

What happens during Phase II of the migrating motor complex?
Acceleration and gallbladder contraction

What happens during Phase III of the migrating motor complex?
Peristalsis

What happens during Phase IV of the migrating motor complex?
Deceleration

What is the primary effect of the hormone gastrin?
Stimulates gastric mucosal growth; stimulates acid and pepsinogen secretion

Location of the cells that release the hormone gastrin:
G cells in the duodenum; antrum

What are the major stimulants for the release of the hormone gastrin?
Amino acids; peptides; antral distention; gastrin-releasing peptide (bombesin); vagal and adrenergic stimulation

What is the primary effect of the hormone cholecystokinin?
Stimulates gallbladder contraction; relaxes sphincter of Oddi; stimulates pancreatic enzyme secretion; inhibits gastric emptying

Location of the cells that release the hormone cholecystokinin:
Duodenum; jejunum (I cells)

What are the major stimulants for the release of the hormone cholecystokinin?
Amino acids; peptides; fats

What is the primary effect of the hormone secretin?
Stimulates flow/alkalinity of bile and release of water and bicarbonate from pancreatic ductal cells; inhibits gastrin releases and gastric acid secretion and motility

Location of the cells that release the hormone secretin:
Duodenum; jejunum (S cells)

What are the major stimulants for the release of the hormone secretin?
Bile salts; fatty acids; luminal acidity

What is the primary effect of the hormone somatostatin?
Inhibits gastric acid secretion, release of gastrointestinal hormones, small bowel water and electrolyte secretion, and secretion of pancreatic hormones (universal "off" switch)

Location of the cells that release the hormone somatostatin:
Pancreatic islets (D cells); antrum; duodenum

What are the major stimulants for the release of the hormone somatostatin?
Pancreas: amino acids, cholecystokinin, and glucose;
Gut: acid, fat, protein, and other hormones (gastrin, cholecystokinin)

What is the primary effect of the hormone gastrin-releasing peptide?
Stimulates release of all gastrointestinal hormones (except secretin), gastric acid secretion and release of antral gastrin, gastrointestinal secretion and motility, and growth of intestinal mucosa and pancreas (universal "on" switch)

Location of the cells that release the hormone gastrin-releasing peptide:
Small bowel

What are the major stimulants for the release of the hormone gastrin-releasing peptide?
Vagal stimulation

What is the primary effect of the hormone gastric inhibitory peptide?
Stimulates pancreatic insulin release in response to hyperglycemia and inhibits gastric acid and pepsin secretion

Location of the cells that release the hormone gastric inhibitory peptide:
Duodenum; jejunum (K cells)

What are the major stimulants for the release of the hormone gastric inhibitory peptide?
Adrenergic stimulation
Glucose
Fat
Protein

What is the primary effect of the hormone motilin?
Stimulates upper gastrointestinal tract motility (may initiate migrating motor complex)

Location of the cells that release the hormone motilin:
Duodenum; jejunum

What are the major stimulants for the release of the hormone motilin?
Gastric distention; fat

What is the primary effect of the hormone vasoactive intestinal peptide?
Potent vasodilator; stimulates pancreatic and intestinal secretion and inhibits gastric acid secretion (primarily functions as a neuropeptide)

Location of the cells that release the hormone vasoactive intestinal peptide:
Neurons throughout the gastrointestinal tract

What are the major stimulants for the release of the hormone vasoactive intestinal peptide?
Vagal stimulation

What is the primary effect of the hormone neurotensin?
Stimulates growth of small and large bowel mucosa

Location of the cells that release the hormone neurotensin:
Small bowel (N cells)

What are the major stimulants for the release of the hormone neurotensin?
Fat

What is the primary effect of the hormone enteroglucagon?
Glucagon-like peptide-1: stimulates insulin release and inhibits pancreatic glucagon release
Glucagon-like peptide 2: potent enterotrophic factor

Location of the cells that release the hormone enteroglucagon:
Small bowel (L cells)

What are the major stimulants for the release of the hormone enteroglucagon?
Glucose; fat

What is the primary effect of peptide YY?
Inhibits gastric and pancreatic secretion and gallbladder contraction

Location of the cells that release peptide YY:
Distal small bowel; colon

What are the major stimulants for the release of peptide YY?
Cholecystokinin; fatty acids

SMALL BOWEL OBSTRUCTION/ILEUS

What are the 3 categories for the causes of small bowel obstruction?
Extraluminal cause of obstruction
Intraluminal cause of obstruction
Obstruction intrinsic to the bowel wall

What is the #1 cause of small bowel obstruction in the world?
Hernia

What is the #1 cause of small bowel obstruction in children?
Hernia

What is the #1 cause of small bowel obstruction in adults?
Postoperative adhesions

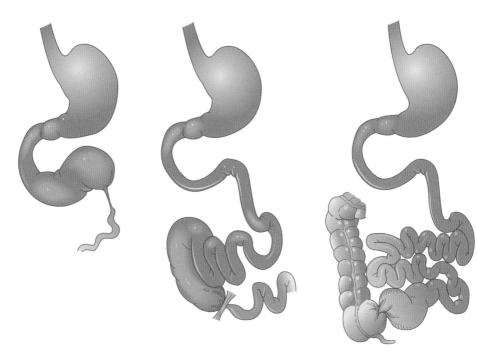

High	**Middle**	**Low**
Frequent vomiting. No distention. Intermittent pain but not classic crescendo type	Moderate vomiting. Moderate distention. Intermittent pain (crescendo, colicky) with free intervals	Vomiting late, feculent. Marked distention. Variable pain; may not be classic crescendo type

FIGURE 19-3. Small bowel obstruction. Variable manifestations of obstruction depend on the level of blockage of the small bowel. *(Reproduced from Gerard M Doherty. CURRENT Diagnosis & Treatment: Suregery. 13th ed. http://www.accessmedicine.com. Copyright © The McGraw-Hill Companies, Inc. All rights reserved.)*

Why can diarrhea accompany early partial or even complete small bowel obstruction?
Intestinal motility and contraction increase both above and below the obstruction in an effort to propel luminal contents past the obstruction

What are the cardinal symptoms of intestinal obstruction?
Abdominal distension; colicky abdominal pain; nausea; vomiting; failure to pass flatus and stool (obstipation)

What must you remember to do on physical exam in a patient with a small bowel obstruction?
Note previous surgical scars; auscultate and palpate the abdomen; perform a careful examination to rule out incarcerated inguinal hernias, femoral hernias, and obturator hernia; perform a rectal exam to assess for intraluminal masses and occult blood

What is the characteristic appearance of a small bowel obstruction on upright abdominal x-ray?
Dilated loops of small bowel with multiple air-fluid levels (often layer in stepwise pattern)

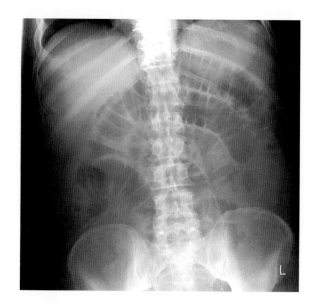

What percentage of plain abdominal radiographs accurately make the diagnosis of small intestinal obstruction?
~60%

What is the usual treatment for a patient with a small bowel obstruction?
Make patient NPO; aggressive intravenous fluid replacement with isotonic solution; monitor urine output with a Foley catheter; decompress with nasogastric suction; follow serial electrolyte measurements and complete blood cell count; perform serial abdominal exams

Reported percentage of patients with small bowel obstruction whose symptoms resolve and get discharged from the hospital without the need for surgery:
60% to 85%

What are the classic signs of intestinal strangulation from obstruction?
Constant, noncramping abdominal pain
Fever
Leukocytosis
Tachycardia

Name CT findings associated with the late stages of irreversible intestinal ischemia:
Pneumatosis intestinalis; portal venous gas

What clinical parameters lower the threshold to operate on a patient with a small bowel obstruction?
Worsening abdominal pain
Fever
Increasing leukocytosis
Tachycardia/tachypnea

Indications for surgery in a patient with a small bowel obstruction:
Fever
Progressive pain
Failure to resolve

Worsening leukocytosis
Signs of strangulation/perforation
Peritoneal signs

What are absolute indications to operate on a patient with a partial small bowel obstruction?
Free air on x-ray; peritoneal signs

What is the usual operative management in a patient with a small bowel obstruction secondary to an adhesive band without evidence of strangulation?
Lysis of adhesions

What is the usual operative management in a patient with a small bowel obstruction secondary to an incarcerated hernia without evidence of strangulation?
Manual reduction of herniated segment of bowel and closure of the defect

What is the usual operative management in a patient with a small bowel obstruction secondary to Crohn disease without evidence of strangulation?
If acute, try conservative management; if chronic fibrotic stricture, perform strictureplasty versus bowel resection (try to conserve bowel if possible)

What is the usual operative management in a patient with a small bowel obstruction secondary to intra-abdominal abscess without evidence of strangulation?
Percutaneous drainage of the abscess (may be sufficient to relieve obstruction)

What is the usual operative management in a patient with a small bowel obstruction secondary to radiation enteropathy without evidence of strangulation?
If acute, try nonoperative management with tube decompression ± corticosteroids; if chronic, will likely require laparotomy with possible resection of the irradiated bowel or bypass.

How can you evaluate the viability of bowel after the release of a strangulation?
Place released bowel in warm, saline-moistened sponge for 15 to 20 minutes and re-examine (normal color and peristalsis indicate viability); Doppler probe; administration of fluorescein and evaluating fluorescence; second-look laparotomy 18 to 24 hours after the initial procedure

What is the most effective means of limiting the number of adhesions?
Good surgical technique: avoidance of unnecessary dissection; adequate irrigation and removal of infectious/ischemic debris; exclusion of foreign material from the peritoneal cavity

What is an ileus?
Slowing/absence of the intestinal passage of luminal contents and distention without a demonstrable mechanical obstruction.

What are the causes of ileus?
Postoperative ; drugs (opiates, psychotropics, anticholinergics); intra-abdominal inflammation; intestinal ischemia; metabolic and electrolyte derangements; retroperitoneal hemorrhage/inflammation; systemic sepsis

What is the treatment for ileus?
Correction of the underlying cause (correction of any metabolic/electrolyte abnormalities, treatment of sepsis, discontinuation of possible ileus-producing medications) and supportive with nasogastric decompression and IV fluids

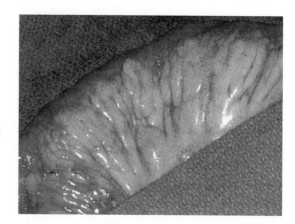

What is the most common primary surgical disease of the small bowel?
Crohn disease

What is the most common reason to operate on a patient with Crohn disease?
Small bowel obstruction

What are the most common sites of occurrence of Crohn disease?
Small intestine; colon

What percentage of Crohn patients present with small bowel involvement alone?
30%

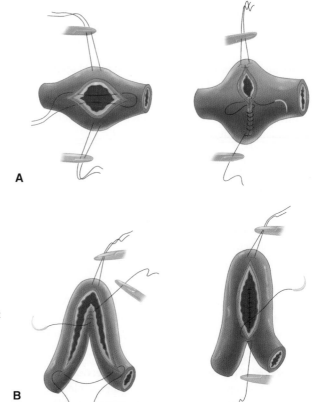

SMALL BOWEL NEOPLASMS

The decreasing frequency of malignant neoplasms of the small bowel:
Adenocarcinoma; carcinoid tumor; malignant GIST; lymphoma

What is the surgical treatment of an adenoma of the small bowel?
Wide resection including regional lymph nodes (may need Whipple for duodenal lesions);
if surgical resection for cure is impossible, perform palliative resection or bypass of the
involved segment.

What is the surgical treatment of a lymphoma of the small bowel?
Wide resection including regional lymph nodes (may need Whipple for duodenal lesions)
with adjuvant chemotherapy and radiation; if surgical resection for cure is impossible,
perform palliative resection or bypass of the involved segment.

What are the most common benign small bowel lesions that produce symptoms?
GISTs

What is the eponym for an intestinal pacemaker cell of mesodermal descent?
Interstitial cell of Cajal

What is the surgical treatment of GIST tumor of the small bowel?
Segmental bowel resection

What cells do carcinoids of the small bowel arise from?
Enterochromaffin cells (Kulchitsky cells/argentaffin cells)

Where can enterochromaffin cells (Kulchitsky cells/argentaffin cells) be found?
The crypts of Lieberkühn

Second most common affected site in the gastrointestinal tract by carcinoid:
Small intestine (ileum 28%)

What percentage of ileal carcinoids metastasize?
~35%

What percentage of small bowel carcinoids are multicentric?
20% to 30%

**What procedure would you perform for a patient with a primary small bowel
carcinoid tumor <1 cm in diameter without evidence of regional lymph node
metastasis?**
Segmental intestinal resection

**What procedure would you perform for a patient with a primary small bowel
carcinoid tumor >1 cm or multiple small bowel carcinoid tumors or primary small
bowel carcinoid tumor with regional lymph node metastasis?**
Search the abdomen thoroughly for multicentric lesions; perform wide excision of bowel
and mesentery; right hemicolectomy for lesions of the terminal ileum; local excision of
small duodenal tumors versus pancreaticoduodenectomy for more extensive lesions

**What would you do if you find a hepatic metastasis from a primary small bowel
carcinoid tumor during abdominal exploration?**
Perform surgical debulking (wedge resection, formal hepatic lobectomy)

What is the most common extra-abdominal malignancy to metastasize to the small intestine?
Cutaneous melanoma

What is the most common benign tumor of the small bowel?
Leiomyoma

What are the 3 primary types of small bowel adenomas?
True adenoma; villous adenoma; Brunner gland adenoma

What is the most common site of cancer in a patient with Peutz-Jeghers syndrome?
The small intestine

DIVERTICULAR DISEASE OF SMALL BOWEL

What are the most common acquired diverticula of the small bowel?
Duodenal diverticula

Where are most duodenal diverticulum found?
Within a 2 cm radius from the ampulla (periampullary)

What is the most common true congenital diverticulum of the small bowel?
Meckel diverticulum

What are the major complications of duodenal diverticula?
Cholangitis from obstruction of the biliary duct; pancreatitis from obstruction of the pancreatic duct; hemorrhage; perforation; blind loop syndrome

Which border of the small bowel are jejunoileal diverticula usually found?
Mesenteric border

What is the treatment of choice for perforated jejunoileal diverticula?
Resection with reanastomosis (simple closure, excision, invagination associated with greater mortality/morbidity); if diffuse peritonitis, may require enterostomies.

What are your surgical options for treating an obstruction caused by a dislodged enterolith formed in a jejunal diverticulum?
Enterotomy and removal of the enterolith; can try to milk the enterolith distally into the cecum; if enterolith causes obstruction at the level of the diverticulum, perform bowel resection with reanastomosis.

What is a Meckel diverticulum?
A remnant of the omphalomesenteric duct (vitelline duct)

What border of the intestine is a Meckel diverticulum found?
Antimesenteric border

What is the most common heterotopic tissue found within a Meckel diverticulum?
Gastric mucosa (50% of all Meckel diverticula)

What percentage of Meckel diverticula contain heterotopic pancreatic tissue?
~5%

What is the most common clinical presentation of Meckel diverticulum?
Gastrointestinal bleeding (accounts for half of all lower GI bleeding in patients <2 years old)

What is the most common complication from a Meckel diverticulitis in an adult?
Obstruction (25%)

Regarding Meckel diverticulum, what is the "rule of twos"?
2% of patients are symptomatic; found ~2 ft from the ileocecal valve; found in 2% of the population; most symptoms occur before age 2; ectopic tissue is found in half of patients (50%); approximately 2 in long; 2:1 male:female ratio

Name the hernia associated with an incarcerated Meckel diverticulum:
Littre hernia

What is the single most accurate diagnostic test for Meckel diverticula in children?
Scintigraphy with sodium 99mTc-pertechnetate (Meckel scan)

What are the reported diagnostic sensitivity, accuracy, and specificity for a Meckel scan in the pediatric age group?
85%; 90%; 95%

What drugs can be given to improve the sensitivity and specificity of 99mTc-pertechnetate scanning in an adult (less accurate secondary to reduced prevalence of ectopic gastric mucosa)?
Pentagastrin (indirectly increases metabolism of mucous-producing cells); glucagon (inhibits peristaltic dilution/washout of intraluminal radionuclide); cimetidine (histamine-2 [H_2]-receptor antagonists result in higher radionuclide concentrations in the wall of the diverticulum)

What is the treatment for a symptomatic Meckel diverticulum?
Diverticulectomy by hand-sewn technique versus stapling at the base of the diverticulum in a diagonal/transverse line (avoid narrowing) versus segmental resection of ileum bearing the diverticulum and reanastomosis

Why is segmental intestinal resection usually required for treatment of patients with a bleeding Meckel diverticulum?
Bleeding site is usually in the ileum adjacent to the diverticulum

What is the general recommendation for an asymptomatic Meckel diverticula found in a child versus an adult?
Child: asymptomatic Meckel diverticula found in children should be resected
Adult: controversial (earlier thought that morbidity > potential for prevention of disease); recent studies suggest prophylactic Meckel diverticulectomy in select asymptomatic adult patients may be beneficial and safer than originally reported.

SMALL BOWEL FISTULA

What does the HIS FRIEND mnemonic regarding the spontaneous closure of an enterocutaneous fistula stand for?
High output (>500 mL/24 h); intestinal disruption (>50% of bowel circumference); short fistula tract (<2.5 cm long); foreign body in the fistula tract; radiation enteritis; inflammatory bowel disease/infection; epithelialization of fistula tract; neoplasm; distal obstruction

How much output must there be for an enterocutaneous fistula to be considered low output?
<200 mL/24 h

What are the major complications associated with small bowel fistulas?
Sepsis; fluid/electrolyte depletion; skin necrosis at the site of external drainage; malnutrition

What does the successful management of a patient with an enterocutaneous fistula entail?
Establishment of controlled drainage; management of sepsis; prevention of fluid/electrolyte depletion; skin protection; adequate nutrition

What is the optimal time period to follow a conservative course in the management of an enterocutaneous fistula before surgical management should be considered?
4 to 6 weeks; if no closure has been obtained, consider surgical management (has been shown that when sepsis was controlled, >90% closed within 1 month, <10% closed after 2 months, none closed spontaneously after 3 months)

What is the preferred operation in the management of an enterocutaneous fistula?
Tract excision and segmental resection of the involved segment of intestine and reanastomosis; if primary anastomosis unsafe (unexpected abscess; long, rigid, distended bowel wall), perform exteriorization of both intestinal ends.

What radiologic studies can be performed to define the precise location of the fistula, possibly surrounding abscess cavity, or disruption of the bowel wall?
Fistulogram; can consider CT scan

MISCELLANEOUS

What is the most common site for pneumatosis intestinalis?
Jejunum

What is the second most common site for pneumatosis intestinalis?
Ileocecal region

What are the causes of pneumatosis intestinalis?
COPD; immunocompromised patients (AIDS; chemotherapy/corticosteroids; transplant patients; patients with leukemia, lymphoma, vasculitis, or collagen vascular disease); inflammatory/obstructive/infectious conditions of the intestine; iatrogenic conditions (endoscopy, jejunostomy placement); ischemia; extraintestinal diseases (diabetes); primary pneumatosis (not associated with any of the aforementioned)

What is the most common cause of small bowel bleeding?
Small bowel angiodysplasia

What study can be performed to further work up a patient with guaiac positive stools and negative upper and lower endoscopy?
Capsule study; small bowel contrast study (enteroclysis)

How does blind loop syndrome manifest?
Abdominal pain; diarrhea; steatorrhea; weight loss; neurologic disorders; megaloblastic anemia; deficiencies of the fat-soluble vitamins (A, D, E, and K)

What tests can be used to diagnose the bacterial overgrowth with blind loop syndrome?
Cultures obtained through an intestinal tube; 14C-xylose or 14C-cholylglycine breath tests

How can blind loop syndrome be differentiated from pernicious anemia with a Schilling test (57Co-labeled vitamin B$_{12}$ absorption)?
A course of broad-spectrum antibiotic (tetracycline) will return vitamin B$_{12}$ absorption to normal and intrinsic factors will have no effect in a patient with the blind loop syndrome.

What is the treatment for patients with blind loop syndrome?
Parenteral vitamin B$_{12}$ therapy and broad-spectrum antibiotics usually for 7 to 10 days (most commonly tetracycline or amoxicillin-clavulanate potassium [Augmentin]; alternative is combination of a cephalosporin [cephalexin {Keflex}] and metronidazole; if ineffective then chloramphenicol); surgery is indicated in those patients who require multiple rounds of antibiotics or are on continuous therapy

What is the treatment of acute noncomplicated radiation enteritis?
Symptom control: antispasmodics/analgesics for abdominal pain and cramping; opiates/antidiarrheal agents for diarrhea; dietary manipulation; ± corticosteroids (questionable benefit)

What are indications for surgery in a patient with radiation enteritis?
Obstruction; fistula formation; perforation; bleeding

What is the most common presentation of radiation enteritis?
Obstruction

What are the surgical options for the treatment of radiation enteritis?
Obstruction: bypass or resection with reanastomosis
Perforation: resection and reanastomosis, if reanastomosis unsafe, exteriorize intestinal ends

What is the most common cause of short bowel syndrome in a pediatric patient?
Bowel resection secondary to necrotizing enterocolitis

What are the clinical hallmarks of short bowel syndrome?
Diarrhea; fluid and electrolyte deficiency; malnutrition (can also see gallstones from disruption of enterohepatic circulation and nephrolithiasis from hyperoxaluria)

How many centimeters of intestine do you need to survive off of TPN with short gut syndrome without an ileocecal valve?
75 cm

How many centimeters of intestine do you need to survive off of TPN with short gut syndrome with an ileocecal valve?
50 cm (can resect up to 70% of the small bowel if terminal ileum/ileocecal valve intact)

What is the usual treatment of short gut syndrome?
Supplementation with TPN; lomotil/codeine/diphenoxylate/cholestyramine/octreotide for diarrhea; H$_2$ blockers for acid reduction; reduce fat with resumption of diet

What surgical strategies are used to treat patients with short bowel syndrome on chronic TPN?
Procedures to delay intestinal transit time (construction of valves and sphincters; antiperistaltic jejunal segment); procedures to increase absorptive area (intestinal tapering and lengthening procedure); small bowel transplantation

What syndrome is characterized by vascular compression of the duodenum?
Wilkie syndrome (SMA syndrome)

What portion of the duodenum is compressed by the SMA with Wilkie syndrome (SMA syndrome)?
Third portion of the duodenum

What studies can be ordered to make the diagnosis of Wilkie syndrome (SMA syndrome)?
Barium upper gastrointestinal series; hypotonic duodenography; CT scan

What is the operative treatment of choice for patients with Wilkie syndrome refractory to conservative management?
Duodenojejunostomy

What organism is responsible for typhoid enteritis?
Salmonella typhosa

How is the diagnosis of typhoid fever confirmed?
Isolating *Salmonella typhosa* from blood, bone marrow, and stool cultures; finding of high titers of agglutinins against the O and H antigens

What is the usual treatment for uncomplicated typhoid enteritis?
Antibiotics (chloramphenicol, ampicillin, amoxicillin, trimethoprim-sulfamethoxazole)

Most common site of protozoal infection *(Cryptosporidium, Isospora, Microsporidium)* causing diarrhea in a patient with AIDS?
The small bowel

Most common site of intestinal involvement with *Mycobacterium tuberculosis:*
Distal ileum and cecum (85%–90%)

MULTIPLE CHOICE QUESTIONS

1. Stricturoplasty is indicated in a Crohn patient with:
   A. Fistula at the level of the stricture
   B. Intra-abdominal abscess
   C. Multiple areas of stenosis
   D. Multiple intestinal fistulas

2. How do adults with Meckel diverticulum usually present?
   A. Hemorrhage
   B. Perforation
   C. Meckel diverticulitis
   D. Obstruction

3. Which of the following forms of calcium supplementation should be administered to gastric bypass patients?
   A. Calcium citrate
   B. Calcium chloride
   C. Calcium oxide
   D. Calcium hydroxide

4. Which of the following is the FIRST to recover from postoperative ileus?

   A. Stomach
   B. Small intestine
   C. Colon
   D. The stomach, small intestine, and colon recover from ileus simultaneously

5. You perform exploratory surgery on a 35-year-old male for presumed appendicitis. The terminal ileum is identified and noted to be edematous, inflamed, and beefy red. The cecum and appendix are normal in appearance. What should you do?

   A. Abort the procedure and close
   B. Perform an ileocecectomy with end ileostomy
   C. Perform a right hemicolectomy
   D. Perform an appendectomy

6. Which of the following is the principal fuel used by the small intestine?

   A. Methionine
   B. Glycine
   C. Glutamine
   D. Melatonin
   E. Tyrosine

7. Which of the following statements regarding short gut syndrome is false?

   A. The diagnosis of short gut syndrome, the inability to absorb enough water and nutritional elements to be off TPN, is clinical
   B. In the absence of an ileocecal valve, the length of bowel generally needs to be 100 cm
   C. In the absence of an ileocecal valve, the length of bowel generally needs to be 75 cm
   D. In the presence of an ileocecal valve, the length of bowel generally needs to be 50 cm

8. A 55-year-old female undergoes liver resection for metastatic carcinoid tumor. Upon induction, she becomes flushed, tachycardic to HR = 120 bpm, and hypotensive with a systolic blood pressure of 70 mm Hg. Her end-tidal CO_2 is normal and she remains normothermic. What is the next best step in management?

   A. Abort the operation
   B. Administer dexamethasone
   C. Administer dantrolene
   D. Administer octreotide
   E. Administer benadryl

9. Which of the following is the strongest layer of the small intestine?

   A. Mucosa
   B. Submucosa
   C. Muscularis propria
   D. Serosa

10. An 80-year-old male on NSAIDs for arthritis presents with 6 hours of severe abdominal pain. He is hypotensive and tachycardic but stabilizes after 2 L of normal saline. He is subsequently diagnosed with a perforated duodenal ulcer. What operation would you perform?

A. Omental patch of the perforation
B. Close the perforation primarily
C. Perform a gastric resection encompassing the perforation
D. Repair the perforation and perform a truncal vagotomy
E. Repair the perforation and perform a highly selective vagotomy

ANSWERS

1. **Answer: C.** Indications for stricturoplasty include the maintenance of intestinal length after previous resection or the identification of single/multiple strictures in diffusely involved bowel.

   Contraindications include the presence of intestinal fistulas or intra-abdominal abscess.

   A Heineke-Mikulicz stricturoplasty can be performed for strictures <12 cm in length, a Finney stricturoplasty can be performed for strictures up to 25 cm in length, and a side-to-side isoperistaltic enteroenterostomy can be used for strictures up to 50 cm in length.

2. **Answer: D.** The most common presentation of Meckel diverticula in adults is intestinal obstruction. Obstruction from a Meckel diverticulum occurs in various ways such as intussusception with the diverticulum as the lead point, stricture from chronic diverticulitis, intestinal entrapment by a mesodiverticular band, and volvulus of the intestine around a fibrous band connecting the diverticulum to the umbilicus.

   The most common presentation of a Meckel diverticulum in children is bleeding.

3. **Answer: A.** Calcium citrate is the supplementation of choice for patients with low acid exposure.

4. **Answer: B.** Small intestine recovers within 24 hours after laparotomy, the stomach recovers by 48 hours, and the colon recovers within 3 to 5 days.

5. **Answer: D.** If the stump of the appendix is not involved by acute regional enteritis, most surgeons perform an appendectomy to eliminate appendicitis from the differential diagnosis should the patient develop right lower quadrant pain at a later date. In the absence of obstruction and fistula formation, the ileum should not be resected in the setting of acute regional enteritis.

6. **Answer: C.** The principal fuel utilized by the small intestine is glutamine.

7. **Answer: B.** In general, the length of bowel needs to be at least 75 cm in the absence of an ileocecal valve and 50 cm with an ileocecal valve to avoid TPN.

8. **Answer: D.** This patient is experiencing carcinoid crisis, which manifests with flushing, tachycardia, hypotension, and bronchospasm. Treatment consists of octreotide 50 to 100 pg administered as an IV bolus.

9. **Answer: B.** The submucosa consists of dense connective tissue and is the strongest layer of the small intestine.

10. **Answer: A.** The perforation is best closed with an omental patch (Graham patch). After surgery, the patient should be taken off of his NSAIDs and treated for *H. pylori*. A definitive operation should only be performed on a hemodynamically stable patient.

CHAPTER 20
Colorectal

Carlos Glanville, Anton Kelly, and Dale A. Dangleben

ANATOMY AND PHYSIOLOGY

Where does the hindgut begin and end?
Hindgut begins at distal third of the transverse colon and extends to the rectum

The hindgut relies on which artery for its blood supply?
Inferior mesenteric artery

What are the white lines of Toldt?
The lateral peritoneal reflections of the ascending and descending colon

What parts of the gastrointestinal (GI) tract do not have a serosa?
Esophagus, middle, and distal rectum

What are the major anatomic differences between the small bowel and colon?
The small bowel is smooth, whereas the colon has fat appendages (appendices epiploicae), haustra, and taenia coli

What is the arterial blood supply to the rectum?
Proximal: superior hemorrhoidal artery (superior rectal artery) from the inferior mesenteric artery
Middle: middle hemorrhoidal artery (middle rectal artery) from the hypogastric artery (internal iliac artery)
Distal: inferior hemorrhoidal artery (inferior rectal artery) from the pudendal artery, which is a branch of hypogastric artery (internal iliac artery)

What is the venous drainage of the rectum?
Proximal: inferior mesenteric vein that joins the splenic vein to drain into the portal vein
Middle: iliac vein into the inferior vena cava
Distal: iliac vein into inferior vena cava

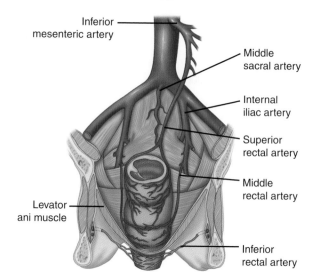

FIGURE 20-1. Arterial supply to the rectum and anal canal. *(Reproduced from Brunicardi FC, Andersen DK, Billiar TR, Dunn DL, Hunter JG, Matthews JB, Pollock RE. Schwartz Principles of Surgery. 9th ed. www.accessmedicine.com. Copyright © The McGraw-Hill Companies, Inc. All rights reserved.)*

What is the purpose of the colon?
Water, sodium, and bile salt absorption and stool storage

What is the main nutrient of a colonocyte?
Short-chain fatty acids (SCFA) (butyrate)

How long is the rectum?
12 to 15 cm

What are the approximate proximal and distal extents of the anal canal/rectum/rectosigmoid junction from the anal verge?
Anal canal: 0 to 5 cm
Rectum: 5 to 15 cm
Rectosigmoid junction: 15 to 18 cm

What 2 points are considered to mark the location of the rectosigmoid junction?
The distal point at which the taeniae converge at the level of the sacral promontory

What do anatomists consider the distal extent of the rectum versus what surgeons consider the distal extent of the rectum?
Anatomists: dentate line
Surgeons: proximal border of the anal sphincter complex

What is the eponym for the extension of the peritoneal cavity between the rectum and back wall of the uterus in the female human body?
Pouch of Douglas (Ehrhardt-Cole Recess/rectouterine excavation/rectouterine pouch)

What is the deepest point of the peritoneal cavity in women?
Pouch of Douglas

What is another name for the rectovesicular fascia in men/rectovaginal fascia in women?
Denonvilliers fascia

What is the eponym for a mass that forms in the pelvic cul-de-sac from a drop metastases from a visceral tumor that may be detected by a digital rectal examination?
Bloomer shelf

What is the thick condensation of endopelvic fascia that connects the presacral fascia to the fascia propria at the level of S4, which then extends to the anorectal ring called?
Waldeyer fascia (rectosacral fascia)

What artery is contained within the lateral rectal stalks?
The middle rectal artery

What muscles make up the pelvic floor (pelvic diaphragm)?
Pubococcygeus, iliococcygeus, puborectalis (which form the levator ani)

Where does the pelvic floor (pelvic diaphragm) lie?
Between the pubis, obturator fascia, sacrum, and ischial spines

What artery runs close to the bowel in the mesentery as part of a vascular arcade that connects the superior mesenteric artery and inferior mesenteric artery?
The marginal artery of Drummond

What artery found low in the mesentery, near the root, is part of a vascular arcade that connects the proximal middle colic artery to the proximal inferior mesenteric artery?
The arc of Riolan (meandering mesenteric artery)

What is the most proximal branch of the inferior mesenteric artery?
Left colic artery

Describe the venous drainage of the colon and rectum?
Right and proximal transverse colon drain into the superior mesenteric vein, which joins with the splenic vein to become the portal vein
Distal transverse colon, descending colon, sigmoid, and most of the rectum drain into the inferior mesenteric vein, which drains into the splenic vein that joins with the superior mesenteric vein to become the portal vein
Anal canal drains by way of the middle and inferior rectal veins into the internal iliac veins, which drain into the inferior vena cava

What nodal chain do lymphatics from the colon and proximal two-thirds of the rectum drain into?
Para-aortic nodal chain

What nodal chains do lymphatics from the distal rectum and anal canal drain into?
Para-aortic nodal chain or superficial inguinal nodal chain

What kind of neurologic injury after rectal surgery generally results in sympathetic dysfunction characterized by retrograde ejaculation and bladder dysfunction?
Severing of the hypogastric nerves near the sacral promontory

What kind of neurologic injury after rectal surgery generally results in impotence and atonic bladder?
Injury to the mixed parasympathetic and sympathetic periprostatic plexus

What is the most prevalent species of bacteria in the colon?
Bacteroides species

What is the most common aerobe in the colon?
Escherichia coli

In what colonic segment are bacteria the most metabolically active?
The cecum

How is diarrhea defined?
>3 loose stools/d

How is constipation defined?
<3 stools/wk

What are absolute contraindications to bowel preparation?
Complete bowel obstruction, free perforation

DIVERTICULITIS

How are the diverticula with colonic diverticulosis formed?
Mucosa herniates through the colon at sites of penetration of the muscular wall by arterioles on the side of the antimesenteric taeniae

What area of the colon is most commonly affected by diverticula?
Sigmoid colon (80%)

What segment of the colon has the smallest intraluminal diameter?
Sigmoid colon

What is the treatment for uncomplicated diverticulitis?
Antibiotics on an outpatient basis; if patient has significant pain (localized peritonitis), admit to the hospital and give intravenous (IV) antibiotics for ~48 hours

How should patients be followed after an episode of uncomplicated diverticulitis?
After symptoms have subsided for at least 3 weeks, a colonoscopic examination should be performed to establish the presence/location of the diverticula and to exclude cancer (mimic diverticulitis)

What is the approximate chance of a patient who recovered from an initial episode of uncomplicated diverticulitis developing a second attack of diverticulitis?
<25%

What is the estimated percentage of patients who recovered from an initial episode of uncomplicated diverticulitis requiring a subsequent emergency colectomy or colostomy?
~5%

Although controversial, what types of patients might you offer an elective sigmoid colectomy?
Young patients with an episode of diverticulitis (<45 years old), patients with 2 episodes of diverticulitis, and immunocompromised patients

What is the treatment for an abscess complicating diverticulitis?
The preferred treatment is computed tomography (CT) or ultrasound-guided percutaneous drainage or drainage of a pelvic abscess into the rectum through a transanal approach followed by elective surgery ~6 weeks after drainage of the abscess when the patient has completely recovered from the infection versus a more undesirable transabdominal approach by laparotomy

What are the 2 causes of generalized peritonitis resulting from diverticulitis?
A perforated diverticulum into the peritoneal cavity that is not sealed by the body's normal defenses; an initially localized abscess that expands and suddenly bursts into the peritoneal cavity

What procedure would you perform for generalized peritonitis from perforated diverticulitis?
A Hartmann procedure: resection of the diseased sigmoid colon; creation of a descending colostomy using noninflamed tissue; closure of the divided end of the rectum with suture/staples

What is the usual time period to wait before restoring intestinal continuity by reversing a Hartmann procedure for perforated diverticulitis?
At least 10 weeks (when patient has completely recovered from their illness)

What is the Hinchey classification grading system for diverticulitis?
Stage I Diverticulitis with associated pericolic abscess
Stage II Diverticulitis associated with distant abscess (retroperitoneal or pelvic)
Stage III Diverticulitis associated with purulent peritonitis
Stage IV Diverticulitis associated with fecal peritonitis

VOLVULUS

What is the most common colonic segment to be involved in a volvulus?
Sigmoid colon

What is the least common colonic segment to be involved in a volvulus?
Transverse colon

What is a cecal bascule?
The cecum folds anteromedial to the ascending colon from the presence of a constricting band across the ascending colon

What findings might you see on plain film, CT scan, and barium enema with a sigmoid volvulus?
Plain film: bent inner tube with apex in the right upper quadrant
CT scan: mesenteric whorl
Barium enema: bird's beak deformity

What is the treatment for sigmoid volvulus?
Appropriate resuscitation; decompression with placement of a soft rectal tube through the proctoscope past the twist of the volvulus and leaving the rectal tube in place
If a rectal tube cannot be passed, detorsion of the volvulus with a colonoscope
If unable to detorse volvulus by rectal tube or colonoscopy, perform Hartmann operation procedure
Confirm the reduction with an abdominal radiograph, attempt a full colonoscopic examination after cleansing the bowel with cathartics, perform an elective sigmoid colon resection

What is the recurrence rate for sigmoid volvulus without surgical intervention?
~50%

What is a cecal (cecocolic) volvulus?
An axial rotation of the terminal ileum, cecum, and ascending colon with concomitant twisting of the associated mesentery from a lack of fixation of the cecum to the retroperitoneum

What might you see on plain abdominal radiographs with a cecal volvulus?
A gas-filled comma shape with the concavity facing inferiorly and to the right (upside down comma sign), a circular shape with a narrow, triangular density pointing to the right and superiorly, a dilated cecum displaced to the left side of the abdomen

What is the treatment for a cecal volvulus?
The procedure of choice is a right colectomy with primary anastomosis; if frankly gangrenous bowel, resect right colon and create an ileostomy; cecopexy is another option (higher recurrence rates)

OBSTRUCTION

What is the most common cause of large intestinal obstruction in the United States?
Colorectal cancer

What is the most common cause of large intestinal obstruction in Russia, Eastern Europe, and Africa?
Colonic volvulus (high-fiber diets)

What is a closed loop obstruction?
An obstruction featuring the occlusion of the proximal and distal parts of the bowel

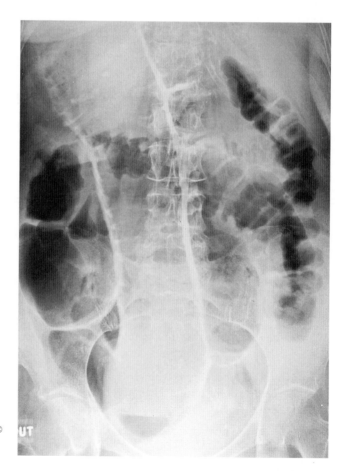

FIGURE 20-2. Acute colonic pseudo-obstruction, with a markedly dilated proximal colon; endoscopy confirmed no distal obstruction. *(Zinner MJ, Ashley SW. Maingot's Abdominal Operations. 11th ed. http://www.accesssurgery.com. Copyright © The McGraw-Hill Companies, Inc. All rights reserved.)*

What is pseudo-obstruction of the colon otherwise known as?
Ogilvie syndrome

What study should be performed in all stable patients with a suspected diagnosis of colonic pseudo-obstruction?
Water-soluble contrast enema can reliably differentiate between mechanical obstruction and pseudo-obstruction; can consider colonoscopy

What is the treatment for Ogilvie syndrome?
Initial treatment with nasogastric decompression, fluid replacement, correction electrolyte abnormalities, discontinuation of all medications that inhibit bowel motility, serial abdominal examinations and radiographs; consider administration of 2.5 mg of neostigmine given intravenously over 3 minutes after ruling out distal obstruction with water-soluble contrast enema or colonoscopy (do not give to patients with significant cardiac history and watch for bradycardia by monitoring patient with telemetry during administration of the drug with atropine immediately available); can consider colonoscopic decompression but high recurrence

What is the Law of Laplace?
Tension is directly proportional to increased pressure times radius. Stated differently, for a given pressure, increased radius requires increased wall thickness to accommodate a stable wall tension; also, increased pressure requires increased thickness to maintain a stable wall tension.
It is remembered by the following equation:
$T = \frac{1}{2} (P \times R)/t$
(T = wall tension, P = pressure, R = radius, T = wall thickness)
The law explains why the cecum, with its largest diameter, is the most common site of colonic rupture secondary to distal obstruction or increased pressure (eg, overzealous insufflations with excessive air during colonoscopy).

ULCERATIVE COLITIS

What layers of the bowel wall are affected by ulcerative colitis?
Mucosa and submucosa

What is the sine qua non of ulcerative colitis?
Rectal involvement (proctitis)

What diagnostic characteristics of ulcerative colitis help differentiate it from Crohn disease?
Continuous, uninterrupted inflammation of the colonic mucosa beginning in the distal rectum and extending proximally (Crohn disease features normal segments of colon [skipped areas] interspersed between distinct segments of colonic inflammation), ulcerative colitis does not involve the terminal ileum, except with backwash ileitis; ulcerative colitis affects the mucosa and submucosa where Crohn can have transmural involvement

What 3 features are suggestive of a malignant stricture in the setting of ulcerative colitis?
Stricture appears later in the course of ulcerative colitis; stricture is proximal to the splenic flexure and causes large bowel obstruction

What are the extraintestinal manifestations of ulcerative colitis?
Arthritis, ankylosing spondylitis, erythema nodosum, pyoderma gangrenosum, primary sclerosing cholangitis

What extraintestinal manifestation of ulcerative colitis does not improve with colectomy?
Primary sclerosing cholangitis, ankylosing spondylitis

What are the American Cancer Society guidelines regarding surveillance colonoscopy for ulcerative colitis patients?
Colonoscopy every 1 to 2 years beginning 8 years after the onset of pancolitis
12 to 15 years after the onset of left-sided colitis

What classes of drugs are used in the treatment of ulcerative colitis?
Aminosalicylates (sulfasalazine, mesalamine)
Corticosteroids (prednisone)
Immunosuppressive agents (azathioprine, cyclosporine)

What are indications for surgery in a patient with ulcerative colitis?
Dysplasia-carcinoma, longstanding disease, intractability, massive colonic bleeding, toxic megacolon (may consider surgery for malnutrition/growth retardation in pediatric/adolescent patients), persistent obstruction or stricture, perforation

What is the treatment for toxic megacolon?
Nasogastric decompression; IV hydration (with consideration given to IV hyperalimentation depending on length of illness before fulminant episode and patient's nutritional status); broad-spectrum IV antibiotics; high-dose IV steroids if patient is steroid-dependent; follow with serial abdominal exams and leukocyte counts, if deteriorates or if lack of improvement with medical therapy for 24–48 hours, perform an urgent procedure

What is the preferred operation for toxic megacolon?
Total abdominal colectomy with ileostomy and preservation of the rectum

What is the procedure of choice in a patient with massive hemorrhage from ulcerative colitis?
Subtotal colectomy; if severe bleeding from rectal mucosa, may also require emergency proctectomy

What are your options for elective surgery in patients with ulcerative colitis?
Total proctocolectomy with ileostomy; restorative proctocolectomy with ileal pouch anal anastomosis; total proctocolectomy with a continent ileal reservoir (Kock pouch)

CROHN DISEASE

What are indications for surgery in a patient with Crohn disease?

Cancer	Intractability
Fistula	Toxic megacolon
Fulminant colitis	Massive bleeding
Growth retardation	Intestinal obstruction
Intra-abdominal abscess	

What operation would you perform for massive bleeding from Crohn disease?
Abdominal colectomy and ileostomy versus ileorectal anastomosis if the rectum is not inflamed

INFECTIOUS AND ISCHEMIC COLITIS

What organisms should be evaluated for in a stool sample from a patient with suspected infectious colitis?
Campylobacter jejuni, Yersinia enterocolitica, Salmonella typhi, Clostridium difficile

What is the most common form of intestinal ischemia?
Colonic ischemia

What sign may be seen on radiographic imaging with intestinal wall edema or submucosal hemorrhage?
Thumb printing

Which colonic segment is the most prone to ischemia?
Splenic flexure and rectosigmoid junction (Griffith and Sudeck point)

What are indications for surgery with acute colonic ischemia?
Peritoneal signs, massive bleeding, universal fulminant colitis with or without toxic megacolon

LYNCH SYNDROMES (HEREDITARY NONPOLYPOSIS COLON CANCER)

What are the Amsterdam criteria for Hereditary Nonpolyposis Colorectal Cancer (HNPCC)?
"3,2,1"
At least 3 first-degree relatives with colon cancer and all of the following:
2 successive generations affected
At least 1 case of colon cancer diagnosed before age 50 years; familial adenomatous polyposis excluded

What is the difference between the Amsterdam criteria and the modified Amsterdam criteria?
The modified Amsterdam criteria is almost the same as the Amsterdam criteria, except that with the modified Amsterdam criteria the cancer must be associated with HNPCC (colon, endometrium, small bowel, ureter, renal pelvis) instead of specifically colon cancer

What are the screening recommendations for patients with HNPCC?
Colonoscopy at age 20 to 25 years and repeat every 1 to 3 years
Transvaginal ultrasound or endometrial aspirate at age 20 to 25 years and repeat annually

What is the mainstay of the diagnosis of HNPCC?
A detailed family history

What is the procedure of choice when colon cancer is detected in a patient with HNPCC?
Abdominal colectomy with ileorectal anastomosis
If the patient is female with no further plans for childbearing, prophylactic total abdominal hysterectomy and bilateral salpingo-oophorectomy are recommended

FAMILIAL ADENOMATOUS POLYPOSIS

What are the screening recommendations for patients with familial adenomatous polyposis(FAP)/Gardner syndrome?
Flexible proctosigmoidoscopy at age 10 to 12 years and repeat every 1 to 2 years until age 35, after age 35 repeat every 3 years
Upper GI endoscopy every 1 to 3 years starting when polyps are first identified

What is the most commonly recommended procedure for the treatment of FAP syndrome?
Restorative proctocolectomy with ileal pouch anal anastomosis with distal rectal mucosectomy
Alternative includes total abdominal colectomy with ileorectal anastomosis

What percentage of patients with the *adenomatous polyposis coli (APC)* mutation express the gene?
100%

Do you have to worry about duodenal and ampullary polyps found in a patient with FAP syndrome?
Yes, because the duodenal and ampullary polyps are usually neoplastic
All large polyps should be removed with endoscopic polypectomy, and pancreatoduodenectomy (Whipple procedure) is indicated with ampullary cancer discovered at an early stage

How many juvenile polyps need to be present to make the diagnosis of familial juvenile polyposis?
10 juvenile polyps

POLYPS AND COLON CANCER

What are the most common colonic polyps?
Hyperplastic polyps

Are hyperplastic polyps considered to have malignant potential?
No, but adenomatous changes can be found in hyperplastic polyps

What autosomal dominant syndrome is characterized by a combination of hamartomatous polyps of the intestinal tract and hyperpigmentation of the buccal mucosa, lips, and digits?
Peutz-Jeghers syndrome

T or F: patients with Peutz-Jeghers syndrome are not at increased risk for the development of cancer?
False; Peutz-Jeghers syndrome is associated with an increased risk for cancer throughout the intestinal tract, from the stomach to the rectum and extraintestinal malignancies (breast, ovary, cervix, fallopian tubes, thyroid, lung, gallbladder, bile ducts, pancreas, testicles)

What is the approximate lifetime risk of colon cancer in the general US population?
6%

The *APC* gene is located on what chromosome?
Chromosome 5q21

What kind of gene is the *APC* gene?
Tumor suppressor gene

What is the most frequently mutated tumor suppressor gene in human neoplasia?
p53

On what chromosome can p53 be found?
Chromosome 17p

On which chromosome can the ras proto-oncogene be found?
Chromosome 12

What do right-sided colon cancers tend to do?
Bleed

What do left-sided colon cancers tend to do?
Obstruct

What is the gold standard for establishing the diagnosis of colon cancer?
Colonoscopy

In patients with colon cancers causing a complete obstruction, what study can you order to establish the anatomic level of the obstruction when colonoscopy cannot be performed?
A water-soluble contrast enema

What is the treatment for an obstructing cancer of the proximal colon?
Right colectomy with primary anastomosis between the ileum and the transverse colon

What is the procedure of choice for a colon tumor involving the cecum, ascending colon, or the hepatic flexure?
Right hemicolectomy

What is the procedure of choice for most transverse colon tumors?
Extended right hemicolectomy

What is the procedure of choice for a descending colon tumor?
Left hemicolectomy

What is the procedure of choice for a sigmoid colon tumor?
Sigmoidectomy

When is abdominal colectomy for colon cancer indicated?
Patients with multiple primary tumors
Individuals with HNPCC
Occasionally for patients with completely obstructing sigmoid cancers

AJCC TNM STAGING

According to the AJCC TNM Staging System for Colorectal Cancer, what is a Tis lesion?
Carcinoma in situ: intraepithelial or invasion of lamina propria

According to the AJCC TNM Staging System for Colorectal Cancer, what is a T1 lesion?
Tumor invades submucosa

According to the AJCC TNM Staging System for Colorectal Cancer, what is a T2 lesion?
Tumor invades muscularis propria

According to the AJCC TNM Staging System for Colorectal Cancer, what is a T3 lesion?
Tumor invades through the muscularis propria into the subserosa, or into nonperitonealized pericolic or perirectal tissues

According to the AJCC TNM Staging System for Colorectal Cancer, what is a T4 lesion?
Tumor directly invades other organs or structures and/or perforates visceral peritoneum

According to the AJCC TNM Staging System for Colorectal Cancer, what is N0 nodal status?
No regional lymph node metastasis

According to the AJCC TNM Staging System for Colorectal Cancer, what is N1 nodal status?
Metastasis in 1 to 3 regional lymph nodes

According to the AJCC TNM Staging System for Colorectal Cancer, what is N2 nodal status?
Metastasis in 4 or more regional lymph nodes

According to the AJCC TNM Staging System for Colorectal Cancer, what does M0 mean?
No distant metastasis

According to the AJCC TNM Staging System for Colorectal Cancer, what does M1 mean?
Distant metastasis

According to the AJCC TNM Staging System for Colorectal Cancer, what is a stage 0 colon cancer?
Tis, N0, M0

According to the AJCC TNM Staging System for Colorectal Cancer, what is a stage I colon cancer?
T1, N0, M0; T2, N0, M0

According to the AJCC TNM Staging System for Colorectal Cancer, what is a stage IIA colon cancer?
T3, N0, M0

According to the AJCC TNM Staging System for Colorectal Cancer, what is a stage IIB colon cancer?
T4, N0, M0

According to the AJCC TNM Staging System for Colorectal Cancer, what is a stage IIIA colon cancer?
T1-2, N1, M0

According to the AJCC TNM Staging System for Colorectal Cancer, what is a stage IIIB colon cancer?
T3-4, N1, M0

According to the AJCC TNM Staging System for Colorectal Cancer, what is a stage IIIC colon cancer?
Any T, N2, M0

According to the AJCC TNM Staging System for Colorectal Cancer, what is a stage IV colon cancer?
Any T, Any N, M1

What is the 5-year survival rate for patients who undergo appropriate resection of a T stage 1 colon cancer?
~95%

What is the 5-year survival rate for a patient with stage II colon cancer treated by appropriate surgical resection?
~80%

What is the survival rate for stage III cancer treated by surgery alone?
~65%

What is the 5-year survival rate for a patient with colon cancer with distant metastatic disease (stage IV)?
<10%

What would you do if you found an isolated hepatic or pulmonary lesion while performing a right colectomy for colon cancer?
Attempt to resect the isolated hepatic/pulmonary metastasis

What stage of colon cancer shows a clear benefit with chemotherapy?
Stage III colon cancer

What is FOLFOX?
Oxaliplatin, 5-fluorouracil, leucovorin regimen

What is Xeloda?
Capecitabine (an oral fluoropyrimidine)

What is bevacizumab (Avastin)?
A monoclonal antibody that is a vascular endothelial growth factor inhibitor

What is cetuximab (Erbitux)?
A monoclonal antibody that binds to and inhibits the epidermal growth factor receptor (EGFR)

What percentage of colon cancer recurrences is detected within 2 years of the time of resection?
~85%

MULTIPLE CHOICE QUESTIONS

1. **Risk factors associated with colorectal cancer include which one of the following?**
   A. Irritable bowel syndrome
   B. Low intake of dietary fiber
   C. Low intake of red meat
   D. Chronic aspirin therapy

2. **Surgery for liver metastases from colorectal cancer is:**
   A. Associated with a 10% mortality
   B. Contraindicated if more than 1 lesion is present

C. Associated with 16% to 40% 5-year survival

D. Usually followed with consolidation radiotherapy

3. **Bevacizumab**

A. Is a monoclonal antibody that targets vascular endothelial growth factor (VEGF)

B. Is a monoclonal antibody that targets EGFR

C. Has no proven survival benefit in the metastatic setting

D. Is standard treatment for metastatic colorectal cancer in the UK

4. **True about ulcerative colitis with malignancy**

A. It has a better prognosis

B. Is related to disease activity

C. Is related to duration of ulcerative colitis

D. Malignancy is more in anorectal ulcerative colitis

5. **Which of the following is false about the physiology of colon?**

A. Colectomy increases Na requirement by 80 to 100 mEq/d

B. SCFA are produced by bacteria from sugar

C. SCFA have nutrient value for colonocytes

D. Motility of colon is 8 to 12 cm/h

E. Colon absorbs Na and water

6. **What is the second most common cause of death in patients with FAP?**

A. Adenocarcinoma of the colon

B. Adenocarcinoma of the stomach

C. Desmoid tumors

D. Adenocarcinoma of the ovaries

E. Adenocarcinoma of the duodenum

7. **What is the most common site of involvement in patients with Crohn disease?**

A. Stomach

B. Isolated small bowel

C. Ileocecal

D. Colon

E. Anus

8. **Which of the following is not considered a tenet of colonic cancer resection?**

A. Proximal and distal resection margins of 5 cm

B. High ligation of the mesentery and vascular structures

C. Negative radial margins of resection

D. Sentinel lymph node assessment prior to mesenteric resection

E. Greater than 12 lymph nodes in the resected specimen

9. **Which of the following patients is at an average risk of colorectal cancer?**

A. 45-year-old female with an aunt and cousin with colorectal cancer

B. 35-year-old female with ulcerative colitis diagnosed at age 25

C. 75-year-old male with a history of recurrent diverticulitis

D. 60-year-old male whose grandfather was diagnosed with colon cancer at age 60

E. 25-year-old male whose older brother had hundreds of polyps on colonoscopy

10. **Which of the following statements regarding *C difficile* colitis is NOT true?**
    A. Endoscopy may demonstrate pseudomembranes on colonoscopy
    B. PO vancomycin is a therapeutic option
    C. IV or PO metronidazole is a therapeutic option
    D. Gel or foam hand cleansing is indicated after contact with a *C difficile*–positive patient
    E. Symptoms are caused by the toxin released with bacterial overgrowth

ANSWERS

1. **Answer: B.** Inflammatory bowel disease is associated with an increased risk of colorectal cancer, but there is no association with irritable bowel syndrome. Other factors associated with increased risk are a low intake of dietary fiber and a high intake of red meat. Risk has been shown to be reduced by regular ingestion of aspirin.

2. **Answer: C.** Surgery for liver metastases from colorectal cancer is associated with a 2% mortality, can be performed if more than 1 lesion is present, and is associated with 16% to 40% 5-year survival. Radiotherapy is not used for liver metastases, as the toxicity to normal liver tissue would be too severe.

3. **Answer: A.** Bevacizumab is a monoclonal antibody that targets VEGF. It has been shown to improve survival in the metastatic setting when used in combination with chemotherapy.

4. **Answer: C.** Carcinoma of the colon afflicts patients with ulcerative colitis 7 to 30 times more frequently than it does the general population.

   The risk of colon cancer in ulcerative colitis is related to 2 factors:

   (1) Duration of the colitis, and (2) extent of colonic involvement. The risk of colon cancer for patients who have had the disease less than 10 years is low, but this risk steadily increases. The cancer risk for patients who have had disease activity for 10 to 20 years is 23 times that of the general population, while disease duration of more than 20 years is associated with a cancer risk 32 times greater than that of the general population. The extent of colonic involvement in colitis also influences the risk of cancer. The incidence of cancer when ulcerative colitis is limited to the rectum or to the left side of the colon is much lower than when ulcerative colitis involves the entire colon.

   The colonic malignancy associated with ulcerative colitis is generally an adenocarcinoma evenly scattered throughout the colon. The adenocarcinoma is often flatter than cancers in the general population and has fewer overhanging margins. It is generally considered extremely aggressive.

5. **Answer: D.** In the proximal colon bacteria ferments organic carbohydrates to SCFA acetate, propionate, butyrate. These SCFA augment Na, Cl, and water absorption and are the fuel for colonocytes. They also regulate proliferation, differentiation gene expression, and immune function in colon.

   Three types of electrical activity in colonic circular smooth muscle are slow wave, 2 to 4/min; membranous potential oscillations (MPO), 18/min; action potential superimposed on slow waves and MPO

   In humans colonic motor activity varies from quiescence to isolated contractions, bursts of contractions, and propagated contractions

   The predominant is irregular contractions

Propagated contractions are low (5–40 mm Hg) and high (75 mm Hg)

High propagated contractions occuring 6 times/d originating in cecum, responsible for mass movement, occur more while awake and after meals

6. **Answer: E.** Colonic adenocarcinoma is the primary cause of death in patients with FAP. If colectomy is not performed, 100% of these patients will progress to cancer of the colon. The second most common cause of death is duodenal adenocarcinoma. These patients develop periampullary and duodenal adenomatous polyps, which present 10 to 15 years after the colonic polyps and will also progress to adenocarcinoma. Surveillance endoscopy is required every 1 to 3 years to excise or fulgurate these polyps. The third most common cause of death in FAP patients is development of desmoid tumors, which can locally expand and involve mesenteric, vascular, or urologic structures, making surgery difficult or impossible.

7. **Answer: C.** Ileocecal Crohn represents the most common site of presentation, occurring in ~40% to 50% of patients. This is followed by colonic disease (which can occur in any segment of the colon) in ~30% of patients. Crohn disease isolated to the small bowel (not including terminal ileum) occurs in approximately another 30%. Oral, gastric, and duodenal diseases are thought to be histologically present in 20% to 40% of patients, but are only symptomatic in about 4%. Perianal involvement occurs in ~15% of patients and presents as abscesses and fistulas.

8. **Answer: D.** Studies have shown that the extent of mural spread from colon cancer is approximately 2 cm. These findings have led to the convention that 5 cm are appropriate proximal and distal margins for colon cancer resection. In patients with mid-to-low rectal cancers, a 2-cm distal margin is considered acceptable if it results in sphincter preservation. High ligation of the main feeding vascular pedicle and mesentery is done because this is the drainage pattern for venous and lymphatic flow from the tumor. Negative radial margins are required to prevent local recurrence of cancer. This means that involved structures should be resected en-bloc if possible. Twelve lymph nodes within a specimen are considered the appropriate number to allow adequate pathologic staging of a tumor. Sentinel lymph node assessment and/or biopsy in colorectal cancer have not been adopted as standard of care.

9. **Answer: C.** Screening and surveillance for colorectal cancer is based on a patient's risk factors. A personal history of adenomas or colorectal cancer, a family history of adenomas or colorectal cancer in 1 first-degree relative or 2 second-degree relatives, hereditary colon cancer syndromes, or IBD places a person at increased risk. Age by itself and diverticulitis do not increase the risk of colorectal cancer above that of the average population. Actual screening and surveillance recommendations vary by organization and have been put forth by the US Preventive Task Force, the NCCN, and the American College of Gastroenterology among others.

10. **Answer: D.** Pseudomembranous plaques are the classic colonoscopic findings in *C difficile* colitis, although inflammation or even normal mucosa can be seen. Patients may present with a variety of clinical signs and symptoms including but not limited to abdominal pain, diarrhea, or sepsis after even a single dose of antibiotics, and a high clinical suspicion is necessary. Clindamycin and cephalosporins are common culprits. Treatment options include IV and oral metronidazole, oral vancomycin, and vancomycin enemas. Gels and foams are NOT sufficient for hand cleansing after coming in contact with *C difficile* spores. Washing the hands with soap and water for at least 60 seconds is necessary and rooms and objects must be disinfected with bleach.

CHAPTER 21
Trauma

Dale A. Dangleben, Rovinder Sandhu, and Firas Madbak

INITIAL MANAGEMENT

When does the first mortality peak for trauma occur?
Within seconds to minutes after injury

The trauma system and acute patient care has the greatest impact on patients in which mortality peak for trauma?
Second mortality peak (golden hour)

Most of the deaths during the second mortality peak for trauma occur from?
Hemorrhage, central nervous system injuries

When does the third mortality peak for trauma occur?
24 hours after injury, from multisystem organ failure and sepsis

How long should the primary survey in the initial evaluation of a trauma patient take?
No more than 5 minutes, unless an intervention is needed.

What mnemonic is used to conduct the primary survey?
ABCDE: Airway, Breathing, Circulation, Disability, Exposure

What are the goals during airway assessment?
Secure the airway, protect the spinal cord

What is required for spinal immobilization?
A rigid cervical collar, use of a full backboard

Contraindications to nasotracheal intubation:
Apnea, maxillofacial fracture

What is the quickest way to test for an adequate airway in an awake, alert patient?
Ask a question, if the patient is able to speak the airway is intact.

Indications for a surgical airway:
Anatomic distortion as a result of neck injury, massive maxillofacial trauma, inability to visualize the vocal cords (blood, secretions, airway edema)

What are the goals during the breathing assessment?
Secure oxygenation and ventilation; treat life-threatening thoracic injuries

What should be done on physical examination to adequately assess breathing?
Inspection (air movement, cyanosis, tracheal shift, JVD, respiratory rate, asymmetric chest expansion, open chest wounds, use of accessory muscles of respiration)
Auscultation/ percussion (hyperresonance or dullness over lung fields)
Palpation (flail segments, subcutaneous emphysema)

What life-threatening conditions must be treated during the breathing assessment if encountered?
Open pneumothorax, tension pneumothorax, massive hemothorax

What is the most common cause for upper airway obstruction?
The tongue

What is the preferred emergency airway procedure?
Cricothyroidotomy

In a patient with poor peripheral upper extremity access, what alternative routes can be considered for intravenous access?
Femoral vein at the groin, venous cutdown on greater saphenous vein at the ankle, subclavian vein, IJ

What are the goals of the circulation assessment?
Treatment of bleeding, assuring adequate tissue perfusion

What is the initial test for adequate circulation?
Palpation of pulses

What systolic blood pressure are you expecting with a palpable radial pulse?
80 mm Hg

What systolic blood pressure are you expecting with a palpable femoral/carotid pulse?
At least 60 mm Hg

What should be done of physical examination to adequately assess circulation?
Obtain heart rate and blood pressure; check peripheral perfusion and capillary refill, mental status; examine the skin

Which patients may not demonstrate tachycardia with hypovolemic shock?
Patients on beta-blockers, well-conditioned athletes, patients with concomitant spinal cord injury

During femoral catheter placement, what is the pneumonic used to remember the anatomy of the groin?
NAVEL (from lateral to medial): Nerve, Artery, Vein, Extralymphatic space, Lymphatics

What is the preferred alternative route if intravenous access cannot be obtained on a small child?
Intraosseous tibial plateau

What are the goals of the disability assessment?
Determination of neurologic injury

What should be performed during the physical examination for an adequate assessment of disability?
Mental status (GCS), pupils for size, appearance, and reactivity, motor/sensory examination for lateralizing extremity movement and sensory deficits

What are the goals during the exposure portion of the primary survey?
Completely disrobe patient and thoroughly inspect and evaluate the patient; keep patient in warm environment.

What 3 elements are measured with the GCS?
Eye opening, best verbal response, best motor response

What does a GCS score with a T signify?
Patient is intubated

What is the highest GCS an intubated patient can have?
4 (eye) + 1 (verbal) + 6 (movement) = 11, GCS 11t

What is the secondary survey?
A complete physical examination, obtain labs and x-rays, place additional lines, tube (foley, ngt), and monitoring devices

When should the tertiary examination be performed?
Another complete head-to-toe physical examination should be performed 12 to 24 hours after the initial trauma and should be aimed at identifying injuries missed during the primary and secondary surveys.

NEURO/SPINE

What are the typical signs of a basilar skull fracture?
Raccoon eyes, Battle sign, clear otorrhea or rhinorrhea, hemotympanum

What is the "halo" sign?
A halo of clear fluid around drainage from nose and ears, representing basilar skull fracture with CSF leakage.

What conditions must be present before a cervical spine can be cleared by physical examination?
No neck pain on palpation or full range of motion without neurologic injury, no ethanol/drug intoxication, no distracting injury, no pain medications

What vertebral bodies must be seen on lateral cervical spine film for adequate evaluation?
C1 to T1

What view on x-ray can help visualize C7 to T1?
Swimmer view

What imaging studies evaluate cervical spine ligamentous injury?
Lateral flexion and extension c-spine films, MRI of c-spine

What is primary brain injury?
Anatomic and physiologic disruption that occurs as a direct result of external trauma

What are the most significant factors leading to poor neurologic outcome or death in patients with traumatic brain injury?
Hypotension and hypoxemia, which can lead to secondary brain injury

What is the Monro-Kellie doctrine?
The doctrine states that the volume inside the cranium is a fixed volume and that the cranial compartment is incompressible.
Blood, CSF, and brain are in a state of volume equilibrium and any increase in volume of one of the cranial constituents is compensated for by a decrease in the volume of another.

How do you calculate the cerebral perfusion pressure (CPP)?
Mean arterial pressure (MAP) — Intracranial pressure (ICP)

What signs of elevated ICP can be seen on imaging studies?
Decrease in ventricular size, loss of sulci, loss of cisterns, midline shift, herniation

Indications for ICP monitoring:
GCS <8
Patient with moderate to severe head injury and inability to follow clinical examination
Suspicion of elevated ICP

What is the normal ICP?
10

What ICP requires treatment?
20

What CPP is desired in a head injured patient?
CPP >60

How is serum osmolarity adjusted in head injured patients?
3% NSS or Mannitol

When do the peak ICPs occur after injury?
48 to 72 hours after injury

What does a unilateral dilated pupil in a head injured patient signify?
Uncal herniation with compression of cranial nerve III

What GCS score indicates moderate head injury?
9> GCS <12

What GCS score indicates severe head injury?
GCS <8

Which component of the GCS is the most predictive of serious anatomic injury to the brain and correlates most strongly with outcome?
The motor component

What does a score of 0 on assessment of motor strength signify?
No contraction of muscle

What does a score of 1 on assessment of motor strength signify?
Palpable muscle contraction without limb movement

What does a score of 2 on assessment of motor strength signify?
Able to move in a gravity-neutral plane

What does a score of 3 on assessment of motor strength signify?
Able to move against gravity

What does a score of 4 on assessment of motor strength signify?
Diminished strength

What does a score of 5 on assessment of motor strength signify?
Normal strength

Table 21-1 Motor Examination	
C5 nerve root	Shoulder abduction (Deltoid)
C6 nerve root	Elbow flexion (Biceps)
C7 nerve root	Elbow extension (Triceps)
C8 nerve root	Wrist flexion (Flexor carpi ulnaris)
T1 nerve root	Finger abduction (Lumbricales)
L2 nerve root	Hip flexion (Iliopsoas)
L3 nerve root	Knee extension (Quadriceps)
L4 nerve root	Ankle dorsiflexion (Tibialis anterior)
L5-S1 nerve root	Great toe extension (Extensor hallucis longus)
S1 nerve root	Ankle plantar flexion (Gastrocnemius)
Sensory Assessment	
C2 nerve root	Occipital region
C3 nerve root	Supraclavicular region, near the head of the clavicle
C4 nerve root	Top of the shoulder, near the acromion
C5 nerve root	Lateral aspect of the arm, just above the elbow
C6 nerve root	Dorsum of the thumb
C7 nerve root	Dorsum of the middle finger
C8 nerve root	Dorsum of the little finger
T1 nerve root	Medial aspect of the arm, just above the elbow
T2 nerve root	Axilla
T4 nerve root	Thorax at the level of the nipples
T10 nerve root	Abdomen at the level of the umbilicus
L1 nerve root	Region of the femoral pulse
L2 nerve root	Medial aspect of the thigh, mid-femur
L3 nerve root	Medial aspect of the knee
L4 nerve root	Medial aspect of the leg, above the medial malleolus
L5 nerve root	Dorsum of the great toe
S1 nerve root	Lateral aspect of the heel
S2 nerve root	Popliteal fossa
S3 nerve root	Medial gluteal region
S4-5 nerve root	Perianal region

What artery is usually responsible for an epidural hematoma?
Middle meningeal artery

What kind of deformity is seen on CT head with an epidural hematoma?
Lenticular (lens-shaped) deformity

What kind of head injury is associated with a lucid interval?
Epidural hematoma

How many mm of shift on CT head is considered significant mass effect?
5 mm

How does a subdural hematoma most commonly occur?
Bridging veins between the dura and arachnoid are torn

What kind of deformity is seen on CT head with a subdural hematoma?
Crescent-shaped deformity

What are indications for drainage of a chronic subdural hematoma?
Significant symptoms, large size

Where do intracerebral hematomas usually occur?
Frontal or temporal lobes

What is the most common site of facial nerve injury with a temporal skull fracture?
Geniculate ganglion

Indications for operative intervention in a patient with skull fracture:
Significant depression (8–10 mm), contaminated, persistent CSF leak not responding to conservative management

What is central cord syndrome?
Hyperflexion or hyperextension of the neck leads to interference with blood flow in the spinal arteries leading to motor weakness and sensory loss primarily affecting the distal muscles of the upper extremities.

What is Brown-Séquard syndrome?
Partial transection of the spinal cord, which results in loss of ipsilateral motor function and loss of contralateral sensory function.

What are the 3 columns of the spinal column?
Anterior spinal ligament/anterior walls of the vertebral bodies, posterior spinal ligament/posterior walls of the vertebral bodies, posterior elements of the vertebral column (facet joints, lamina, spinous processes, interspinous ligaments)

How many columns need to be involved for a spinal column injury to be considered unstable?
≥2 columns

How are stable spinal column injuries treated?
Immobilization (collar for cervical spine, molded jacket for thoracic and lumbar spine)

How are unstable spinal column injuries treated?
Surgical stabilization (placement of hardware posteriorly, use of hardware and bone grafting anteriorly, both techniques simultaneously (3-column injury)

If you were going to give steroids to treat a spinal cord injury, what drug, dose, and schedule should be used?
If within a few hours of injury: bolus with 30 mg/kg of methylprednisolone over a 1-hour period, followed by 5.4 mg/kg/h for next 23 hours.
If injury is greater than 3 hours old but less than 8 hours old continue the steroids for a total of 48 hours—controversial and no longer recommended by ATLS.

What is the eponym for a C1 burst fracture?
Jefferson fracture

What is a type I odontoid fracture?
A stable fracture that occurs above the base

What is a type II odontoid fracture?
An unstable fracture that involves the base that is treated with immobilization or fusion

What is a type III odontoid fracture?
Fracture extends into the vertebral body that is treated with immobilization or fusion

What is known as SCIWORA?
Spinal Cord Injury Without Radiologic Abnormality—usually transient motor/sensory symptoms attributable to spinal cord distribution but without injury noted by x-ray, CT scan, or MRI.

What study should be obtained in patients without bony injury to the spine with neurologic deficits?
MRI, look for ligamentous injury

HEAD AND NECK

What is the #1 indicator of mandibular injury?
Malocclusion

What injury is not to be missed during examination of nose?
Septal hematoma

Where are the major vascular and aerodigestive structures in the neck, in the anterior triangle or the posterior triangle?
Anterior triangle

Which zone of the neck extends from the sternal notch to the cricoid cartilage?
Zone I

Which zone of the neck extends from the cricoid cartilage to the angle of the mandible?
Zone II

Which zone of the neck extends from the angle of the mandible to the base of the skull?
Zone III

What are the clinical indications for neck exploration with neck trauma?
Airway: dysphonia/voice changes, hemoptysis, hoarseness, stridor, subcutaneous air
Digestive tract: blood in oropharynx, dysphagia/odynophagia, subcutaneous air
Neurologic: altered state of consciousness not caused by head injury, lateralized neurologic deficit consistent with injury
Vascular: diminished carotid pulse, expanding hematoma, external hemorrhage

What is the most commonly injured vascular structure in the neck?
Internal jugular vein

How should you treat an actively bleeding unstable patient with a penetrating neck injury?
Take immediately to operating room for neck exploration

How would you manage an asymptomatic patient with a penetrating injury to the base of the neck (zone I)?
CT neck/chest or 4-vessel arch angiography; bronchoscopy; rigid esophagoscopy; barium swallow

How would you manage an asymptomatic patient with a penetrating midcervical injury (zone II)?
Neck exploration
An acceptable alternative is 4-vessel angiography, bronchoscopy, esophagoscopy, and barium swallow.

How would you manage an asymptomatic patient with a penetrating injury above the angle of the mandible (zone III)?
CT neck, 4-vessel arch angiography, laryngoscopy, rigid esophagoscopy, barium swallow

In a patient with an expanding neck hematoma, how do you perform a safe exploration of an anatomically hostile neck?
Follow the "trail of safety": make a standard cervical incision along the anterior border of the sternocleidomastoid muscle, divide the platysma, identify the anterior border of the sternocleidomastoid muscle (first key structure), dissect and identify the internal jugular vein (second key structure), dissect along the anterior border of the internal jugular vein until you find the facial vein (marks the carotid bifurcation), ligate and divide the facial vein to gain access to the carotid bifurcation.

During a neck exploration for neck trauma, you encounter an injury to the internal carotid artery, how would you repair the artery?
Debridement and primary repair if possible.
If primary repair not possible because of loss of length perform a bypass with a short interposition graft (PTFE).

What would you do if during neck exploration for trauma you encountered a major injury to the left common carotid artery with uncontrollable hemorrhage making repair technically impossible?
Ligate the common carotid artery (same goes for internal carotid and external carotid arteries), approximately 50% stroke rate, high mortality.

What methods have been described to control bleeding from the distal stump of an injured internal carotid artery at the base of the neck?
Interventional angiography, place balloon catheter through the missile tract and tamponade bleeding, ligate and divide the internal carotid artery at the carotid bifurcation, and remove the balloon 3 days later, insert a balloon catheter into the distal stump of the internal carotid, and clip and cut the catheter, leaving the balloon inside the artery.

What would you do if during a neck exploration for trauma, you encountered hemorrhage emanating from a hole between the transverse processes of the cervical vertebrae, posterolateral to the carotid sheath?
Tightly fill the bleeding hole in the transverse process with bone wax.

What are the typical mechanisms for blunt traumatic injury to the carotid/vertebral arteries?
Direct blow to neck, hyperextension with contralateral neck rotation

What is the clinical hallmark of blunt carotid artery injury?
Hemispheric neurologic deficit that is incompatible with CT findings

What is the treatment of blunt carotid/vertebral artery injury?
Antiplatelet agents for low-grade injuries.
Systemic anticoagulation for higher-grade injuries (if not prohibited by associated injuries).
Consider endovascular techniques for inaccessible pseudoaneurysm or hemodynamically significant dissection or inaccessible pseudoaneurysm but controversial.

What percentage of asymptomatic minimal arterial injuries (small false aneurysms, and small arteriovenous fistulas, nonocclusive intimal flaps, segmental arterial narrowing) progress to require surgical or endovascular repair?
~10%

How should initial control of hemorrhage be obtained?
Direct pressure over bleeding site with digital or manual compression

Under what 3 clinical situations can a temporary intraluminal shunt be used to maintain distal perfusion through an injured artery?
Situations where skeletal alignment is accomplished before vascular repair in an ischemic limb in a patient with combined vascular and orthopedic extremity injuries.
Transport of a patient from the field/remote facility with a peripheral arterial injury for vascular reconstruction at a trauma center.
Damage control technique in a critically injured patient unlikely to survive a complex repair because of exhausted physiologic reserve.

Using damage control techniques for vascular injuries, how is hemorrhage control and distal perfusion maintained?
Hemorrhage is controlled with balloon tamponade or ligation.
Distal perfusion is maintained with temporary intra-arterial shunt.

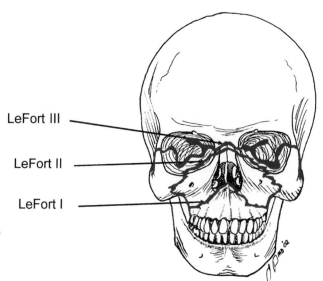

LeFort III

LeFort II

LeFort I

FIGURE 21-2. LeFort classification of maxillary fractures. *(Reproduced from Feliciano DV, Mattox KL, Moore EE. Trauma. 6th ed. http://accesssurgery.com. Copyright © The McGraw-Hill Companies, Inc. All rights reserved.)*

How would you repair a simple laceration to the trachea?
Debridement and primary repair with absorbable suture.
If loss of more than 2 tracheal rings, may require tracheostomy/complex reconstructive procedures.

How would you repair a laryngeal injury?
Closure of mucosal lacerations and reduction of cartilaginous fractures

How would you manage a facial fracture with significant hemorrhage?
Secure the airway, obtain initial control with anterior and posterior nasal packing and direct packing of the oropharynx, then proceed to angiography and selective embolization versus ligation of external carotid artery.

When should sutures be removed from the face to prevent cross-hatching of the scar?
~3 days

What elements should be obtained with a functional eye examination?
Visual acuity; pupillary response; assessment of extraocular eye movements, globe pressure (palpation or tonopen)

What procedure is performed if high intraocular pressure due to retrobulbar hematoma?
Lateral canthotomy

CHEST

What is the major morbidity and mortality associated with esophageal injuries?
Delay in diagnosis

Describe how you would repair a traumatic esophageal perforation found in the upper two-thirds of the esophagus <24 hours old?
Perform right thoracotomy, debride nonviable tissue, perform myotomy to define extent of mucosal injury, close in 2 layers over a nasogastric tube, cover repair with tissue flap

(pleural/pericardial/intercostal muscle), place a chest tube (consider J tube), keep patient NPO and on TPN or feeds through J tube, and on IV antibiotics.

Describe how you would repair a traumatic esophageal perforation found in the lower one-third of the esophagus <24 hours old?
Perform left thoracotomy, debride nonviable tissue, perform myotomy to define extent of mucosal injury, close in 2 layers over a nasogastric tube, cover repair with Thal patch/diaphragm/or fundoplication, place a chest tube (consider J tube), keep patient NPO and on TPN or feeds through J tube, and on IV antibiotics.

How you would manage a traumatic esophageal perforation in an unstable patient >24 hours old?
Wide debridement and exclusion with cervical esophagostomy, wide drainage, possible T-tube in perforation, make patient NPO, feed with TPN or J tube feeds, continue antibiotics, high mortality.

What are the most frequent injuries leading to mortality after motor vehicle accident?
Blunt cardiac injuries with chamber disruption, injuries to the thoracic aorta

Most frequent injury after blunt thoracic trauma:
Chest wall trauma

Describe where to place a chest tube:
The fifth or sixth intercostal space in the midaxillary line

General criteria for chest tube removal:
Absence of air leak, <100 mL of fluid drainage over a 24-hour period

In regards to penetrating trauma, what are the borders of the "box"?
Clavicles, xiphoid process, nipples

What injury must be ruled out in a penetrating "box" injury?
Pericardial tamponade—cardiac injury

Indications for emergency thoracotomy after blunt chest trauma:
Witnessed cardiac arrest (resuscitative thoracotomy), massive hemothorax (>1500 mL blood immediately after chest tube insertion or >200–300 mL/h after initial drainage)

What is the usual primary clinical manifestation after rib fracture?
Pain on inspiration

How should you control the pain from rib fracture?
Attempted control initially with oral or IV analgesics, consider intercostal nerve blocks with bupivacaine versus epidural analgesia

What is a flail chest?
Two or more fractures in 3 or more consecutive ribs that causes instability of the chest wall

What are the most important components in the pathophysiology of the respiratory failure associated with flail chest?
Underlying pulmonary contusion, pain during inspiration—leading to progressive atelectasis

Treatment for a sternal fracture:
Conservative
If significant chest wall instability/debilitating chest pain, open reduction and internal fixation

What is a pulmonary contusion?
Hemorrhage and edema of the lung parenchyma in the absence of parenchymal disruption

Most common complication of a pulmonary contusion:
Pneumonia

What clinical findings are suggestive of a pneumothorax?
Decreased breath sounds, decreased expansion of the affected lung during inspiration, hyperresonance to percussion

Clinical signs and symptoms of a tension pneumothorax:
Diaphoresis, dyspnea, distended neck veins, hypotension, tachypnea

How is a tension pneumothorax diagnosed?
Clinically

Treatment for a tension pneumothorax:
Chest decompression with a large-bore needle inserted in the second intercostal space, midclavicular line with subsequent tube thoracostomy (test answer)
If you are a surgical resident/surgeon perform immediate tube thoracostomy (hard to get needle into pleural space, especially in the obese)

What is an open pneumothorax?
A large defect in the chest wall (> laryngeal cross-sectional area) allows external air to enter into the pleural cavity resulting in lung collapse from rapid equilibration between intrathoracic (pleural) and atmospheric pressures.

Treatment for an open pneumothorax:
Treat initially by sealing the defect with petroleum gauze and leave 1 side of the gauze unsecured to allow escape of air under pressure then perform a tube thoracostomy. Operative repair of the chest wall defect can be performed after other life-threatening injuries are addressed.

How many liters of blood can the pleural space accumulate?
3 L blood

Treatment options for massive hemorrhage from an extensive lung injury:
Attempt oversewing or stapling of the wound.
If initial measures fail, consider performing wedge or lobar resection.
Pneumonectomy is a last resort.

What is hemodynamic consequence on traumatic pneumonectomy?
Acute right heart failure

How would you manage hemorrhage from a gunshot wound causing through-and-through injury to the lung?
Tractotomy (opening up the missile trajectory by making a communication between the entrance and exit wounds), anatomic resection is also an option.

What injury might you suspect if a trauma patient is noted to have continuous flow of air from his chest tube with inability to adequately ventilate, oxygenate, or re-expand his lung?
Major tracheobronchial injury

How would you manage the chest tube in a patient with a major tracheobronchial injury? Why?
Disconnect the suction apparatus on the collection system and leave the tube to water seal; minimizes air leak and allows egress of air under pressure

Treatment for a minor tracheobronchial injury:
Perform bronchoscopy (before intubation if possible), place an endotracheal tube (ET) beyond the injury; if endotracheal intubation not possible, perform a tracheostomy

How would you treat a tracheobronchial injury > one-third the circumference of the airway?
Perform bronchoscopy to determine site of injury and appropriate operative approach, selectively intubate the contralateral bronchus, make a posterolateral thoracotomy on the affected side and primarily repair.

Which chamber of the heart is most commonly ruptured with blunt chest trauma?
Right ventricle (close to sternum)

Time period for a patient with blunt cardiac injury will develop a complication:
Within 24 hours (if abnormal ECG: admit for 24 hours; if normal EKG: discharge)

What tests can rule out significant blunt cardiac injury?
ECG and serum troponin I levels at admission and 8 hours after injury
If normal at both time points, the patient can be safely discharged

What is the most frequent arrhythmia seen on ECG with blunt cardiac injury?
Sinus tachycardia

What is cardiac tamponade?
Bleeding into the pericardial sac with subsequent constriction of the heart, which results in decreased inflow and decreased cardiac output

What are the signs/symptoms of cardiac tamponade?
Tachycardia and shock with Beck triad
Kussmaul sign, pulsus paradoxus

What is Beck triad?
Muffled heart tones, distended neck veins, and hypotension

How does the blood from pericardiocentesis differ from blood drawn from a peripheral artery/vein?
Blood from pericardiocentesis does not form clot

What is Kussmaul sign?
JVD with inspiration

Treatment for cardiac tamponade:
Immediate IV fluid bolus and pericardiocentesis, followed by surgical exploration

What various methods are used to control hemorrhage with a penetrating cardiac injury?
Skin staples for the temporary control of hemorrhage
If cardiac hole small: accept the blood loss while you suture the hole versus place a peanut sponge (on a hemostat) into the wound while you repair.
If cardiac hole is large: insert a 16-French Foley catheter with a 30-mL balloon into the wound and inflate with 10 mL of saline and apply gentle traction on the catheter while progressively closing the ends of the wound toward the middle of the wound until the amount of blood loss is acceptable without the balloon (can clamp superior and inferior vena cavae for short periods to control inflow).

What is the approach for injuries of the posterior trachea or mainstem bronchi near the carina?
Right posterolateral thoracotomy

What is the approach for a tear of the descending thoracic aorta?
Left posterolateral thoracotomy

What side are diaphragmatic injuries after blunt trauma usually found?
Left side

How would you repair an acute diaphragmatic injury?
Perform a midline laparotomy, grab the torn edges of the diaphragm with a clamp (Allis clamps) to make injury more accessible for repair, repair the diaphragmatic defect primarily (if large defect may need prosthetic mesh)

How would you approach a chronic (months to years after the initial trauma) diaphragmatic rupture?
Transthoracic secondary to adhesions (can perform combined approach with laparotomy)

What is the classic mechanism of blunt aortic injury?
Sudden deceleration resulting from a fall from height or frontal impact motor vehicle collision

Radiographic findings on supine chest radiograph to suggest aortic transection:
Widened mediastinum (>8 cm), obscured/indistinct aortic knob, deviation of left main-stem bronchus, off-midline position of nasogastric tube, obliteration of aortopulmonary window, apical capping, first rib/scapula fractures, loss of aortic contour, left hemothorax, tracheal deviation to the right

Gold standard imaging modality to identify blunt aortic injury:
Aortography

What is the estimated risk of free aortic rupture with blunt aortic injury?
1% per hour

What is the reported operative mortality following open repair of a blunt descending thoracic aorta injury?
5% to 25%

What is the rate of paraparesis/paraplegia in patients undergoing open repair of a blunt descending thoracic aorta injury?
5% to 10%

What is the second most common blunt thoracic vascular injury?
Tear of the innominate artery at its origin

ABDOMEN

Where is the most expedient place to clamp the supraceliac aorta via a laparotomy?
At the diaphragmatic hiatus

How is supraceliac clamping of the aorta performed?
An opening in the lesser omentum is created using rapid blunt dissection, the left diaphragmatic crus is opened longitudinally in the direction of its fibers with finger dissection, the minimal required space is created on both sides of the aorta to accommodate the aortic clamp or manual compression.

What kind of injuries does abdominal CT scan miss?
Hollow viscous injury, diaphragm injury

What kind of injuries does focused abdominal sonography for trauma (FAST) miss?
Retroperitoneal bleeds, hollow viscous injury, diaphragm

What does diagnostic peritoneal lavage (DPL) miss?
Retroperitoneal bleeds/injury, contained hematomas, diaphragm

How would you rule out intra-abdominal injury in a hemodynamically stable patient after blunt trauma?
CT scan of the abdomen and pelvis (vs abdominal ultrasound)

How would you rule out intra-abdominal injury in a hemodynamically unstable patient with multiple other injuries?
FAST, DPL, laparotomy

How would you manage a patient with an isolated penetrating abdominal trauma with hypotension/shock?
Take patient to operating room

How would you manage a stab wound victim without peritoneal signs, evisceration, or hypotension?
Local wound exploration and DPL versus diagnostic laparoscopy to check for violation of posterior sheath versus observation and serial examinations.

What are the standard criteria for a positive DPL in blunt trauma?
Aspiration of at least 10 mL of gross blood, a bloody lavage effluent, a red blood cell count >100,000/mm^3, a white blood cell count >500/mm^3, amylase level >175 IU/dL, or detection of bile, bacteria, or food fibers

Contraindications for DPL:
Clear indication for exploratory laparotomy

What injuries are frequently underdiagnosed by DPL alone?
Diaphragmatic tears, retroperitoneal hematomas, and renal, pancreatic, duodenal, minor intestinal, and extraperitoneal bladder injuries

What red blood cell count is usually used to determine a positive DPL in a patient with a stab wound?
Red blood cell count 1000 to 5000/mm^3, but no real consensus

What are the zones of retroperitoneal hemorrhage?
I, II, III

Which Zone is bilateral, and what structures are at risk?
II—kidney, adrenals, renal vasculature

What is Zone III usually associated with?
Pelvic fractures, iliac artery, and vein injuries

What is Zone I?
Central hematoma—can be supramesocolic involving—pancreas, SMV, SMA, portal vein, aorta, cava, or inframesocolic—aorta, IVC

How do you fix a penetrating gastric wound?
Debridement of the wound edges and primary closure in layers
If major tissue loss, may need to perform gastric resection

What is the most common mechanism of blunt duodenal injury?
Impact of the steering wheel on the epigastrium from a motor vehicle accident

Most portion of the duodenum to be injured with trauma:
Second portion of the duodenum

What findings on abdominal x-ray might you see with a duodenal injury?
Absence of air in duodenal bulb, mild scoliosis, obliteration of the right psoas shadow, retroperitoneal air outlining the kidney

What studies will provide diagnosis in a hemodynamically stable patient with suspected duodenal injury?
CT scan of the abdomen with oral and IV contrast, gastrografin upper gastrointestinal series

What is the test of choice with equivocal CT findings in a hemodynamically stable patient with a suspected duodenal injury?
Upper gastrointestinal series with diluted barium

What injury must you have a high suspicion for if you encounter a retroperitoneal hematoma around the duodenum?
Pancreatic injury

According to the duodenum injury scale, what is a grade I duodenal injury?
Hematoma: involving a single portion of the duodenum
Laceration: partial thickness, no perforation

According to the duodenum injury scale, what is a grade II duodenal injury?
Hematoma: involving more than 1 portion
Laceration: disruption <50% of the circumference

According to the duodenum injury scale, what is a grade III duodenal injury?
Laceration: disruption 50% to 75% of the circumference of D2 or disruption 50% to 100% of the circumference of D1, D3, D4

According to the duodenum injury scale, what is a grade IV duodenal injury?
Laceration: disruption >75% of the circumference of D2 and involving the ampulla or distal common bile duct

According to the duodenum injury scale, what is a grade V duodenal injury?
Laceration: massive disruption of the duodenopancreatic complex
Vascular: devascularization of the duodenum

Treatment for grades I and II duodenal injuries diagnose within 6 hours of injury:
Primary repair

Treatment for grades I and II duodenal injuries diagnose after 6 hours of injury:
Repair and duodenal decompression (transpyloric nasogastric tube, tube jejunostomy, or tube duodenostomy) because of increased risk of leakage

Treatment for a grade III duodenal injury:
Primary repair, pyloric exclusion, and drainage versus Roux-en-Y duodenojejunostomy

Treatment for a grade IV duodenal injury:
Primary repair of the duodenum, repair of the common bile duct, and placement of a T-tube with a long transpapillary limb versus choledochoenteric anastomosis. If repair of common bile duct impossible, perform ligation and a second intervention for a biliary enterostomy

Treatment for a grade V duodenal injury:
Pancreaticoduodenectomy (trauma whipple) versus closure of the duodenal wound, debridement of pancreas if necessary, and pyloric exclusion with wide drainage

What is the most significant complication after duodenal injury?
The development of a duodenal fistula

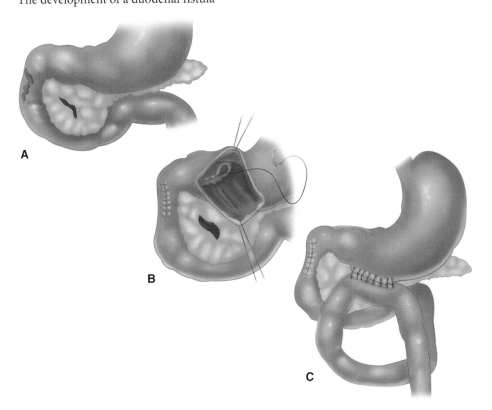

FIGURE 21-3. (**A**) Pyloric exclusion is used to treat combined injuries of the duodenum and the head of the pancreas as well as isolated duodenal injuries when the duodenal repair is less than optimal. (**B**) and (**C**). The pylorus is oversewn through a gastrotomy, which is subsequently used to create a gastrojejunostomy. The authors frequently use needle-catheter jejunostomy tube feedings for these patients. *(Reproduced from Brunicardi FC, Andersen DK, Billiar TR, et al. Schwartz's Principles of Surgery. 9th ed. http://www.accessmedicine.com. Copyright © The McGraw-Hill Companies, Inc. All rights reserved.)*

How do you manage a duodenal fistula?
Nonoperatively with nasogastric suction, IV nutrition, and aggressive stoma care (usual closure within 6–8 weeks)
Percutaneously drain any abscesses that develop or perform surgical drainage if multiple abscesses present or if abscesses located between small bowel loops.

Treatment for a distal pancreatic injury with suspected ductal injury:
Distal pancreatectomy ± splenectomy

Most frequent complications after pancreatic trauma:
Pancreatic fistula and peripancreatic abscess

What is the most frequently injured organ after penetrating trauma?
Small bowel

What are suggestive findings on CT scan for small bowel injury?
Free fluid without solid organ injury, free air, thickening of the small bowel wall or mesentery

How would you repair a small injury to the small bowel caused by a firearm?
Debridement and primary repair

How are extensive lacerations, devascularized segments, or multiple lacerations in a short segment of mall intestine repaired?
Small bowel resection and primary anastomosis

What are the general criteria for primary closure of a traumatic colon injury?
Absence of prolonged shock/hypotension, absence of gross contamination, absence of associated colonic vascular injury, early diagnosis (within 4–6 hours), <6 units of blood transfused, no requirement for the use of mesh

How should stab and low-velocity wounds to the colon with minimal contamination in a hemodynamically stable patient be repaired?
Primary repair versus resection with primary anastomosis

How should traumatic colon injuries at high-risk or associated with other severe injuries be repaired?
Colonic resection and colostomy

How would you manage an extraperitoneal rectal injury (distal one-third of the rectum)?
Attempt primary closure of the extraperitoneal rectal injury but not necessary, create a diverting colostomy, wash out the distal rectal stump with +/- wide presacral drainage.

How would you manage an intraperitoneal rectal injury?
Primary closure with a diverting colostomy

How would you control the bleeding from a small superficial hepatic laceration?
Simple suture repair, argon beam coagulator, electrocautery, topical hemostatic agents, fibrin glue

How would you control the bleeding from a severe hepatic laceration that continues to bleed despite attempts at local control?
Finger fracture hepatotomy along nonanatomic planes with direct ligation of any bleeding vessels with placement of an omental flap in the laceration, Pringle maneuver, pack the

liver wound, consider angiography with second look operation in 48 to 72 hours, if multiple lacerations and no major vascular injury mesh hepatorrhaphy (wrap each lobe of liver individually with absorbable mesh and attach to falciform ligament), less attractive options include formal hepatic resection and hepatic artery ligation.

What injury might you suspect if bleeding continues after performing a Pringle maneuver in a patient with traumatic hepatic injury?
Hepatic vein or retrohepatic vena cava injury

How would you control the bleeding from a hepatic vein injury?
Perform a pringle maneuver, place a rummel tourniquet around infrahepatic IVC, perform a median sternotomy, open the pericardium; place a rummel tourniquet around intrapericardial IVC ± atriocaval shunt (total hepatic isolation)

Reported incidence of biliary fistula after hepatic trauma:
7% to 10%

Usual treatment for hemobilia:
Angiographic embolization

How would you manage a blunt hepatic injury in hemodynamically stable patient without extravasation on the arterial phase of CT scan?
Nonoperatively: follow with serial hematocrit, vital signs, serial abdominal examinations, repeat CT scan to evaluate and quantify hemoperitoneum if the hematocrit drops, angiography with superselective embolization with persistent bleeding/fluid requirement

What procedure would you perform for an obvious traumatic injury to the gallbladder?
Cholecystectomy

How would you repair a minor injury to the common bile duct <50% of the duct's circumference?
Primary repair and placement of a T-tube with a closed suction drain in the vicinity of the repair

How would you repair a major injury to the common bile duct >50% of the duct's circumference?
Choledochoenteric anastomosis with placement of a closed suction drain near the anastomosis

What is the commonly used estimation of the incidence of overwhelming post splenectomy sepsis (OPSI) in children and in adults?
0.6% in children and 0.3% in adults

How would you manage a hemodynamically stable patient with a splenic injury with contrast extravasation on the arterial phase of abdominal CT scan?
Controversial: operative intervention versus angiographic embolization versus observation

How would you manage a hemodynamically stable patient with a splenic injury without contrast extravasation on abdominal CT scan?
Admission to ICU, serial hematocrit, vital signs, serial abdominal examinations, bed rest, NPO

What classic criteria are used for the nonoperative management of splenic injury?
Absence of contrast extravasation on CT, absence of other associated injuries requiring surgical intervention, absence of health conditions with an increased risk for bleeding (coagulopathy, hepatic failure, anticoagulants, specific coagulation factor deficiency), hemodynamic stability, negative abdominal examination, splenic injury grade I to III

How long will you tell your patient with a splenic injury treated nonoperatively to avoid intense physical activity/contact sports?
3 months

After performing an exploratory laparotomy for trauma, you incidentally discover a capsular tear of the spleen; how should you control the bleeding?
With compression or with topical hemostatic agents.

What are your options for controlling bleeding from a splenic laceration?
Closing the laceration with horizontal absorbable mattress sutures, argon beam coagulator/fibrin glue
If major laceration involving <50% of splenic parenchyma and not extending into hilum, can perform segmental or partial splenic resection
Splenectomy/splenorrhaphy

How should you manage a patient with an injury to the central portion of the spleen extending into the hilum?
Splenectomy

What measures are taken to help prevent OPSI
Vaccinate against *Streptococcus pneumoniae*, *Hemophilus influenzae*, and *Neisseria meningitidis*; prophylactic penicillin for all minor illnesses/infections; immediate medical evaluation if febrile

What is abdominal compartment syndrome?
Increasing intra-abdominal pressure that reduces blood flow to abdominal organs leading to impaired pulmonary, cardiovascular, renal, and gastrointestinal function causing multiple organ dysfunction syndrome and death.

Which physiologic parameters are decreased with abdominal compartment syndrome?
Renal blood flow, cardiac output, central venous return, glomerular filtration, visceral blood flow

Which physiologic parameters are increased with abdominal compartment syndrome?
Central venous pressure, heart rate, intrapleural pressure, peak inspiratory pressure, pulmonary capillary wedge pressure, systemic vascular resistance

What is the treatment for abdominal compartment syndrome?
Decompressive laparotomy

UROLOGIC

What is the most frequent sign associated with a urinary tract injury?
Gross hematuria

What are the usual manifestations of a lower urinary tract injury?
Blood in the urethral meatus; floating or displaced prostate on rectal examination; distended bladder; inability to void; large perineal hematoma/perineal injury

Usual manifestation of upper urinary tract injury:
Gross or microscopic hematuria

What is your workup to rule out urethral/bladder injury in a blunt trauma patient with blood at the urethral meatus?
Urethrocystography before bladder catheterization (rule out urethral injury)
If negative, perform cystography by injecting 250 to 300 mL of contrast through foley to maximally distend bladder and obtain films with the bladder fully distended and empty

When performing cystography to rule out bladder injury, why do you need to obtain a postvoid film?
To rule out posterior extravasation of contrast not seen on AP films with the bladder maximally distended

What is the most commonly injured part of the urinary tract?
Kidney

Usual treatment for a small parenchymal injury to the kidney caused by a penetrating wound:
Debridement, primary repair, and drainage

Usual treatment for an extensive hilar injury to the kidney caused by a penetrating wound:
Total nephrectomy

What should you do before opening a major perinephric hematoma?
Obtain proximal control of the renal pedicle before opening Gerota fascia

What surgery would you perform for a ureteral injury located in the upper (or middle) third of the ureter with minimal tissue loss?
Ureteroureterostomy with placement of a double-J stent

What surgery would you perform for a ureteral injury located in the distal third of the ureter with minimal tissue loss?
Ureteral implantation into the bladder

What are your surgical options for a patient with a ureteral injury where primary repair is not possible (long segment of ureter lost; poor clinical condition of patient)?
Percutaneous nephrostomy with delayed repair, transureteroureterostomy if possible, kidney autotransplantation into iliac fossa

Approximate percentage of patients with bladder rupture that have an associated pelvic fracture:
~70%

How would you repair an intraperitoneal bladder rupture?
Using a transabdominal approach, perform a primary repair with a 3-layer closure leaving a Foley catheter in place for decompression (if large defect, consider suprapubic cystostomy).

What is the usual management of an extraperitoneal bladder rupture?
Nonoperative: leave Foley catheter in place for 10 to 14 days

What is the study of choice to diagnose a urethral injury?
Retrograde urethrogram

What physical examination findings can be associated with urethral injuries?
High riding prostate on rectal, blood at meatus, perineal or scrotal hematoma/ecchymosis

Usual management for a patient with a urethral injury:
Bladder decompression with suprapubic cystostomy and delayed urethroplasty

ORTHOPEDICS

What kind of bone fracture involves young, soft bone that bends and leads to an incomplete disruption of the bone?
Greenstick fracture

What types of bone fracture occur when a bending moment is applied to the bone?
Transverse and oblique fractures

What type of bone fracture generally results from a rotational force about the long axis of the bone?
Spiral fracture

What fracture results bone be stressed beyond its failure point from chronic, repetitive trauma resulting in microscopic disruption?
Stress fracture

Term for a fracture that occurs through an area weakened by pre existing disease?
Pathologic fracture

What is an open fracture?
A fracture with a communication between the fracture site and the outside environment from an overlying wound

What are the 3 main mechanisms leading to cervical spine injury?
Direct trauma to the neck, motion of the head relative to the axial skeleton, direct axial load imparted on the cranium causing axial compression forces across the cervical vertebrae

How can a burst fracture be differentiated from a compression fracture?
Burst fractures involve injury to the middle column (posterior third of vertebral body)
Compression fractures involve injury to the anterior column only (anterior two-thirds of vertebral body)

When filming long bone injuries, what must be done to assess the integrity of adjacent limb segments?
Include the joints above and below the level of injury
If the joint is injured, image the long bones above and below the joint injury

Why do you immobilize a fracture?
Splinting reduces bleeding, helps avoid additional soft tissue injury (prevents conversion of a closed fracture to an open fracture), reduces patient discomfort, and facilitates transportation and radiographic evaluation of the injury.

What should you do for a patient with a clear indication for abdominal exploration with a bleeding pelvic fracture with a ruptured retroperitoneum?
Pack the pelvis (can pack space of Retzius), temporarily close the abdomen, follow with external fixation and angiography as needed

If you are to perform a DPL on a patient with an obvious pelvic fracture, where should you place your incision?
Supraumbilical

Rotational instability of a pelvic ring disruption is defined as:
Widening of the pubic symphysis; displacement of pubic rami fractures >2.5 cm

Vertical instability of a pelvic ring disruption is defined as:
Superior translation of a hemipelvis through fractures of the sacrum or ilium with disruption of the sacroiliac joint >1 cm

What type of compression injury to the pelvis has the greatest risk of retroperitoneal hemorrhage?
Anteroposterior compression

What is the most common cause of death in a patient with a lateral compression injury of the pelvis?
Associated closed head injury

In a patient with an unstable pelvic ring disruption and a positive abdominal study, what must you do before laparotomy?
Stabilize the pelvis (external fixation, C clamp), if still hemodynamically unstable after pelvic stabilization perform arteriography

What are indications for performing an arteriogram in patients with suspected vascular trauma?
Any pulse deficit, ankle-brachial index <0.90

What are the hallmarks of successful treatment of an open femoral fracture?
Antibiotic prophylaxis, irrigation and debridement, compartment decompression, stabilization, and early wound coverage

What kind of complications can arise from prolonged joint dislocation?
Ankylosis, avascular necrosis, cartilage cell death, neurovascular injury, posttraumatic arthritis

What position does the thigh assume with a posterior hip dislocation?
Flexed and internally rotated

What position does the arm assume with an anterior shoulder dislocation?
Adducted and externally rotated

If the hip remains dislocated for 24 hours, what percentage of patients will develop avascular necrosis of the femoral head?
100%

What is the treatment of choice for closed femoral fractures and type I to IIIA open femoral fractures?
Closed, locked intramedullary nailing

What is the most common fractured diaphyseal long bone?
Tibia

What nerve is evaluated by testing sensation of the first dorsal web space and foot and toe dorsiflexion?
Deep peroneal nerve

What nerve is evaluated by testing sensation along the dorsum of the foot and foot eversion strength?
Superficial peroneal nerve

What nerve is evaluated by testing sensation of the sole of the foot and motor function to the foot and toe plantar flexors?
Tibial nerve

What nerve is evaluated by testing sensation to the lateral aspect of the heel?
Sural nerve (purely sensory)

How is a closed tibial fracture with minimal displacement treated?
Cast immobilization and functional bracing

What is the treatment of choice for open moderate and severe tibial fractures?
Open reduction and internal fixation; use of reamed intramedullary nailing debatable

What is entailed in the typical nonoperative treatment of a humeral fracture?
Application of a coaptation splint in the acute setting with subsequent replacement by a functional fracture brace 3 to 7 days later when the pain from the initial fracture has passed.

Indications for operative intervention in patients with humeral shaft fractures:
Concomitant neurologic/vascular injury, failed closed reduction, intra-articular fractures, ipsilateral forearm or elbow fractures ("floating elbow"), open fractures, polytrauma patients, segmental fractures

Surgical options for a humeral shaft fracture include:
Intramedullary nailing, plate and screw fixation, external fixation

What 3 conditions must be met before a patient can be allowed to bear weight on an injured extremity?
There must be bone-to-bone contact at the fracture site, demonstrated intraoperatively or on postreduction radiographs, stable fixation of the fracture must be achieved, the patient must be able to comply with the weight-bearing status

MULTIPLE CHOICE QUESTIONS

1. **The correct treatment for an intraperitoneal bladder rupture:**
   A. Foley catheter drainage
   B. Suprapubic drainage
   C. Suprapubic drainage with Foley catheter drainage
   D. Bladder drainage, percutaneous paravesical drainage and antibiotics
   E. Laparotomy with open bladder exploration and repair, paravesical drainage, and Foley catheter drainage

2. **A passenger was involved in a high-speed head on motor vehicle collision and sustained severe hyperflexion injury of the lumbar region. She was wearing a seat belt. The most important abdominal injury to exclude would be:**
   A. Pancreatic neck transection
   B. IMV transection
   C. Gastric rupture
   D. Duodenal transection
   E. Gallbladder rupture

3. A hypotensive patient had sustained multiple stab wounds to the abdomen. In the operating room, a through-and-through laceration to the stomach and a pancreatic and a low-grade splenic injury. How would you manage the gastric perforations?
   A. Gastric resection with primary closure
   B. Primary closure of both wounds
   C. A posterior gastrojejunostomy with primary repair of the anterior injury
   D. Resection with Roux-en-Y reconstruction
   E. Subtotal gastrectomy with gastrojejunostomy

4. Which of the following scenarios requires immediate operative intervention?
   A. A stab wound to zone II of the that violates the platysma
   B. A grade III splenic injury in a stable 7-year-old girl
   C. A nonexpanding retroperitoneal zone II hematoma
   D. A distal femur fracture with overlying palpable thrill
   E. Extraperitoneal bladder rupture

5. Regarding cervical spine injury, which of the following statements are true?
   A. Hangman fractures are very unstable and are best managed with operative spinal fusion
   B. Type II dens (odontoid) fractures are stable
   C. C1 fractures are usually caused by an axial load and involve a blowout of the ring
   D. Radiographic assessment of the cervical spine is recommended in trauma patients who are awake, alert, and not intoxicated, who are without neck pain or tenderness, and who do not have significant associated injuries that detract from their general evaluation

6. Which one of the following is an indication for immediate ventriculostomy in head trauma?
   A. 1 mm subdural hematoma, GCS 14
   B. 5 cm epidural hematoma, GCS 5
   C. Multiple hemorrhagic contusions, GCS 13
   D. Mild global cerebral edema, GCS 7
   E. Normal CT scan, with serum alcohol of 250, GCS 9

7. A 20-year-old male involved in high-speed motor vehicle collision arrives to the emergency department. He was intubated at the scene, arrives with oxygen saturation of 80%, systolic blood pressure is 90 mm Hg with 1 L of crystalloid infusing, and he has near amputation of left leg. What is the first most appropriate step in treatment?
   A. Infuse PRBC
   B. Reasses airway and listen to breath sounds
   C. Amputate left leg
   D. Place a large-bore central line
   E. Check CXR

8. An obese 40-year-old female arrives to the ED after a motor vehicle collision awake but confused and complaining of abdominal pain with a systolic BP of 80 after 2 L of crystalloid infusion. She also has crepitus due to bilateral

pneumothoraces s/p chest tube placement. FAST is positive in RUQ. What is the next step?

A. Operative exploration
B. Aggressively resuscitate
C. CT scan of abdomen and pelvis
D. DPL
E. Check Stat H/H

9. A 30-year-old male patient complains of abdominal pain after a snowboarding accident. He is hemodynamically stable. A CT scan of the abdomen and pelvis shows a grade III spleen with moderate hemoperitoneum and an IV contrast blush. What is the appropriate treatment?

A. Observation and serial H/H
B. Laparotomy
C. Angioembolization
D. DPL
E. Laparoscopic exploration

10. A motorcyclist crashes and arrives to the emergency department intubated, hypotensive despite 2 L of crystalloid infusion, with a fixed and dilated pupil on the right. His chest and pelvic x-rays are unremarkable, and his FAST is positive. What is the first priority in management?

A. CT head
B. Right-sided craniotomy
C. Ventriculostomy
D. Laparotomy
E. Mannitol

11. An 18-year-old male arrives to the emergency department after sustaining a stab wound to left chest, just below the nipple and parasternal. His blood pressure is normal and his heart rate is 110. There are no other wounds on examination. A chest x-ray is normal, and a FAST examination shows fluid in the pericardium. A subxiphoid pericardial window is performed and is positive for blood in the pericardium. The patient remains hemodynamically stable. What is the next step in management?

A. TEE
B. Exploration
C. Observation
D. CT Chest/abdomen

ANSWERS

1. **Answer: E.** An intraperitoneal bladder rupture must be operatively repaired. Drainage of the paravesical space at laparotomy as well as Foley catheter drainage is essential. Any option that suggests drainage without exploration would be inadequate.

2. **Answer: A.** A missed pancreatic injury could have devastating consequences. Hyperflexion injuries while wearing a seat belt trap abdominal viscera and cause severe deceleration injuries that could result in pancreatic neck transection. Interestingly, falling over bicycle handlebars in pediatric trauma is associated with pancreatic injury.

All the other listed injuries are exceedingly rare with this mechanism; a duodenal hematoma is more commonly associated with a pancreatic injury.

3. **Answer: B.** This patient is a candidate for rapid primary closure of both wounds. There is no need for pyloric exclusion, resection, or gastrojejunostomy.

4. **Answer: D.** This question covers a lot of ground: Distal femur fractures are frequently associated with vascular injury. A thrill is a hard sign of vascular injury, which mandates immediate surgery. Other hard signs of vascular injury are arterial bleeding, pulsatile hematoma, bruit, and obvious arterial occlusion (pulselessness). In cases where there are so-called soft signs (diminished pulses, proximity of wound to vessels, small nonpulsatile hematoma, an ankle brachial index of <0.9, neurologic deficit, or history of arterial bleeding at the scene), further evaluation with arteriography or serial examinations is warranted in respect to penetrating neck trauma; the paradigm has shifted from mandatory exploration of deep zone II injuries after literature showed that many explorations were unnecessary and did not demonstrate any clinically significant injury. If associated with hard signs of neck injury or hemodynamic instability, then exploration should be pursued. Hard signs include respiratory, digestive, or vascular findings: dyspnea, hoarseness, stridor, dysphagia, odynophagia, pulsatile hematoma, thrill/bruit, or neurologic deficit. Particularly in children, because of the slightly higher incidence of postsplenectomy sepsis, splenic preservation should be attempted. This is acceptable in a stable patient.

All zone I retroperitoneal hematomas should be explored. Retroperitoneal hematomas secondary to penetrating trauma should be explored; however, recent evidence has demonstrated that observation of nonexpanding zone II hematomas is safe.

Extraperitoneal bladder rupture does not lead to intra-abdominal urine extravasation and are managed with transurethral (Foley) catheter drainage for 7 to 10 days. No surgery is usually required.

5. **Answer: C.** Jefferson (C1 burst) fractures are considered stable and are treated with a rigid collar. Hangman fractures involve the posterior elements of C2 and are unstable. They are treated with traction for displacement and a halo for immobilization lasting 3 months. Odontoid fractures are subdivided into 3 types. Type I involve the odontoid above the base and are stable. Type II fractures occur at the base of C2 and are usually unstable. They are treated with a halo for 3 months if the displacement is less than 5 mm. If greater than 5 mm, then posterior fusion of C1 and C2 or screw fixation is generally required. Type III extend into the C2 body and are treated with a halo or rigid collar. Per nexus criteria, a patient with the above findings could have his cervical spine clinically cleared without imaging.

6. **Answer: C.** If you can follow a neurologic examination and it is adequate, there is no need for ICP monitoring. If the alcohol level is high with a normal CT scan, then it is reasonable to allow the intoxicating drugs to metabolize. A patient with a large epidural hematoma should undergo emergent neurosurgical intervention with evacuation in the operating room.

7. **Answer: B.** While these are likely all important in the care of this patient, one must always remember to reevaluate the ABCs, and always double check the ET whenever a patient arrives or is transferred. This patient may have a right mainstem intubation, malpositioned ET, tension hemo/pneumothorax, or massive lung contusions to account for the desaturation and the blood pressure may respond to securing the airway or decompressing the chest.

8. **Answer: A.** This patient is still in hypotensive despite initial resuscitation and chest tube placement. While further resuscitation is ongoing with likely colloid or blood product infusion, the patient's abdomen should be explored. The FAST is positive in this case; however, if the FAST were negative or equivocal due to obesity/subcutaneous air, one should also obtain a pelvis x-ray and perform a DPL. Since the patient is unstable, a CT scan would not be appropriate as the next step.

9. **Answer: C.** While this is dependent on resources at your hospital, angioembolization is associated with high splenic salvage rates. Findings on CT associated with failure of pure observation and nonoperative management are high grade of injury, amount of hemoperitoneum, and presence of blush. If there is no interventional radiology capabilities available, this patient can be observed closely with an expected high failure rate or nonoperative management or alternatively taken for a laparotomy and either a splenectomy or splenorraphy. Laparoscopic splenectomy has no role in the acute setting.

10. **Answer: D.** This is a multitrauma patient with multiple life-threatening issues. Thus, it is important to prioritize and start with the primary survey. Airway must be secured and adequate ventilation ensured. Next, circulation is assessed—as this patient is hypotensive despite initial fluid resuscitation, a source of ongoing hemorrhage that needs to be identified or excluded controlled. Given a positive FAST, negative plain films, and the mechanism, the abdomen is the most likely source. While the presence of a lesion with mass effect on the brain is a true emergency, the most important way to prevent secondary brain injury is to prevent hypotension and hypoxia. If simultaneous craniotomy and laparotomy is feasible, this too could be considered.

11. **Answer: B.** A positive pericardial window in this setting mandates exploration to evaluate for a cardiac injury. While the method is dependent on comfort level of the surgeon, a median sternotomy is preferred over left anterolateral thoracotomy. However, if the patient arrives unstable or becomes hypotensive during initial assessment then more urgent exploration (left anterolateral thoracotomy or sternotomy) without confirmatory tests is appropriate.

    If a pulseless penetrating chest trauma victim arrives with CPR in progress, within 15 minutes a left anterolateral thoracotomy is indicated. It is also appropriate to proceed with exploration with a positive ultrasound examination (FAST, TTE, TEE) without pericardial window in the hemodynamically stable patient. Remember, penetrating injuries to the mediastinal "box" have to be evaluated either with a pericardial window or with ECHO ultrasonography to exclude tamponade.

CHAPTER 22
Critical Care

Dale A. Dangleben, Firas Madbak, and Jayme Lieberman

HEMODYNAMIC PARAMETERS

What is the formula for mean arterial pressure (MAP)?
$MAP = DBP + 1/3 \times (SBP - DBP)$

What is the normal range for cardiac output (CO)?
4 to 8 L/min

What is the normal range for cardiac index (CI)?
2.5 to 4 L/min

What is the normal range for systemic vascular resistance (SVR)?
800 to 1400 dyn · s/(cm⁵)

What is the normal range for SVR index (SVRI)?
1500 to 2400 dyn · s/(cm⁵)

What is the normal range for pulmonary capillary wedge pressure (PCWP)?
7 to 15 mm Hg

What is the normal range for central venous pressure (CVP)?
2 to 6 mm Hg

What is the normal range for pulmonary artery (PA) pressure?
20 to 30/6 to 15 mm Hg

What is the normal range for mixed venous oxygen saturation (SvO_2)?
70% ± 5%

What is SvO_2?
The oxygen saturation of blood in the right ventricle/pulmonary artery that serves as an indirect measure of peripheral oxygen supply and demand

What factors influence SvO_2?
Oxygen delivery and oxygen extraction

Approximate percentage of CO that goes to the kidney:
25%

Approximate percentage of CO that goes to the brain:
15%

Approximate percentage of CO that goes to the heart:
5%

INVASIVE MONITORING

What complications can occur during central venous catheter placement?
Arterial puncture, air or catheter embolism, dysrhythmias, hemorrhage or arteriovenous fistulization, pneumothorax, pseudoaneurysm formation

What should you immediately do if a patient receives an air embolus?
Roll the patient to the left and place head down to keep air in right atrium/ventricle; attempt to aspirate air with central catheter/pulmonary artery catheter

Relative contraindications for pulmonary artery catheter placement:
Left bundle branch block, previous pneumonectomy

Treatment for hemoptysis after pulmonary artery catheter placement:
Immediately pull the pulmonary artery catheter slightly back and reinflate balloon, increase positive end expiratory pressure (PEEP) to help tamponade the bleeding, mainstem intubate the nonaffected side; attempt can be made to place a fogarty catheter down the affected side; if recalcitrant, may need thoracotomy and lobectomy

What West zone of the lung is the desired location for a pulmonary artery catheter?
Zone III (Pa > Pv > PA); pressure in the arteries (Pa), pressure in the veins (Pv), pressure in the alveoli (PA)

Which portion of the lung has the highest V/Q ratio and which portion has the lowest V/Q ratio?
V/Q ratio highest in upper lobes
V/Q ratio lowest in lower lobes

At what point in the respiratory cycle is the PCWP most accurate in a ventilated patient?
End expiration

At what point in the respiratory cycle is the PCWP most accurate in a nonventilated patient?
Peak inspiration

What conditions may make the wedge pressure unreliable?
Aortic regurgitation, high PEEP, mitral stenosis, mitral regurgitation, poor left ventricular compliance, pulmonary hypertension, pulmonary disease (acute respiratory distress syndrome [ARDS]), tamponade, pneumothorax

Pulmonary artery catheters allow the direct measurement of which physiologic parameters?
CVP, right atrial pressure, pulmonary arterial pressure, right ventricular end-diastolic pressure, pulmonary artery wedge pressure, SVO_2

What complications are associated with pulmonary artery catheter placement?
Arrhythmias and conduction defects, knotting or catheter entrapment, pulmonary infarction, pulmonary artery rupture, valvular damage.

What is an intra-aortic balloon pump?
A mechanical device that consists of a cylindrical balloon that actively deflates in systole increasing forward blood flow by reducing afterload, and actively inflates in diastole increasing blood flow to the coronary arteries resulting in decreased myocardial oxygen demand and increased CO

When does the balloon from an intra-aortic balloon pump inflate on ECG?
T wave (diastole)

When does the balloon from an intra-aortic balloon pump deflate on ECG?
P wave or start of Q wave (systole)

Indications for intra-aortic balloon pump placement:
Bridge to heart transplant for patients with left ventricular failure; cardiogenic shock, percutaneous coronary angioplasty, post cardiothoracic surgery, preoperative use for high-risk patients (unstable angina with stenosis >70% main coronary artery), reversible intracardial mechanical defects complicating infarction, unstable angina pectoris, ventricular dysfunction with ejection fraction <35%

Absolute contraindications to intra-aortic balloon pump placement:
Aortic regurgitation, aortic dissection, severe aortoiliac occlusive disease

Relative contraindications to intra-aortic balloon pump placement:
Prosthetic vascular grafts in the aorta, aortic aneurysm, aortofemoral grafts

Desired location for the tip of the intra-aortic balloon pump catheter?
1 to 2 cm below the top of the aortic arch just distal to the left subclavian

CARDIAC PHYSIOLOGY

What is preload?
End diastolic length of cardiac myocytes, which is linearly related to end-diastolic volume (EDV) and filling pressure

What is afterload?
Resistance against ventricular contraction (SVR)

What is contractility?
The force of myocardial contraction

What 3 things determine stroke volume?
Left ventricular EDV (LVEDV) (preload), contractility, afterload

How is stroke volume calculated?
LVEDV – left ventricular end-systolic volume

How is the ejection fraction calculated?
Stroke volume/EDV

What is the normal O_2 delivery to consumption ratio?
5 to 1

What are the primary determinants of myocardial O_2 consumption?
Heart rate (HR), increased ventricular wall tension

What is the normal range for the alveolar:arterial gradient?
10 to 15 mm Hg

What shifts the oxygen-hemoglobin dissociation curve to the left?
Decrease temperature
Decrease 2,3-diphosphoglycerate (DPG)
Decrease pCO_2
Increase pH

What shifts the oxygen-hemoglobin dissociation curve to the right?
Increase temperature
Increase 2,3-DPG
Increase pCO_2
Decrease pH

SHOCK

What is the definition of shock?
Inadequate perfusion to meet the body's metabolic needs

What are the 5 broad categories of shock?
Hypovolemic, obstructive, neurogenic, septic, cardiogenic

Table 22-1	Signs and Symptoms of Advancing Stages of Hemorrhagic Shock			
	Class I	Class II	Class III	Class IV
Blood loss (mL)	Up to 750	750–1500	1500–2000	>2000
Blood loss (%BV)	Up to 15	15–30	30–40	>40
Pulse rate (bpm)	<100	>100	>120	>140
Blood pressure	Normal	Normal	Decreased	Decreased
Pulse pressure (mm Hg)	Normal or increased	Decreased	Decreased	Decreased
RR (breaths/min)	14–20	20–30	30–40	>35
Urine output (mL/h)	>30	20–30	5–15	Negligible
CNS/mental status	Slightly anxious	Mildly anxious	Anxious and confused	Confused and lethargic

BV, blood volume; CNS, central nervous system; RR, respiratory rate.
Reproduced from Brunicardi FC, Andersen DK, Billiar TR, et al. *Schwartz's Principles of Surgery.* 9th ed. http://www.accessmedicine.com. Copyright © The McGraw-Hill Companies, Inc. All rights reserved.

What is the formula for the O_2 content of blood (CaO_2)?
$CaO_2 = [Hb \times SaO_2 \times 1.34] + [0.003 \times PaO_2]$; Hb is hemoglobin in g/dL, SaO_2 is arterial O_2 saturation (%), PaO_2 is partial pressure of O_2 (mm Hg) in arterial blood

What is the formula for O_2 delivery (DO_2)?
$DO_2 = CaO_2 \times CO$; $[(Hb \times SaO_2 \times 1.34) + (0.003 \times PaO_2)] \times (HR \times SV)$; Hb is hemoglobin in g/dL, SaO_2 is arterial O_2 saturation (%), PaO_2 is partial pressure of O_2 (mm Hg) in arterial blood, HR is heart rate (beats/min [bpm]), SV stroke volume (mL)

What is the formula for O_2 consumption (VO_2)?
$VO_2 = CO \times (CaO_2 - CVO_2) \times 10$
(This can be rearranged to estimate the mixed venous saturation; the Fick equation)

How many milliliters of oxygen will a gram of hemoglobin bind when hemoglobin is fully saturated with oxygen?
1.34 mL of oxygen is bound to each gram of hemoglobin. (1.39 mL of oxygen is normally bound to hemoglobin, but you subtract the 3%–5% of circulating hemoglobin present as methemoglobin and carboxyhemoglobin.)

What does the solubility coefficient of 0.03 mL/L/mm Hg in the oxygen delivery equation signify?
0.03 mL of O_2 dissolves in 1 L of water when the PO_2 is 1 mm Hg at normal body temperature (37°C)

Manipulation of what factors can increase oxygen delivery?
Greatest increase of oxygen delivery with increasing hemoglobin content and SaO_2; can also increase oxygen delivery by raising CO by increasing either HR or stroke volume

What is the equation for oxygen extraction ratio?
$O_2ER = VO_2/DO_2$
Usually expressed as a percentage; the normal value is 0.25 to 0.3 or 25% to 30%

ARRHYTHMIAS

Treatment for ventricular fibrillation/pulseless ventricular tachycardia:
1 shock (monophasic 360 J; biphasic, 100–200 J); cardiopulmonary resuscitation with additional countershocks if shockable rhythm obtained; epinephrine 1 mg IV and repeat every 3 to 5 minutes, or vasopressin, 40 units IV (to replace the first or second dose of epinephrine); consider amiodarone (300 mg IV), lidocaine (1–1.5 mg/kg), magnesium (1–2 g IV); if no shockable rhythm, revert to asystole/pulseless electrical activity algorithm

Treatment for asystole/pulseless electrical activity:
Verify with lead rotation; epinephrine 1 mg IV and repeat every 3 to 5 minutes, or vasopressin 40 units IV (to replace the first or second dose of epinephrine); consider atropine 1 mg IV every 3 to 5 minutes, up to 3 doses; if shockable rhythm, revert to ventricular fibrillation/ventricular tachycardia algorithm

Treatment for an unstable patient with bradycardia (HR <60 bpm):
Transcutaneous pacing; if transcutaneous pacing not immediately available, give atropine 1 mg and epinephrine 2 to 10 mg/min

In which patients with atrial fibrillation is anticoagulation unnecessary?
Patients who had atrial fibrillation for <48 hours

What is the treatment for atrial fibrillation with hemodynamic instability?
Cardioversion and anticoagulation

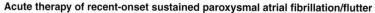

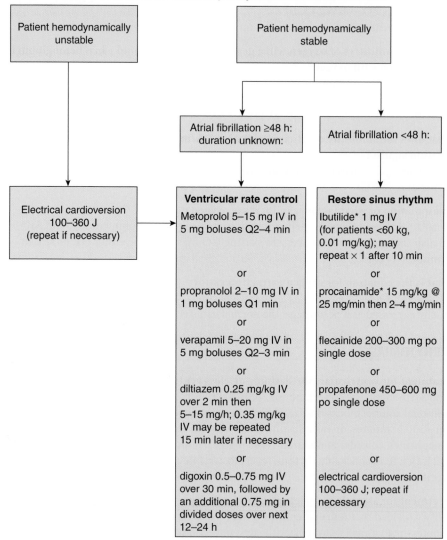

*Procainamide or ibutilide is the drug of choice for Wolff-Parkinson-White syndrome.

FIGURE 22-1. Management algorithm for atrial fibrillation (AF) or flutter. *(Reproduced from Hall JB, Schmidt GA, Wood LDH. Principles of critical care. 3rd ed. http://www.accessmedicine.com. Copyright © The McGraw-Hill Companies, Inc. All rights reserved.)*

What is the treatment for atrial fibrillation without hemodynamic instability?

Rate control (amiodarone, calcium channel blockers, β-blockers, digoxin) and correction of the underlying cause (fluid overload, electrolyte imbalance, MI, hypoxemia, acidosis, PE); anticoagulation

ACID/BASE PHYSIOLOGY

Formula for anion gap:
$Na^+ - (Cl^- + HCO_3^-)$

What is the normal range for the anion gap?
10 to 14

What is the "10 for 0.08" rule of acid base balance?
The pH falls by 0.08 for every increase of $PaCO_2$ by 10 mm Hg

What pH, $PaCO_2$, and bicarbonate will you see with a pure respiratory acidosis?
↓ pH; ↑ $PaCO_2$; normal bicarbonate

What pH, $PaCO_2$, and bicarbonate will you see with a pure metabolic acidosis?
↓pH; normal $PaCO_2$; ↓ bicarbonate

What pH, $PaCO_2$, and bicarbonate will you see with a pure respiratory alkalosis?
↑pH; ↓$PaCO_2$; normal bicarbonate

What pH, $PaCO_2$, and bicarbonate will you see with a pure metabolic alkalosis?
↑pH; normal $PaCO_2$; ↑ bicarbonate

What is the 35-45 rule of blood gas values?
pH = 7.35 to 7.45 corresponds to pCO_2 = 35 to 45

RENAL PHYSIOLOGY

What is the most common cause of postoperative renal failure?
Hypotension

What laboratory results suggest a prerenal cause of acute renal failure?
BUN/Cr ratio >20, fractional excretion of sodium (FENa) <1%, urine Na^+ <20 mEq/24 h, urine osmolality >500 mOsm

What is the formula for the FENa?
(Urine sodium × plasma creatinine/plasma sodium × urine creatinine) × 100

What does a FENa <1.0 % indicate?
Prerenal cause of renal failure, from decreased renal blood flow

What does a FENa >3.0 % indicate?
Intrinsic kidney damage (acute tubular necrosis, severe obstruction of both the kidneys)

What are indications for dialysis?
Fluid overload, metabolic acidosis, hyperkalemia, poisoning, uremic coagulopathy, uremic encephalopathy

What are the advantages of intermittent hemodialysis over continuous renal replacement therapy?
Lower cost, lower risk of systemic bleeding, facilitates transport for other interventions, more suitable for severe hyperkalemia

What are the advantages of continuous renal replacement therapy over intermittent hemodialysis?
Better fluid control, better hemodynamic stability, fewer cardiac arrhythmias, improved nutritional support, better pulmonary gas exchange

What are the disadvantages of intermittent hemodialysis over continuous renal replacement therapy?
Availability of dialysis staff, inadequate fluid control, inadequate dialysis frequency, inadequate nutritional support, more difficult hemodynamic control, potential complement activation by nonbiocompatible membranes, not suitable for patients with intracranial hypertension

What are the disadvantages of continuous renal replacement therapy over intermittent hemodialysis?
Greater cost, greater vascular access problems, higher risk of systemic bleeding, long-term immobilization of patient, more filter problems (clotting, rupture)

How does acute adrenal insufficiency present?
Cardiovascular collapse unresponsive to fluids and pressors

How much steroids should a patient be on preoperatively to have presumed hypothalamic-pituitary-adrenal axis suppression?
20 mg of prednisone or equivalent per day for 3 weeks or longer

How much perioperative steroid supplementation should you give a patient with hypothalamic-pituitary-adrenal axis suppression undergoing a moderate operation (open cholecystectomy, lower extremity revascularization)?
50 to 75 mg/d of hydrocortisone equivalent for 1 to 2 days

How much perioperative steroid supplementation should you give a patient with hypothalamic-pituitary-adrenal axis suppression undergoing a major operation (colectomy, cardiac surgery)?
100 to 150 mg/d of hydrocortisone equivalent for 2 to 3 days

How much perioperative steroid supplementation should you give a patient with acute adrenal insufficiency?
100 mg of hydrocortisone IV Q6 to 8 hours tapered as the patient's condition stabilizes

What steroid can you give to treat suspected acute adrenal insufficiency without interfering with the rapid adrenocorticotropic hormone (ACTH) stimulation test?
Dexamethasone

How do you interpret the results of the rapid ACTH stimulation test?
Normal response if baseline cortisol doubles, if baseline cortisol is >34 µg/dL, or incremental increase >9 µg/dL in patients with a baseline cortisol level between 15 to 34 µg/dL. (Note that most recent surviving sepsis guidelines suggest that the ACTH stimulation test not be used to identify the subset of adults with septic shock who should receive hydrocortisone. Instead, steroids should be empirically administered to septic patients with hypotension that is refractory to fluid and vasopressor infusion).

VASOACTIVE AGENTS

What is the role of α-1 receptors?
Vascular smooth muscle constriction, gluconeogenesis, glycogenolysis

What is the role of α-2 receptors?
Venous smooth muscle constriction

What is the role of β-1 receptors?
Myocardial contraction and rate

What is the role of β-2 receptors?
Relaxes bronchial smooth muscle, relaxes vascular smooth muscle, insulin secretion

What is the role of dopamine (DA) receptors?
Relaxation of renal and splanchnic smooth muscle

What is the site of action of intermediate dose (4–10 μg/kg/min) dopamine?
++β1, +α1 (increase inotropy with some vasoconstriction)

What is the site of action of high dose (>10 μg/kg/min) dopamine?
+++ α-1 agonist (marked arteriolar vasoconstriction increasing afterload)

What is the site of action of epinephrine?
Low-dose β1 and β2 ($\uparrow$ contractility, $\uparrow$ vasodilation) and high-dose α1 and α2 (vasoconstriction)

What is the site of action of norepinephrine?
Low-dose β1 ($\uparrow$ contractility) and high-dose α1 and α2 (vasoconstriction)

What is the site of action of vasopressin?
V-1 receptors: vasoconstriction of vascular smooth muscle
V-2 receptors: water reabsorption in the collecting ducts of the kidney
V-3 receptors: mediate release of von Willebrand factor and factor VIII

What is the site of action of phenylephrine?
α1 (vasoconstriction)

What is the site of action and effect of dobutamine?
β1 (5–15 μg/kg/min) and β2 agonist (>15 μg/kg/min), $\uparrow$ inotropy, $\uparrow$ chronotropy, $\downarrow$ SVR

What is the site of action and effect of isoproterenol?
β1 and β2 agonist, $\uparrow$ inotropy, $\uparrow$ chronotropy. $\uparrow$ vasodilation of skeletal and mesenteric vascular beds, extremely arrhythmogenic

What is milrinone?
A phosphodiesterase inhibitor that causes vasodilation, vascular smooth muscle relaxation, and leads to $\uparrow$ cAMP $\rightarrow$ $\uparrow$ calcium flux $\rightarrow$ $\uparrow$ myocardial contractility

Which cardiovascular drug is an arterial and venous dilator: nipride or nitroglycerine?
Nipride is an arterial and venous dilator; nitroglycerine is predominately a venodilator.

What is the treatment for cyanide toxicity?
Inhaled amyl nitrite then IV sodium nitrite followed by thiosulfate

Table 22-2 Dosage, Mechanism, and Actions of Pharmacologic Agents Commonly Used in the Treatment of Cardiovascular Failure

Agent	Typical Dosage	HR	MAP	CO	SVR	α_1	β_1	β_2	DA1	DA2
Catecholamines:										
Dopamine	3–5 µg/kg/min	+	+	++			++		+	+
	10–20 µg/kg/min	++	++	+	+++	++	+		+	+
Dobutamine	2–20 µg/kg/min	+	+/–	++	–		++	+		
Epinephrine	0.5–2 µg/kg/min	++	+	+	–		++	++		
	2–10 µg/kg/min	++	++	+	++	++	++	+		
Norepinephrine	0.5–30 µg/kg/min	+	++	+	++	++	+			
Vasopressin	0.01–0.04 U/min	–	++		++					
Phosphodiesterase Inhibitors:										
Amrinone	5–10			++	–					
Milrinone	0.3–1.5			+++	–					
Nitrovasodilators:										
Sodium nitroprusside	0.1–5 µg/kg/min			+	–					
Nitroglycerin	10–20 µg/min		–	+	–					

CO, cardiac output; DA1, dopamine receptor 1; HR, heart rate; MAP, mean arterial pressure; SVR, systemic vascular resistance.

What is atrial natruretic factor?
A vasodilator that is released from the atrial wall with atrial distension that inhibits sodium and water resorption in the collecting ducts

SEPSIS

What are the criteria to diagnose systemic inflammatory response syndrome (SIRS) in an adult?
2 or more of the following criteria present: body temperature <36°C or >38°C, HR >90 bpm, respiratory rate (RR) >20 breaths/min or $PaCO_2$ <32 mm Hg, white blood cell count <4000 cells/mm^3 or >12,000 cells/mm^3 or >10% bands

What is the most potent stimulus for SIRS?
Endotoxin (lipopolysaccharide-lipid A)

What happens to insulin and glucose with early Gram-negative sepsis?
↓ Insulin, ↑ glucose, impaired utilization

What happens to insulin and glucose with late Gram-negative sepsis?
↑ Insulin, ↑ glucose, insulin resistance

What is the early sepsis triad?
Confusion, hyperventilation, respiratory alkalosis

PULMONARY PHYSIOLOGY AND VENTILATOR MANAGEMENT

What is the P/F ratio?
The ratio of PaO_2 to FiO_2

What is the diagnostic triad of ARDS?
Capillary wedge pressure <18 mm Hg, x-ray of chest with bilateral infiltrates, ratio of PaO_2 to FiO_2 <200

What does the classic chest x-ray in a patient with ARDS look like?
Bilateral fluffy infiltrates

What concentration of oxygen leads to oxygen toxicity?
FiO_2 >60% for 48 hours

What are the main causes of carbon dioxide retention?
Increased dead space ventilation, hypoventilation, increased carbon dioxide production

What is total lung capacity (TLC)?
Lung volume after maximal inspiration; TLC = forced vital capacity (FVC) + residual volume (RV)

What is FVC?
Volume of air maximally exhaled after maximal inhalation

What is RV?
Lung volume after maximal exhalation

What is tidal volume?
Volume of air with normal inspiration and expiration

What is functional residual capacity (FRC)?
Lung volume after normal exhalation, FRC = expiratory reserve volume (ERV) + RV

What is ERV?
The volume of air that can be forcefully expired after normal expiration

What is inspiratory capacity?
The maximal amount of air that inspired from the FRC

What is the FEV1?
The forced expiratory volume after maximal inhalation in 1 second

What is PEEP?
Positive end expiratory pressure, positive pressure maintained at the end of a breath that keeps alveoli open

What is normal "physiologic" PEEP?
5 cm H_2O, postulated to be the normal pressure caused by the closed glottis in a nonventilated patient

What are the presumed advantages of PEEP?
Prevention of alveolar collapse/atelectasis, decreased shunt fraction, improved gas exchange, increased pulmonary compliance

What are the side effects of excessive PEEP?
↓ Preload leading to decreased CO, barotrauma (pneumothorax), increased intracranial pressure, decreased compliance, decreased gas exchange, fluid retention

What is dead space?
The portion of inspired air that does not participate in gas exchange (large airways/endotracheal [ET] tube)

What increases dead space?
Underperfusion (PE, pulmonary artery vasoconstriction, low CO), overventilation (excessive PEEP, emphysema)

What is shunt fraction?
Portion of pulmonary venous gas that does not participate in gas exchange

Name some clinical situations that can cause increased airway resistance:
Airway/ET tube obstruction, ARDS, bronchospasm, congestive heart failure (pulmonary edema), mucus plug

What 2 conditions must you worry about in a patient with low urinary output and increased peak airway pressures?
Abdominal compartment syndrome, tension pneumothorax

How can you manipulate ventilation to decrease pCO_2?
Increase minute ventilation

How can you increase PO_2 in a ventilated patient?
↑PEEP, ↑FiO_2

Why does increasing the FiO_2 in a patient with a high shunt fraction has minimal effect on the arterial PO_2?
If >50% shunt fraction, the oxygenated blood is already at maximal oxygen absorption hence the minimal effect

What is minute ventilation?
Total lung ventilation per minute
Tidal volume × RR
Can be measured by expired gas collection for a period of 1 to 3 minutes

What is the normal range of minute ventilation?
5 to 10 L/min

What is CPAP mode on the ventilator?
Continuous positive airway pressure: patient breathes on their own with continuous positive pressure delivered during inspiration and expiration with no volume breaths given by the ventilator

What is pressure support ventilation?
A mode that overcomes the resistance of the ventilator circuit to decrease the work of breathing; the ventilator only delivers pressure during an initiated breath

What is IMV mode on the ventilator?
Intermittent mandatory ventilation: patient can breathe on their own above the mandatory rate without assistance from the ventilator, otherwise the ventilator will deliver a mandatory breath at the predetermined rate

What is SIMV mode on the ventilator?
Synchronous intermittent mandatory ventilation: delivers a mandatory breath synchronously with the patient's initiated breath; if the patient does not initiate a breath, the ventilator delivers a predetermined mandatory breath

What is A-C mode on the ventilator?
Assist-control ventilation: the ventilator "assists" the patient by delivering a breath when the patient initiates a breath, otherwise the ventilator takes "control" if the patient does not initiate a breath and delivers a breath at a predetermined rate.

What medications can be delivered through an ET tube?
Narcan, atropine, vasopressin, epinephrine, lidocaine (NAVEL) along with acetylcysteine, albuterol

What parameters are evaluated when deciding to extubate a patient on the ventilator?
Awake, alert patient able to protect airway (absence of correctible comorbid conditions (afebrile, no significant electrolyte abnormalities), no evidence of myocardial ischemia, HR ≤140 bpm, normotensive without vasopressors or with minimal vasopressor support), RR <35, PaO_2 ≥60 mm Hg on FiO_2 ≤40% to 50% and PEEP ≤5 to 8 cm H_2O, pCO_2 <50 mm Hg, tidal volume >5cc/kg, minute ventilation <10 L/min, negative inspiratory pressure <−20 cm H_2O, pH >7.25, rapid shallow breathing index (RSBI) ≤105

What adjustment should you make to the diet/total parenteral nutrition (TPN) in a patient with hypercapnia, a respiratory quotient >1.0, and difficulty getting off of the ventilator?
Decrease the amount of carbohydrates in the diet/TPN; carbohydrates have the highest CO_2 production

MULTIPLE CHOICE QUESTIONS

1. **What is the most sensitive predictor for successful extubation?**

    A. NIF <−20 cm H_2O
    B. RR <35
    C. RSBI <100
    D. Minute ventilation <10 L/min
    E. PEEP <8 cm H_2O

2. **A 68 year old female is postoperative day 3 status post a pancreaticoduodenectomy. Her post-extubation arterial blood gas shows: pH 7.58, pCO_2 30, HCO_3 26, O_2Sat 94%, and BE 2.2. Based solely on this ABG, what is her underlying acid-base disturbance?**

    A. Metabolic alkalosis
    B. Compensated metabolic alkalosis
    C. Normal
    D. Respiratory alkalosis

3. **Which is not indicative of ARDS?**

    A. Acute onset
    B. Bilateral infiltrates
    C. Wedge pressure <18 mm Hg
    D. P/F ratio <300

4. **Which of the following ventilation modes is more likely to cause increased auto-PEEP?**

    A. Pressure support ventilation
    B. Airway pressure release ventilation
    C. Assist control ventilation
    D. Pressure-controlled inverse ratio ventilation
    E. Continuous positive pressure ventilation

5. **A normotensive bleeding patient is mildly anxious with a HR of 110 and an RR of 25. What class of hemorrhagic shock is she in?**

    A. I
    B. II
    C. III
    D. IV

6. **Approximately 5 hours after ruptured AAA repair, you are called to see a patient with only 15 cc of urine for the past 2 hours. Intraoperatively, she received 9 L of crystalloid and 4 units of pRBC. At the bedside, you are also informed that his peak airway pressure on the ventilator is 42 mm Hg. His BP is 90/52, HR 115 bpm. What is an appropriate next step?**

    A. Diuresis with furosemide
    B. Increase PEEP
    C. Check bladder pressure
    D. Start inotropic agent

7. **Which of the following is most likely suggestive of hypovolemic shock?**

	CVP	PCWP	CI	SVR	VO_2	DO_2
A.	Low	Low	High	Low	Low/normal	High
B.	High	High	Low	High	Low	Low
C.	Low	Low	Low	High	High	Low
D.	Normal	Low	Normal	High	High	Normal

8. **The formula for oxygen extraction ratio is:**
   A. DO_2/VO_2
   B. VO_2/DO_2
   C. $1/VO_2$
   D. CO_x oxygen content
   E. MAP-CVP/CO

9. **Use the equation below to calculate the respiratory quotient:**
   $$C_6H_{12}O_6 + 6O_2 \rightarrow 6CO_2 + 6H_2O$$
   A. 1.00
   B. 0.90
   C. 0.85
   D. 0.65
   E. 0.75

ANSWERS

1. **Answer: C.** The rapid shallow breathing index (RSBI) is the ratio of the respiratory frequency (f) and the tidal volume (VT). An RSBI <105 has been shown to be the most sensitive criteria for weaning patient to extubation.

2. **Answer: D.** First, look at the pH; in this case it is alkalotic. You must now distinguish if this is respiratory, mixed, or metabolic. So pay attention to the pCO_2 and the HCO_3 and note that the HCO_3 is normal but the pCO_2 is low. The characteristic of respiratory alkalosis is increase in pH with decrease in pCO_2. In the acute setting, note that HCO_3 typically decreases by 2 mEq/L for every 10 mm Hg drop in pCO_2. In chronic respiratory alkalosis, HCO_3 typically increases by 4 mEq/L of HCO_3 for every 10 mm Hg drop in pCO_2.

3. **Answer: D.** The distinction between ALI and ARDS is the degree of hypoxemia defined by the P/F ratio. In ALI the ratio is less than 300 mm Hg and for ARDS it is 200 mm Hg or less.

4. **Answer: D.** Normal respiration typically has an inspiration to expiration ratio of 1:2. This means that inverse ratio makes inspiration time longer than expiration time. High inverse ratios do not allow adequate expiration time and patients usually stack their breaths. Thus, every inspiration occurs before expiration is complete resulting in auto-PEEP.

5. **Answer: B.** In Class I hemorrhagic shock, the patient has normal mental status. Class II is defined as 750- to 1500-mL blood loss; 15% to 30% blood loss; HR >100 bpm; normal blood pressure; decreased pulse pressure; RR 20 to 30 breaths/min; urinary output 20 to 30 mL/h and mildly anxious.

6. **Answer: C.** The oliguria, low CVP, and hypotension could be suggestive of underresuscitation. However, the very high peak airway pressure in conjunction with the other findings plus the fact he had very large fluid resuscitation in the operating room should increase the suspicion for abdominal compartment syndrome. Measuring the bladder pressure would be the next best decision since the other choices would not be beneficial in this scenario.

7. **Answer: C.** Choice A is more descriptive of distributive shock with high CI and lower SVR. Overall, B would most likely represent cardiogenic shock with the lower than normal CI and high wedge pressure. In hypovolemic shock preload (CVP) is decreased, leading to decreased PCWP and CO.

8. **Answer: B.** The oxygen extraction ratio (O_2ER) is the ratio of oxygen consumed to that delivered (VO_2/DO_2). It represents the amount of oxygen delivered via the circulation that is taken up by the tissues. Normal O_2ER is 0.2 to 0.3, indicating that only 20% to 30% of the delivered oxygen is utilized.

9. **Answer: A.** The respiratory quotient is the ratio of the volume of carbon dioxide produced to the volume of oxygen consumed per unit of time by the body. The equation above illustrates the utilization of glucose. Six molecules of carbon dioxide are produced for the 6 molecules of oxygen used up.

CHAPTER 23
Burns

Karin McConville

CLASSIFICATION

What are the 5 different causal categories for burns?
1. Flame: damage from superheated, oxidized air
2. Scald: damage from contact with hot liquids
3. Contact: damage from contact with hot or cold solid materials
4. Chemical: contact with noxious chemicals
5. Electrical: conduction of electrical current through tissues

What is a 1st-degree burn?
Injury localized to the epidermis

What is a superficial 2nd-degree burn?
Injury to the epidermis and superficial dermis

What is a deep 2nd-degree burn?
Injury through the epidermis and into the deep dermis

What is a 3rd-degree burn?
Full-thickness injury through the epidermis and dermis into the subcutaneous fat

What is a 4th-degree burn?
Injury through the skin and subcutaneous fat into underlying muscle or bone

Identify the depth of the burn:
A painful, erythematous burn with an intact epidermal barrier that blanches to the touch?
1st degree
Painful burn with blebs and blisters; hair follicles intact; blanches to the touch?
Superficial 2nd degree
Sensation decreased; loss of hair follicles?
Deep 2nd degree
Leathery feeling, no sensation?
3rd degree

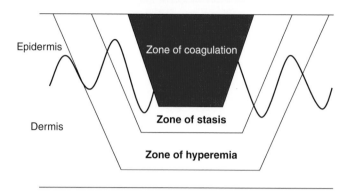

FIGURE 23-1. Illustration of the zones of injury after burn. Factors likely to affect the zone of stasis determine the extension of injury from the original zone of coagulation. *(Reproduced from Felliciano DV, Mattox, Moore EE. Trauma. 6th ed. http://www.accesssurgery.com. Copyright © The McGraw-Hill Companies, Inc. All rights reserved.)*

PATHOPHYSIOLOGY

What are the 3 zones of injury from a burn?
Zone of coagulation, zone of stasis, zone of hyperemia

Define the zone of coagulation:
Irreversibly damaged necrotic area of a burn where cells have been disrupted

Define the zone of stasis:
Area associated with vascular damage and leakage that is immediately adjacent to the necrotic zone with a moderate degree of insult and decreased tissue perfusion that can either survive or progress to coagulative necrosis

Zone of hyperemia:
Area of vasodilation from inflammation surrounding the burn with viable tissue where the healing process begins

EVALUATION OF BURN WOUNDS

How can you differentiate a superficial 2nd-degree from a deep 2nd-degree burn?
Superficial 2nd-degree burn will blanch to the touch, whereas deep 2nd-degree burn will not

Where does a superficial 2nd-degree burn re-epithelialize from?
Rete ridges; hair follicles; sweat glands (7–14 days)

Where does a deep 2nd-degree burn re-epithelialize from?
Hair follicles; sweat gland keratinocytes (14–35 days)

Where does a 3rd-degree burn re-epithelialize from?
Wound edges

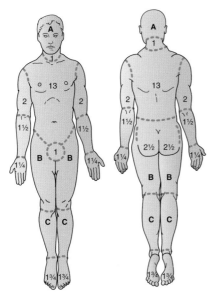

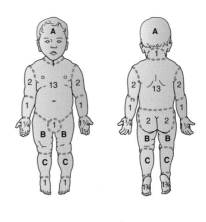

Relative percentages of areas affected by growth

Area	Age		
	10	15	Adult
A = half of head	5 ½	4 ½	3 ½
B = half of one thigh	4 ¼	4 ½	4 ¾
C = half of one leg	3	3 ¼	3 ½

Relative percentages of areas affected by growth

Area	Age		
	0	1	5
A = half of head	9 ½	8 ½	6 ½
B = half of one thigh	2 ¾	3 ¼	4
C = half of one leg	2 ½	2 ½	2 ¾

FIGURE 23-2. Table for estimating extent of burns. In adults, a reasonable system for calculating the percentage of body surface burned is the "rule of nines": Each arm equals 9%, the head equals 9%, the anterior and posterior trunk each equal 18%, and each leg equals 18%; the sum of these percentages is 99%. *(Reproduced from Doherty GM. Current Diagnosis and Treatment: Surgery. 13th ed. http://www.accessmedicine.com. Copyright © The McGraw-Hill Companies, Inc. All rights reserved.)*

According to the rules of nines, what percentage of total body surface area (TBSA) do these regions represent in an adult?

Each upper extremity?
9% TBSA

Head and neck?
9% TBSA

Each lower extremity?
18% TBSA

Anterior torso?
18% TBSA

Posterior torso?
18% TBSA

Perineum and genitalia?
1% TBSA

What percentage of TBSA does the open hand (palm with fingers extended) of the patient account for?
1%; this area can be visually transposed onto the burn for an estimation of size.

What percentage do the head and neck account for in the TBSA of an infant?
21%

What percentage does each leg account for in the TBSA of an infant?
13%

FLUID RESUSCITATION

What formula estimates the amount of fluid needed for the resuscitation of a burn patient?
Parkland Formula: give 4 mL/kg × % burn in first 24 hours
Give ½ in first 8 hours, the rest in next 16 hours
Use for burns ≥20%
Use lactated Ringer solution

What is the best measure of adequate resuscitation?
Urine output
Adults: 0.5 to 1.0 mL/kg/h
Children <6 months: 2 to 4 mL/kg/h

How do you calculate the Galveston formula for maintenance fluid in the first 24 hours for a pediatric burn patient?
5000 mL/TBSA burned (in m^2) + 1500 mL/m^2 total area

Table 23-1 Resuscitation Formulas			
Formula	Crystalloid Volume	Colloid Volume	Free Water
Parkland	4 mL/kg/% TBSA burn	None	None
Brooke	1.5 mL/kg/% TBSA burn	0.5 mL/kg/% TBSA burn	2.0 L
Galveston (pediatric)	5000 mL/m^2 burned + 1500 mL/m^2 total	None	None

TBSA, total body surface area.
Reproduced from Felliciano DV, Mattox, Moore EE. *Trauma*. 6th ed. http://www.accesssurgery.com. Copyright © The McGraw-Hill Companies, Inc. All rights reserved.

TREATMENT OF BURNS

What is the treatment for a 1st-degree burn?
Topical soothing salves; oral nonsteroidal anti-inflammatory agents

What is the treatment for a superficial 2nd-degree burn?
Clean wound with antiseptic soap to remove dead skin and foreign material
Unroof blisters
Apply topical antibiotic and dress wound

What is the treatment for a deep 2nd- and 3rd-degree burns?
Initially treat like superficial 2nd-degree burns
Follow with early excision and grafting (within 72 hours)
Lower mortality rate
Can mobilize early (improved joint function and short hospitalization)

What is an autograft?
Skin graft from the patient

What is an allograft?
Skin graft from same species (cadaver); allows for temporary wound coverage until autograft can be done

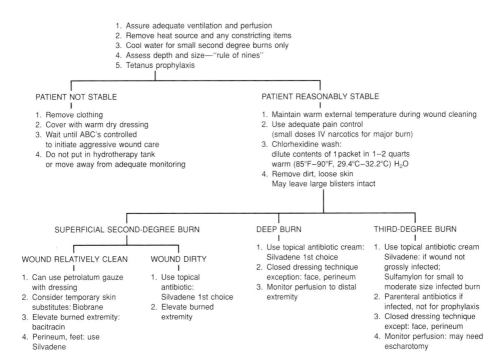

1. Assure adequate ventilation and perfusion
2. Remove heat source and any constricting items
3. Cool water for small second degree burns only
4. Assess depth and size—"rule of nines"
5. Tetanus prophylaxis

PATIENT NOT STABLE

1. Remove clothing
2. Cover with warm dry dressing
3. Wait until ABC's controlled
   to initiate aggressive wound care
4. Do not put in hydrotherapy tank
   or move away from adequate monitoring

PATIENT REASONABLY STABLE

1. Maintain warm external temperature during wound cleaning
2. Use adequate pain control
   (small doses IV narcotics for major burn)
3. Chlorhexidine wash:
   dilute contents of 1 packet in 1–2 quarts
   warm (85°F–90°F, 29.4°C–32.2°C) H_2O
4. Remove dirt, loose skin
   May leave large blisters intact

SUPERFICIAL SECOND-DEGREE BURN

WOUND RELATIVELY CLEAN

1. Can use petrolatum gauze
   with dressing
2. Consider temporary skin
   substitutes: Biobrane
3. Elevate burned extremity:
   bacitracin
4. Perineum, feet: use
   Silvadene

WOUND DIRTY

1. Use topical
   antibiotic:
   Silvadene 1st choice
2. Elevate burned
   extremity

DEEP BURN

1. Use topical antibiotic cream:
   Silvadene 1st choice
2. Closed dressing technique
   exception: face, perineum
3. Monitor perfusion to distal
   extremity

THIRD-DEGREE BURN

1. Use topical antibiotic cream
   Silvadene: if wound not
   grossly infected;
   Sulfamylon for small to
   moderate size infected burn
2. Parenteral antibiotics if
   infected, not for prophylaxis
3. Closed dressing technique
   except: face, perineum
4. Monitor perfusion: may need
   escharotomy

FIGURE 23-3. Treatment summary (0–24 hours). Wound management. *(Reproduced from Hall JB, Schmidt GA, Wood LDH. Principles of Critical Care. 3rd ed. http://www.accessmedicine.com. Copyright © The McGraw-Hill Companies, Inc. All rights reserved.)*

What is a homograft?
Same as allograft

What is a xenograft?
Skin graft from a different species (porcine)

What antimicrobial soak can cause methemoglobinemia?
0.5% Silver nitrate

What antimicrobial soak can cause metabolic acidosis?
5% Mafenide acetate inhibits carbonic anhydrase.

What topical antibiotic can cause a transient leukopenia?
1% Silver sulfadiazine (aka Silvadene)

What topical antibiotic can penetrate eschar?
11% Mafenide acetate (aka Sulfamylon)
Other characteristics: pain when applied to skin, allergic rash, carbonic anhydrase inhibition

What antimicrobial soak can stain surface a gray or black color when dry?
0.5% Silver nitrate solution

INHALATION INJURY

What causes most of the damage with inhalation injury?
Inhaled toxins

What is an abnormal carboxyhemoglobin?
>10% in nonsmokers
>20% in smokers

What is the treatment for carbon monoxide poisoning?
100% oxygen; possibly hyperbaric oxygen

What is the substance in Hurricane spray that causes methemoglobinemia?
Nitrites

What is the treatment of methemoglobinemia?
Methylene blue

What are the 3 stages of the clinical course for patients with inhalation injury?
Acute pulmonary insufficiency
Hypoxia and development of diffuse lobar infiltrates (72–96 hours after injury)
Clinical bronchopneumonia with expectoration of large mucous casts formed in the tracheobronchial tree (3–10 days after injury)

What is the dose and schedule for nebulized heparin given for inhalation injury?
5000 to 10,000 U with 3 mL normal saline every 4 hours

What is the dose and schedule for nebulized acetyl cysteine given for inhalation injury?
3 mL of a 20% solution every 4 hours

MISCELLANEOUS

What is the formula to calculate the daily nutritional needs of a burn patient?
Curreri formula: 25 kcal/kg/d + 40 kcal/%TBSA

What is the major tissue through which electrical current flows, thus sustaining the most damage?
Muscle

As a good rule of thumb, how many liters of tap water should be used to lavage a chemical burn?
15 to 20 L

What 3 factors are involved in the mechanism of alkali burns?
Saponification of fat
Massive extraction of water from cells
Alkali dissolves and combines with proteins to form alkaline proteinates
Contains hydroxide ions, which induce further chemical reactions

What is the strongest inorganic acid?
Hydrofluoric acid

What is the treatment of hydrofluoric acid burn?
Copiously irrigate with water
Apply 2.5% calcium gluconate gel, changing the gel at 15-minute intervals until pain subsides
If pain persists or symptoms recur, give intradermal injection of 10% calcium gluconate (0.5 mL/cm^2 affected) or give intraarterial injection of calcium gluconate into the affected extremity

How does calcium gluconate work in treating hydrofluoric acid burn?
Fluoride ion complexes with bivalent cations (calcium, magnesium) to form insoluble salts; systemic absorption of the fluoride ion results in hypocalcemia from intravascular calcium chelation causing life-threatening arrhythmias.

MULTIPLE CHOICE QUESTIONS

1. A 45-year-old female presents to the hospital after falling into a fire and suffering 2nd-degree burns to her right hand and entire arm. What is the percent of TBSA burned for this patient?
   A. 20%
   B. 10
   C. 5%
   D. 15%

2. A 76-year-old male who weighs 80 kg suffered a 25% TBSA 2nd-degree scald burn when a large pot of boiling water spilled onto his torso and lower extremities. He was immediately transferred to the hospital. He has been given 200 mL of lactated Ringer thus far. What is the amount of fluid needed to resuscitate this patient in the first 8 hours?
   A. 5000 mL
   B. 4300 mL
   C. 3800 mL
   D. 3500 mL

3. A 16-year-old female is admitted to the hospital after suffering a 36% 2nd- and 3rd-degree burns to the face and torso after being involved in a house fire. She is intubated. On the 2nd day of hospitalization, her morning arterial blood gas shows a metabolic acidosis. What is most likely the cause of her lab abnormality?
   A. Respiratory rate of 14
   B. Silver nitrate
   C. Silver sulfadiazine
   D. Mafenide acetate

4. A 43-year-old male suffers a 5% TBSA 2nd-degree burn to his right leg. He is treated with topical ointment and discharged from the emergency room. He returns to the hospital on the 3rd day complaining of increased pain at the burn site. On examination, there is a dark brown discoloration of the wound and presence of blood below the eschar. A biopsy of viable tissue near the eschar is taken, which shows >100,000 microbial organisms per gram. What is the most appropriate treatment?
   A. IV antibiotics only
   B. IV antibiotics and application of Silvadene
   C. Application of Dakin solution
   D. Surgical excision of infected tissues

5. A 23-year-old male spills hydrofluoric acid on the dorsum of his left hand. What is the most appropriate treatment?

   A. Copious irrigation with water
   B. Copious irrigation with water and application of calcium gluconate gel
   C. Copious irrigation with normal saline and application of mafenide acetate
   D. Immediate surgical excision

6. A 4-year-old male presents to the emergency department after knocking over a cup of hot soup onto himself. On examination, he has an area of erythema with visible blisters over his right forearm. There is blanching with palpation. He cries with examination of the burned arm. What is the degree of his burn?

   A. 1st Degree
   B. Superficial 2nd degree
   C. Deep 2nd degree
   D. 3rd Degree

7. A 45-year-old woman is brought to the trauma bay after being rescued from a burning house. She was intubated at the scene due to obvious burns to the face and decreased oxygen saturation. During primary survey, you note that the ET tube is 24 cm at the lip, and she has bilateral breath sounds on auscultation. Her heart rate is 104 and BP is 100/78. However, her saturation is 89% with 100% FiO2. She is noted to have 1st- and 2nd-degree burns to the face and both arms. She also has deep 2nd- and 3rd-degree burns to the torso. A chest x-ray shows endotracheal tube in good position above the carina and no pneumothoraces. What is the next step in improving oxygenation of this patient?

   A. Change mode of ventilation to high-frequency percussive ventilation
   B. Insertion of bilateral chest tubes
   C. Escharotomies of torso
   D. Frequent suctioning and observation

8. A 17-year-old male presents to the emergency department after spilling hot coffee onto his lap. He is found to have 5% TBSA 1st-degree burn to the right thigh and treated with topical 0.5% silver nitrate. He is brought back to the hospital by his mother after a "fainting spell." On examination, he appears to be cyanotic and short of breath. However, his oxygen saturation is 100% on 2 L. What is the most likely cause of his symptoms?

   A. Pulmonary embolism
   B. Pneumonia
   C. Inhalation injury
   D. Methemoglobinemia

9. How would you treat the patient described in the previous question?

   A. Supplemental oxygen and 1% methylene blue
   B. Supplemental oxygen and IV vitamin C
   C. Transfusion of packed red blood cells
   D. IV NADH methemoglobin reductase

10. A 56-year-old male brought to the emergency department by his friends after being found in a stranded vehicle during a snow storm. He denies having any pain but on examination, the toes on both feet are noted to be white and waxy in appearance. There is no capillary refill. What is the appropriate treatment?

A. IV antibiotics
B. Rewarming with warm blankets
C. Rewarming with a warm water bath
D. Immediate amputation

ANSWERS

1. **Answer: B.** According to the rule of nines, an upper extremity is 9% TBSA. Also, the patient's hand is considered 1% of TBSA.

2. **Answer: C.** The Parkland formula for burn patient fluid resuscitation is: total volume 4 mL/kg/%TBSA, which should be given in the first 24 hours after a burn. Half of this volume should be given in the first 8 hours after the burn injury, which includes prehospital/preadmission time. The remainder is given in the remaining 16 hours. Thus, this 80-kg patient with 25% TBSA 2nd-degree burn should receive a total of 8000 mL of volume in the first 24 hours and 4000 mL in the first 8 hours. He received 200 mL by prehospital personnel, and should receive 3800 mL for a total 4000 mL in the first 8 hours.

3. **Answer: D.** Mafenide acetate can cause metabolic acidosis by inhibiting carbonic anhydrase. Silver nitrate is used for treatment of burns and can cause methemoglobinemia. It also does not penetrate eschars. Silver sulfadiazine is known to cause transient leucopenia.

4. **Answer: D.** Dark brown discoloration of the wound and the presence of blood below the eschar are indicative of a burn wound infection. Also, the presence of >100,000 microbial organisms per gram in nonnecrotic tissue is the most important factor in the diagnosis of a burn infection. The treatment of burn wound infection is surgical excision of infected tissues.

5. **Answer: B.** Hydrofluoric acid is the strongest inorganic acid and the treatment of a burn from it is to first thoroughly irrigate the burn with water. Then, calcium gluconate gel should be applied. The gel should be changed every 15 minutes until the pain resolves. If pain does not subside, or if it recurs, an intradermal injection of 10% calcium gluconate or an intraarterial injection of calcium gluconate can be given in the affected extremity. Calcium gluconate treats hydrofluoric acid burns by forming insoluble salts when the fluoride ion complexes with the calcium (bivalent cation). If the fluoride ions were absorbed systemically, intravascular chelation of calcium would result in hypocalcemia and subsequent life-threatening arrhythmias.

6. **Answer: B.** 2nd-degree burn is a partial-thickness burn that involves the epidermis as well as the dermis. They vary from superficial to deep depending on the amount of dermis that is injured. Superficial 2nd-degree burn affects the epidermis and superficial dermis and is characterized by erythema that blanches to the touch, blisters, and pain.

7. **Answer: C.** A 3rd-degree (full-thickness) burn of the torso does not allow the chest to expand and leads to compromised blood flow as the subcutaneous edema increases. Thoracic compartment syndrome can be characterized by decreased ventilation, increased airway pressures, and hypotension. Escharotomies should be performed to decompress the thoracic cavity and allow the chest to expand.

8. **Answer: D.** Methemoglobinemia is a disorder that increases the level of methemoglobin in the blood, which results in decreased affinity for oxygen. Thus, there is a higher affinity for oxygen at other heme sites that leads to decreased tissue oxygenation. The oxygen-hemoglobin dissociation curve is shifted to the left. Signs and symptoms of moderate methemoglobinemia include dyspnea, headache, and fatigue. If levels increase to greater than 60%, confusion, seizures, and death can occur. 0.5% Silver nitrate can cause methemoglobinemia as well as other oxidizing drugs such as local anesthetics, Hurricane spray (nitrates), and aniline dyes.

9. **Answer: A.** Treatment for methemoglobinemia is supplemental oxygen and 1% methylene blue (10 mg/mL) given intravenously. Methylene blue restores the iron in hemoglobin to its reduced state. The dose is 1 to 2 mg/mL given over 5 minutes and can be repeated every 5 minutes to treat symptoms. Do not exceed maximum dose of 7 mg/kg.

10. **Answer: C.** Treatment for frostbite is rewarming in a warm water bath at 40°C to 42.2°C for 20 to 30 minutes. Immersion in warm water is the best method of warming the affected region and minimizing further injury.

CHAPTER 24

Vascular

Samuel N. Steerman and Jason Davis

- Vascular emergency questions are asked twice as much as elective vascular reconstruction. Acute ischemia and traumatic injury are favorite topics along with management. If in doubt, perform fasciotomy. Other common topics are risk factor modification, vascular lab testing (ABI), and visceral aneurysm. Endovascular choices are often wrong; be careful not to select an answer just because you don't fully understand it.

PERIPHERAL ARTERIAL OCCLUSIVE DISEASE

Describe the risk factors associated with atherosclerosis:
Smoking, diabetes, hyperlipidemia, obesity, HTN, sedentary lifestyle

Differentiate between the following:
Arterial ulcers and venous ulcers
Arterial ulcers—painful and usually occur on toes or foot
Venous ulcers—commonly broad-based, shallow at medial malleolus
Claudication and rest pain
Claudication—cramping ischemic muscle pain with exertion that occurs distal to arterial stenosis, associated with 1% risk of limb loss and 5% mortality.
Rest pain—also due to ischemia, arises without exertion and classically wakes patients from sleep (often over distal metatarsals). The pain may resolve with standing or placing foot over side of bed (dependent position, gravity). >50% patients eventually require amputation.
Wet gangrene and dry gangrene
Dry gangrene—dry necrotic "mummified" tissue without signs of infection—not a surgical emergency
Wet gangrene—moist necrotic tissue indicative of active infectious process—requires aggressive debridement or amputation to avoid sepsis

How are ankle brachial index/digital brachial index (ABIs/DBIs) and segmental pressures measured? Pulse volume recordings (PVRs)? What is their significance?
Normal ABI at rest: 1.0 to 1.2, mild arterial insufficiency: 0.7 to 0.9, claudication: 0.5 to 0.7, rest pain and ultimately tissue necrosis: <0.4 (falsely elevated ABIs may be seen in diabetic patients or those with chronic renal disease due to extensive vascular calcification).
PVRs analyze the waveforms at sequential sites along patient's leg—triphasic or biphasic waveforms, indicates more perfusion than monophasic.

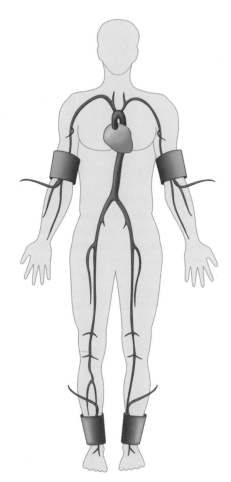

Right ABI = ratio of

Higher of the right ankle systolic pressures (posterior tibial or dorsalis pedis)

———

Higher arm systolic pressure (left or right arm)

Left ABI = ratio of

Higher of the left ankle systolic pressures (posterior tibial or dorsalis pedis)

———

Higher arm systolic pressure (left or right arm)

FIGURE 24-1. Calculating the ankle-brachial index. *(Reproduced from Brunicardi FC, Andersen DK, Billiar TR, et al. Schwartz's Principles of Surgery. 9th ed. http://www.accessmedicine.com. Copyright © The McGraw-Hill Companies, Inc. All rights reserved.)*

What is the half-life of heparin? Intraoperative therapeutic dosing? How is it reversed?
Half-life is 60 to 90 minutes. Intraoperative dosing is 70 to 100 units/kg (activating clotting time of 250 to 350 seconds if measured). Protamine sulfate: 1 mg/100 units of heparin.

What are the 5-year patencies of common and external iliac percutaneous transluminal angioplasty (PTA) without stenting?
Common iliac: 70% to 80%
External iliac: 50% to 60%

What are the classic signs/symptoms of acute arterial occlusion? In what order do they present?
The "6 P's" include: Paresthesias, Pain, Pallor, Poikilothermia, Pulselessness, Paralysis

What percentage of emboli originate in the heart? First and second most common causes?
80% of peripheral emboli are due to cardiac etiology (First—atrial fibrillation, Second—acute MI)

At what anatomic sites do atherosclerotic lesions most commonly occlude?
Atherosclerosis forms at branch points such as carotid bifurcation, bends, and tethered segments such as superficial femoral artery as it passes through Hunter canal
Emboli lodge at arterial bifurcation—that is, femoral bifurcation, brachial bifurcation

How can a peripheral venous embolus cause occlusion in the peripheral arterial circulation?
A "paradoxical embolus" occurs when a peripheral venous thromboembolus crosses into the peripheral arterial circulation through a patent foramen ovale in the heart.

What is the risk of limb loss associated with acute thromboembolic disease? What is the associated mortality?
Risk of limb loss: 8% to 22%
Thromboembolic perioperative mortality: 10% to 17%

Name some of the indications to operate for peripheral arterial occlusive disease:
Tissue necrosis, rest pain, infection, debilitating claudication refractory to nonoperative management (Pentoxifylline, Aspirin, Cessation of smoking, Exercise—PACE pneumonic)
NOTE—claudication is not an indication for surgery; it is best treated with supervised exercise training.

What is 5-year patency rate of Fem-Pop vein grafts versus prosthetic grafts
5-year patency of an above-the-knee vein graft is 75% (no difference between in situ or reverse); prosthetic is 40% to 50%.
5-year patency of a below-the-knee vein graft is 65%, prosthetic is 30%.

What do early (<30 day), intermediate, and late (>2 year) bypass graft failures generally represent?
Early—Use of small, poor-quality vein; anastomosis to inadequate outflow artery or technical error (kink/twist of graft; incomplete lysis of valves) at the time of surgery
Intermediate—Intimal hyperplasia at anastomotic sites or valve sites within the graft
Late—Progression of atherosclerotic disease within the inflow or outflow vessels

Name the 4 calf compartments in order of compartment syndrome probability:
Anterior, lateral, deep posterior, superficial posterior compartment

What is the first sign of compartment syndrome? How long after revascularization is greatest risk?
Numbness of great toe webbing is an early sign of compartment syndrome due to deep peroneal nerve compression (anterior). Greatest risk occurs 4 to 6 hours after revascularization along with release of intracellular ions/proteins/enzymes from damaged sarcolemma.

What is the most common iatrogenic injury during anterior compartment fasciotomy?
Injury to the lateral peroneal nerve in the superior aspect of the incision

Table 24-1 Conditions Qualifying Patients as "High Surgical Risk" for Carotid Endarterectomy	
Anatomical Factors	Physiologic Factors
• High carotid bifurcation (above C2 vertebral body) • Low common carotid artery (below clavicle) • Contralateral carotid occlusion • Restenosis of ipsilateral prior carotid endarterectomy • Previous neck irradiation • Prior radical neck dissection • Contralateral laryngeal nerve palsy • Presence of tracheostomy	• Age ≥80 y • Left ventricular ejection fraction ≤30% • New York Heart Association Class III/IV congestive heart failure • Unstable angina: Canadian Cardiovascular Society Class III/IV angina pectoris • Recent myocardial infarction • Clinically significant cardiac disease (congestive heart failure, abnormal stress test, or need for coronary revascularization) • Severe COPD • End-stage renal disease on dialysis

Brunicardi FC, Andersen DK, Billiar TR, Dunn DL, Hunter JG, Matthews JB, Pollock RE. *Schwartz Principles of Surgery*. 9th ed. www.accessmedicine.com. Copyright © The McGraw-Hill Companies, Inc. All rights reserved.

CEREBROVASCULAR DISEASE

Name the structures that correspond to the following descriptions:
Contents of carotid sheath
Carotid artery, internal jugular vein, vagus nerve, and deep cervical lymph nodes
Vein crosses over carotid at level of bifurcation
Facial vein
Muscle crosses distal carotid arteries
Digastric muscle
Muscle that crosses proximal common carotid artery
Omohyoid muscle
Nerve that is deep to the facial vein and crosses ~1 cm distal to carotid bifurcation
Hypoglossal nerve
Nerve that branches from hypoglossal nerve and can help locate hypoglossal nerve
Ansa cervicalis

Compare and contrast the terms: stroke, TIA, cerebrovascular attack (CVA), and amaurosis fugax.
Stroke refers to acute brain injury with neurologic deficits lasting >24 hours. The neurologic impairment associated with transient ischemic attacks resolves within <24 hours.
CVA indicates permanent ischemic brain damage.
Amaurosis fugax is transient monocular vision loss attributed to ophthalmic artery. Microemboli can be related to carotid artery stenosis.

What underlying conditions and risk factors predispose strokes?
Atrial fibrillation, atherosclerosis at common carotid artery bifurcation, and HTN

True or False: An audible bruit over the carotid bifurcation indicates significant carotid stenosis.
False—an audible carotid bruit does not correlate well with significant carotid stenosis.

What is the gold standard for identifying carotid artery stenosis? What is the best screening test?
Carotid artery angiography is considered the gold standard to diagnose ICA stenosis. It is, however, invasive (1% risk of stroke) and rarely necessary. Duplex ultrasound is the

best test to screen for ICA stenosis. CT angiogram (CTA) or magnetic resonance imaging (MRA) can be used to further characterize.

What are the indications for surgical treatment of cerebrovascular disease?
>50% symptomatic ICA stenosis, <70% asymptomatic ICA stenosis with ulcerated plaque or failure of medical therapy, >80% asymptomatic ICA stenosis, or crescendo TIAs

What are the risks and most common complications of carotid endarterectomy?
0.3% to 1.6% MI, 1% to 4.5% hematoma, restenosis at 2 to 3 years after carotid endarterectomy (CEA) (neointimal hyperplasia) + 3 years after CEA (recurrent atherosclerosis at bifurcation)
Risk of perioperative stroke is 1% for asymptomatic patients and 5% for symptomatic, most often due to a technical defect created at the time of arterial reconstruction (if focal neurologic change occurs in PACU, return to OR for re-exploration)
Cerebral edema +/- headache and/or seizures (due to cerebral *hyper*perfusion syndrome)

A patient presents with left arm claudication, syncope, and ataxia. What might this be?
More common on the left and due to subclavian or innominate stenosis, subclavian steal syndrome is characterized by upper extremity claudication and signs of vertebrobasilar insufficiency (vertigo, syncopal attacks, confusion, blindness, ataxia, dysarthria)

THORACIC AORTA

What are the branches of the thoracic aorta?
Bronchial, esophageal, intercostal arteries

What artery supplies the lower anterior spinal artery and from where does it originate?
The artery of Adamkiewicz usually originates from an aortic intercostal artery between the 9th and 12th intercostal spaces and can be associated with anterior cord syndrome.

What size defines an aorta as aneurysmal, and at what size is intervention indicated?
Localized or diffuse aortic dilation >50% of normal aortic diameter (1.5–2 cm)
Thoracic aortic aneurysms >7 cm or enlargement >0.5 cm/6 mo warrant surgical intervention (>6 cm for patients with connective tissue disorders).

Name 6 risk factors associated with aneurysm formation.
Age, arteriosclerosis, connective tissue disorder, smoking, HTN, dissection

Differentiate between Crawford stages I to IV of thoracoabdominal aneurysms.
Type I—Involve descending thoracic aorta from left subclavian to suprarenal aorta
Type II—Extend from left subclavian to renal arteries (may continue to aortic bifurcation)
Type III—Mid/distal descending thoracic aorta to most abdominal aorta until bifurcation
Type IV—Includes upper abdominal aorta through all or none of the infrarenal aorta

How is management for Stanford type A aortic dissections different from that for type B?
Dissections involving the ascending aorta (type A) require surgery, whereas dissections not involving the ascending aorta (type B) require tight BP control (Esmolol, etc) in the absence of aortic rupture, intractable pain, malperfusion of branches of aorta, or uncontrollable HTN. Follow-up CT scans are recommended at 1.5, 3, and 6 months, and then annually.

Differentiate between Debakey types I to III aortic dissections:
Type I—Ascending and descending aorta
Type II—Ascending aorta only, proximal to left subclavian

I II IIIa IIIb

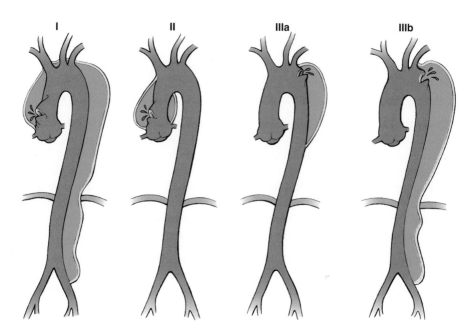

FIGURE 24-2. Classification of aortic dissection. DeBakey type I and Stanford type A include dissections that involve the proximal aorta, arch, and descending thoracic aorta. DeBakey type II only involves the ascending aorta; this dissection is included in the Stanford type A. DeBakey type III and Stanford type B include dissections that originate in the descending thoracic and thoracoabdominal aorta regardless of any retrograde involvement of the arch. These are subdivided into subtypes a and b, depending on abdominal aortic involvement. *(Reproduced from Cohn LH. Cardiac Surgery in the Adults. 4th ed. www.accesssurgery.com. Copyright © The McGraw-Hill Companies, Inc. All rights reserved.)*

Type IIIa—Descending aorta, involves above diaphragm only
Type IIIb—Descending aorta, extends below diaphragm

What genetic defect is most commonly associated with aortic dissections and aneurysms?
Marfan syndrome is caused by a mutation of the fibrillin-1 gene (FBN1).

What are the minimum lengths required distal to the left common carotid artery for the proximal landing zone and proximal to the celiac axis for the distal landing zone when performing a thoracic EVAR (TEVAR)?
Both proximal and distal graft landing zones are required to be 20 mm for TEVAR.

Describe the recommended follow-up for a patient status post-TEVAR:
Lifelong surveillance CTA performed at 1, 6, and 12 months, and yearly thereafter.

Left subclavian revascularization is reserved for which patients during TEVAR with a covered arch?
Patients with a dominant left vertebral artery develop left upper extremity ischemic symptoms, or those who've undergone a previous bypass requiring left subclavian flow, some say all nonemergent patients.

What are the 5-year risks of rupture for thoracic aortic aneurysms of 6 cm, 7 cm, and 8 cm?
5-year risks of rupture for thoracic aorta aneurysm (TAAs) are ~31% for 6 cm, ~43% for 7 cm, and ~100% for 8 cm.

What laboratory test should be sent after clamping the supraceliac aorta?
Amylase, lipase, liver function tests

Table 24-2	Annualized Risk of Rupture of Abdominal Aortic Aneurysm (AAA) Based on Size		
Description	Diameter of Aorta (cm)	Estimated Annual Risk of Rupture (%)	Estimated 5-year Risk of Rupture (%)*
Normal aorta	2–3	0	0 (unless AAA develops)
Small AAA	4–5	1	5–10
Moderate AAA	5–6	2–5	30–40
Large AAA	6–7	3–10	>50
Very large AAA	>7	>10	Approaching 100

*The estimated 5-year risk is more than 5 times the estimated annual risk because over that 5 y, the AAA, if left untreated, will continue to grow in size.
Brunicardi FC, Andersen DK, Billiar TR, Dunn DL, Hunter JG, Matthews JB, Pollock RE. *Schwartz Principles of Surgery*. 9th ed. www.accessmedicine.com. Copyright © The McGraw-Hill Companies, Inc. All rights reserved.

INFRARENAL AORTA

Name the following anatomic structures:
Vein that crosses the proximal abdominal aorta
Left renal vein
Vein that runs posterior to the right common iliac artery
Left common iliac vein
Artery with its origin midway along the abdominal aorta, exiting leftward
Inferior mesenteric artery
Can be injured during dissection/clamping along anterior iliac artery near iliac bifurcation?
Ureter and parasympathetic nerve plexus (results in sexual dysfunction)

Place the following aneurysms in decreasing order of frequency: aorta, iliac, femoral, popliteal.
Aorta > Iliac > Popliteal > Femoral artery aneurysms

At what rates do (cm) abdominal aortic aneurysms (AAAs) grow?
The rate of growth for AAAs <5 cm is ~0.32 cm/y, while that for >5 cm is ~0.4 to 0.5 cm/y.

What is the survival rate for ruptured AAAs? What symptoms indicate rupture?
50% of ruptured AAAs reach the hospital, of which only 50% survive (mortality > in winter).
Classic triad of symptoms includes sudden abdominal/flank pain, shock, and pulsatile mass.

What is the best screening test used for AAAs and in what population?
Abdominal ultrasound at age 65 for males who've smoked more than 100 cigarettes in their life or anyone with family history.

What are the indications for surgical repair of AAAs, and what is the risk of repair?
AAA diameter >5.5 cm for men or 4.5 to 5.0 cm for women and patients with connective tissue disorders, AAA expansion >0.5 cm/6 mo, AAA symptoms (chronic abdominal/back pain), patient preference for smaller AAA (4.5–5.4 cm) if young low-risk patient, or atypical aneurysms (dissecting, pseudoaneurysm, mycotic, saccular, penetrating ulcers). Mortality risk of open repair is quoted to be <5% (1%–3% for high-volume centers).

What does testicular pain in a patient with abdominal aortic aneurysm classically signify?
Retroperitoneal rupture with ureteral stretch and referred testicular pain

Which bacteria are thought to be an infectious cause of aneurysm formation? Graft infection?
Chlamydia pneumoniae
Staphylococcus aureus (and *Staphylococcus epidermidi*s, usually late)

Describe the early and late complications of open AAA repair? Endovascular aneurysm repair (EVAR)?
Early—Most frequent cause of death after open AAA repair is myocardial dysfunction, but sexual dysfunction (up to 25% males), nonfatal MI, and renal failure are most common.
Late—Upper and lower GI bleed due to aortoenteric fistula (fourth portion of duodenum as it crosses anterior to aorta) can be reduced by wrapping the graft with the aneurysm sac.
EVAR—Groin and wound complications related to vascular access sites early (bleeding, hematomas, pseudoaneurysm formation, wound infections) and endoleaks late.

What are endoleaks type I to V and how are they managed differently?
Type I: Occurs at proximal (Ia) or distal (Ib) landing zones, requires immediate repair with balloon dilatation, placement of additional stents/cuffs, or conversion to open repair
Type II: Retrograde flow from branches into sac (lumbar, intercostal arteries)—closely observe and embolize (coils, glue) or laparoscopic branch ligation if sac growth observed
Type III: Structural failure of graft or component separation, requires immediate repair
Type IV: Due to graft porosity (rare with newer grafts), reverse heparin and observe
Type V: Idiopathic aneurysm expansion without identifiable endoleak also known as endotension

What is the recommended follow-up following open repair of abdominal aortic aneurysms? EVAR?
Open: Follow-up appointment 2 weeks after discharge, but no follow-up studies required
EVAR: Baseline CT scan 3 months after graft implant, then 6, 12, 18 months, and annually

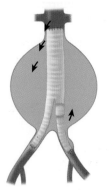 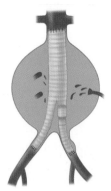 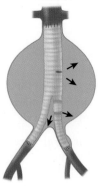 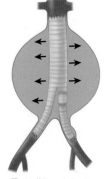

Type I endoleak   Type II endoleak   Type III endoleak   Type IV endoleak

FIGURE 24-3. Four types of endoleak that include type I endoleak, attachment site leak; type II endoleak, side branch leak caused by lumbar or side branches; type III endoleak, endograft junctional leak due to overlapping device components; type IV endoleak, endograft fabric or porosity leak. (Reproduced from Brunicardi FC, Andersen DK, Billiar TR, et al. Schwartz's Principles of Surgery. 9th ed. http://www.accessmedicine.com. Copyright © The McGraw-Hill Companies, Inc. All rights reserved.)

When might a retroperitoneal approach to AAAs be preferred over anterior? Disadvantages?
A retroperitoneal approach can sometimes be preferable in the contexts of ascites, horseshoe kidney, multiple prior abdominal surgeries, radiation, and peritoneal dialysis. Poor accessibility to right renal artery and distal right iliac arteries are disadvantages.

What must workup and management for bloody diarrhea include after AAA repair?
Ischemia of the left colon and rectum occurs in 0.6% to 2% of cases and may initially present as substantial IV fluid requirement within 8 to 12 hours postoperatively or bloody diarrhea in 48 hours. Diagnosis is confirmed with immediate sigmoidoscopy. Treatment requires urgent resection of ischemic bowel and stoma creation. Antibiotics, bowel rest, and resuscitation may be considered for limited mucosal necrosis, although full-thickness necrosis can lead to gross contamination mandating removal of aortic graft and extra-anatomic bypass.

After AAA repair, what can cause small patchy ischemia on bilateral plantar feet with pedal pulses?
Microembolization (also known as "trash foot")

What is the incidence of spinal cord ischemia following AAA repair and why does it occur?
Spinal cord or lumbosacral plexus ischemia occurs after 0.30% of aortic reconstructions with loss of bladder/bowel control, loss of pain/temperature sensation below the level of injury, and paraplegia, but sparing of proprioception due to disruption of flow to the artery of Adamkiewicz between the 9th and 12th intercostal spaces.

What anatomic properties/criteria must be met for EVAR to be considered?
Minimum length of neck: 15 mm, minimum proximal neck diameter: 28 mm
Distal landing zone (iliac arteries) length: ~2 cm and diameter: <18 mm
Access vessels (femoral and external iliac arteries) diameter: >7 mm

Relative to prepping and draping for repair of ruptured AAA, when should anesthesia be induced?
Not until operative site is prepped and draped due to risk of sudden, severe hypotension

SPLANCHNIC, ILIAC, AND PERIPHERAL ARTERY ANEURYSMS

At what diameter is repair of an isolated iliac aneurysm indicated? How are they treated?
Isolated unilateral iliac artery aneurysms >3 cm can be treated with open graft placement, endovascular covered stent graft placement, or bifurcated aortoiliac graft for bilateral. Close observation with semiannual ultrasound or CT is indicated for those <3 cm.

How are internal iliac aneurysms treated?
Embolization coils, plugs, or glue into the aneurysm sac and its branches

What is the most common peripheral artery aneurysm?
Popliteal artery aneurysms account for 70% of peripheral artery aneurysms

Do patients with popliteal aneurysms commonly have other aneurysms? Where? How often?
50% of patients with popliteal artery aneurysms have contralateral popliteal aneurysms
75% of patients with popliteal artery aneurysms have aneurysms elsewhere (aorta/iliacs)

What risk do popliteal artery aneurysms pose? When is intervention indicated? How?
Rupture is RARE! Concern is for embolization or thrombosis. Asymptomatic aneurysms >2 cm, symptomatic aneurysms, and those with evidence of thrombus in aneurysm should be excluded open or endovascularly.

What is the most common splanchnic artery aneurysm and who is at greatest risk of rupture?
Splenic aneurysms >2 cm, any symptomatic, women of child-bearing age need repair
Repair includes embolization (most common), proximal + distal ligation, or splenectomy
Young multiparous pregnant females are at greatest risk for splenic aneurysm rupture (5% rupture overall: mortalities 75% maternal, 95% fetal, 50% transplant recipients)

MESENTERIC ARTERIAL DISEASE

What is the typical history of acute mesenteric ischemia? Chronic mesenteric ischemia?
Acute onset of pain, vomiting/diarrhea, history of atrial fibrillation, or heart disease
Postprandial abdominal pain, fear of eating due to pain (food fear), and weight loss

What's the most common angiographic finding for mesenteric ischemia?
Acute: embolic occlusion distal to the origin of the superior mesenteric artery
Chronic: occlusion of 2 of 3 mesenteric arteries with stenosis of the third patent artery

What is the treatment for acute mesenteric ischemia?
Embolectomy preferable to bypass, possible bowel resection, may require second look laparotomy.

What is the treatment for chronic mesenteric ischemia? How is it diagnosed?
Treatment options include PTA +/- stent at time of diagnostic arteriogram, anterograde branched bypass from supraceliac aorta to celiac and superior mesenteric arteries, or retrograde bypass from infrarenal aorta to SMA distal to occlusion.

What is the treatment for mesenteric venous occlusion?
Anticoagulation, hemodynamic support, and serial abdominal exams.
Laparotomy with segmental bowel resection sometimes needed.

Describe median arcuate ligament syndrome. How is it usually diagnosed? What is treatment?
Chronic intermittent mesenteric ischemia caused by extrinsic compression of celiac axis by median arcuate ligament. Audible abdominal bruit is often reported to be heard. Workup includes CTA/arteriography; treatment is by release of median arcuate ligament.

RENAL ARTERIAL STENOSIS

What degree of renal artery stenosis (RAS) is required to increase renin levels and cause HTN?
60% stenosis of the main renal artery

What are the first and second most common causes of RAS? Other causes?
90% of RAS is caused by atherosclerosis, followed by fibromuscular dysplasia (medial fibroplasias is most common of 3 subtypes). Other causes include neurofibromatosis, radiation vasculitis, Takayasu arteritis, and renovascular thromboembolism.

Table 24-3 Indications for Renal Artery Revascularization	
Angiography Criteria	Clinical Criteria
• Fibromuscular dysplasia lesion • Pressure gradient >20 mm Hg • Affected/unaffected kidney renin ratio >1.5:1	• Refractory or rapidly progressive HTN • HTN associated with flash pulmonary edema without coronary artery disease • Rapidly progressive deterioration in renal function • Intolerance to antihypertensive medications • Chronic renal insufficiency related to bilateral renal artery occlusive disease or stenosis to a solitary functioning kidney • Dialysis-dependent renal failure in a patient with RAS but without another definite cause of end-stage renal disease • Recurrent congestive heart failure or flash pulmonary edema not attributable to active coronary ischemia

How is RAS diagnosed and treated?
Diagnostic arteriogram with or without angioplasty and stenting (PTA only for fibromuscular dysplagia (FMD)).
Renal vein renin ration of >1.5 is diagnostic for unilateral RAS.

What are the 5-year patency and restenosis rates for renal artery stenting?
5-year patency after renal artery stenting is 84.5%, and restenosis occurs 15% to 17%

What antihypertensive is contraindicated in renovascular stenosis?
ACE inhibitors (causes renal insufficiency)

VASCULAR ACCESS (DIALYSIS, ETC)

What are the tenets of vascular access?
Autologous tissue is preferred to prothetic. Start creating access in nondominant arm as distal as possible (to preserve proximal superficial venous system) and move proximal as access failures occur.

What is the most common early complication following AV fistula placement? Late?
Early: failure of the fistula to mature (enlarge). Late: proximal venous limb stenosis (48%)

What percentage of subclavian veins develop stenosis after placement of a subclavian catheter enough to cause fistula clotting or arm swelling? After internal jugular vein catheter?
Up to 50% subclavian vein catheters may cause clinically significant stenosis versus <10% IJs

What is and what percentage of AV fistulas cause arterial steal syndrome? Treatment?
~1.6% of AV fistulas created cause symptoms of ischemia (pain, etc) distal to the fistula. Ligation, banding of conduit, PAI (proximalization of the arterial inflow), RUDI (revision using distal inflow), DRIL procedure (distal revascularization with interval ligation)

What fistula flow rate is needed for a thrill to be palpable?
A thrill indicates flow >450 mL/min (through 6 mm diameter or 4–7 mm rapid taper graft).

For what reasons might removal of an infected arteriovenous fistula be indicated?
Suture line involvement, tunnel infection, thrombosis, failure to improve with local tx

What is the only absolute indication for peritoneal dialysis? Contraindications? (absolute/relative)
Inability to undergo hemodialysis (bleeding diathesis, poor access, unstable cardiovascular system)
Contraindications (absolute): lack of diaphragmatic integrity, obliteration of the peritoneal space due to previous surgery, inadequate peritoneal clearance
Contraindications (relative): large abdominal hernia, respiratory insufficiency secondary to dialysate infusion, or malignant peritoneal disease

What is the most common reason for discontinuation of peritoneal dialysis? Other complications?
Infection most commonly due to coagulase negative staphylococcus
Early complications: Bowel/bladder perforation; subcutaneous bleeding/hematoma formation from tunnel construction; intraperitoneal bleeding; leakage of dialysate; ileus
Late complications: Exit-site infection; mechanical failure; peritonitis

What is the expected 3-year peritoneal dialysis catheter survival rate?
80%

PERIPHERAL VENOUS DISEASE

What are risk factors for venous insufficiency? Name 2 sources of venous HTN?
Age >50 years, heredity, female (hormones), lifestyle (sedentary), gravity (standing)
Hydrostatic pressure (gravitational)—weight of blood from the right atrium to foot and high pressures transmitted to superficial venous system if perforating veins fail

Describe symptoms of venous insufficiency.
Leg heaviness, fatigue, itching, pain with standing (relieved by elevation/compression)

What are the indications for treatment of primary venous insufficiency? How initially treated?
Pain, bleeding, superficial thrombophlebitis (recurrent), cosmesis, heaviness, fatigability
Initial treatment includes limb elevation and compressive garments (20–30 mm Hg)

What surgical options are available for venous varicosities?
Radiofrequency or LASER ablation of GSV +/- microphlebectomy

What is Virchow triad?
Venous stasis, endothelial injury, and hypercoagulable state (DVT risk factors)

What is Homan sign?
Pain in the calf on dorsiflexion of the foot, suggesting the possibility of a DVT

What percentage of venous thromboses are clinically evident?
40%

What is the most common site of venous thrombosis initiation?
The soleal sinuses

What's the difference between phlegmasia cerulea dolens and phlegmasia alba dolens?
Phlegmasia alba dolens—Iliofemoral DVT causes swelling + blanching, pain, pitting edema
Phlegmasia cerulea dolens—Major ileofemoral DVT causes a massively swollen blue leg with pain and edema that compromises arterial inflow and can cause venous gangrene

A hypercoagulability profile includes tests for what abnormalities?
Antithrombin III deficiency, antiphospholipid syndrome, Factor V Leiden mutation, protein C deficiency, protein S deficiency, prothrombin gene mutation, homocysteine

In the absence of surgery, what is the negative predictive value of D-dimer test for suspected DVT?
97% to 99%

What venous duplex ultrasound findings suggest venous thrombosis? Chronic thrombus?
Failure to demonstrate augmentation of flow on compression; resistance to compression. Increased heterogeneity and echogenicity suggests chronic venous thrombus.

What is the recurrence rate for an untreated DVT? What is the duration of treatment for DVT?
30% risk of recurrence if untreated, 15% risk of PE, and 3% risk of PE-related mortality. 3 to 6 months anticoagulation for first DVT secondary to reversible risk factors, 6 to 12 months anticoagulation for first idiopathic DVT, lifetime anticoagulation for 2 DVTs or PE, and compression stocking x1 year to reduce 23% to 60% risk of postthrombotic syndrome (pain, itching, swelling, varicose veins, ulcers, limb heaviness, and skin discoloration)

What are the indications for placement of an IVC filter? Potential complications?
Recurrent thromboembolism on adequate anticoagulation, contraindications to anticoagulation for DVT
Migration of the device to pulmonary artery, device fracture, Caval perforation or occlusion, and 4% rate of recurrent embolism

What is Paget-Schroetter syndrome, and how is it treated?
Upper extremity effort thrombosis due to subclavian vein compression by a cervical rib or myofascial band with repetitive motion. Patients are young (often pitchers/swimmers). Treatment is with thrombolysis followed by first rib resection.

What are the respective treatments for localized, uncomplicated thrombophlebitis, and thrombophlebitis involving clusters of varicosities? Is septic thrombophlebitis treated different?
Anti-inflammatory medications (NSAIDs), heating pads, and compression stockings
Selective removal of the entire vein along its course

VASCULAR TRAUMA

In what 3 situations can an intraluminal shunt be used to maintain temporary distal perfusion?
Skeletal realignment prior to subsequent vascular repair in a fractured ischemic limb
During transport to trauma center for vascular reconstruction of peripheral arterial injury
Damage control for a patient unlikely to survive immediate complex repair

How are penetrating injuries to zones I, II, and III of the neck managed differently?
Zone I (base of neck): CT, 4-vessel arch angiography, bronchoscopy, EGD, barium swallow
Zone II (midcervical neck): Neck exploration if bleeding or unstable; if stable can perform complete imaging
Zone III (above mandible): CT, angiogram, laryngoscopy, esophagoscopy, barium swallow

What percentage of patients manifest deficits hours to days after blunt carotid injury (carotid dissection)? How is it treated?
~50% demonstrate hemispheric neurologic deficits incompatible with CT findings.
Treatment is systemic anticoagulation (if not prohibited by comorbid injuries)

What incisions are indicated: pleural bleed in unstable patient, penetrating injury to base of right neck in unstable patient, penetrating injury to left proximal subclavian, and distal subclavian? How can subclavian vessels exposure be expedited in a bleeding patient with a swollen upper chest?
Anterolateral thoracotomy on the side of injury is indicated in this patient
Median sternotomy accesses innominate, proximal carotid, and subclavian arteries
Left anterolateral thoracotomy at the third intercostal space (above the nipple)
Supraclavicular incision (must identify phrenic nerve on anterior scalene). Subperiosteal resection of the medial half of the clavicle can be performed to expedite access.

What radiographic findings on supine chest film suggest aortic disruption?
Widened mediastinum (>8 cm), obscured/indistinct aortic knob, apical capping, loss of aortic contour, obliteration of aortopulmonary window, left hemothorax, off-midline nasogastric tube, tracheal deviation towards right, left mainstem bronchus deviation

What branch of the aorta is not exposed with the Mattox maneuver?
Right renal artery

What is the management for zone I, II, and III retroperitoneal hematomas?
Zone I (midline)—Exploration for blunt and penetrating injuries (suprarenal aorta, celiac axis, proximal SMA, proximal renal artery injuries with supramesocolic zone I hematomas; infrarenal aorta, IVC injuries with a inframesocolic zone I retroperitoneal hematomas)
Zone II (perinephric)—*Penetrating:* exploration to assess damage and repair injuries versus may observe if severely injured patient with little reserve with stable hematoma, *Blunt:* observe if nonexpanding hematoma (opening Gerota fascia can worsen kidney)
Zone III (pelvic)—*Penetrating:* exploration because probable iliac vessel injury. *Blunt:* observe because usually associated with pelvic fracture, treat with external fixation or angiographic embolization of the bleeding vessels, but may need to explore if rapidly expanding hematoma with suspicion of major iliac vascular injury.

Angiography is indicated for what difference in BP at the ankles?
>10 mm Hg difference between ipsilateral and contralateral ankles

LYMPHATICS

What are the first and second most common etiologies of bilateral extremity edema?
First—Cardiac failure, Second—Kidney failure (ESRD)

What pressure compression should garments provide patients with lymphedema?
30 to 60 mm Hg

What are the 3 stages of lymphedema progression?
Stage 1: Impaired lymphatic drainage causes interstitial accumulation of protein-rich fluid.
Stage 2: Accumulation of adipocytes causes local inflammatory response. Fibroblasts and macrophages deposit connective tissue with progression to spongy nonpitting edema.
Stage 3: Remaining lymphatic channels are further damaged by local inflammation and recurrent episodes of infection with subcutaneous fibrosis and scarring.

What 2 categories of surgery are available for the treatment of lymphedema?
Excisional: a large segment of subcutaneous lymphedematous tissue + skin are excised
Reconstructive: residual dilated lymphatics are anastomosed to nearby veins/lymphatics

How is treatment for lymphangiosarcoma different from that for lymphangioma?
Lymphangiosarcoma requires neoadjuvant chemoradiation before surgical excision

How can lymphedema be differentiated from lipedema? (excessive subcutaneous fat in the obese)
Lymphedema presents with swelling of foot dorsum, but lipedema spares feet

MULTIPLE CHOICE QUESTIONS

1. You are called to the emergency department for what is described as cellulitis and find a 78-year-old male with a history of diabetes, coronary artery disease, an irregular heart rate with an international normalized ratio (INR) of 1.1, and a tobacco abuse history of 2 packs per day for 60 years. He reports severe right foot pain started suddenly while he was watching television 3 hours before presenting at the emergency department, where he's waited to be seen another 3 hours. On exam, his right foot is pale and cooler than the left with no palpable right dorsalis pedis or posterior tibial pulses and decreased sensation. What is the next step in your management?
   A. STAT duplex ultrasound
   B. Immediate heparin anticoagulation and admit to the floor
   C. Heparin, immediate thromboembolectomy and fasciotomy
   D. Routine arteriogram with possible lysis the following morning
   E. Thromboembolectomy with heparin drip anticoagulation

2. An obese 63-year-old male is admitted to the medical service for pneumonia with a history significant for diabetes, HTN, and end-stage renal disease on hemodialysis. You are consulted for nonhealing ulcers and asked to evaluate the patient for peripheral arterial bypass. On exam, you find him sitting in a chair with severely edematous legs and chronic bilateral shallow, nontender medial malleolar ulcers. Though difficult to examine, dorsalis pedis and posterior tibial pulses are palpable bilaterally. How should you explain to the patient and his medical team why arterial bypass is not indicated at this time?
   A. Despite progression of his peripheral arterial disease to ulceration, his disease is not severe enough to warrant urgent revascularization
   B. Peripheral arterial bypass is not indicated for venous disease
   C. Pneumonia is an absolute contraindication to anesthesia and surgery
   D. Because his ulcers are chronic, revascularization can be performed electively following appropriate cardiopulmonary optimization
   E. His disease is too far progressed and requires bilateral amputation

3. A 39-year-old female undergoes a normal cardiac catheterization via left radial artery access. Following the procedure and removal of the access sheath, her arm is noted by her nurses to have "doubled in size", and a hematoma is observed at the access site. Distal pulses are palpable with sensory and motor function intact. The patient is anxious, and you are consulted to evaluate for compartment syndrome. As the vascular surgeon on call, what are your recommendations?

A. Consent patient for urgent fasciotomy
B. Agree with cardiology discharge orders and follow-up in 1 week
C. Return to catheterization suite for urgent arteriogram and embolization
D. Direct pressure for hemostasis, elevate arm, serial neurovascular exams
E. Immediate surgical cut down and ligation of bleeding radial artery

4. A 69-year-old man is seen in the office to discuss management options for his abdominal aortic aneurysm. His medical history includes coronary artery disease, poorly controlled HTN, COPD, and he continues to smoke 1 pack per day. A previous CT scan showed his aneurysm to be 4.5 cm 3 years ago. He was then lost to follow-up until a recent CT performed in the emergency department found it to be 6.5 cm. Which of the findings below would preclude endovascular repair?

A. Contained rupture
B. 1 cm infrarenal aortic neck
C. 3 cm diameter at iliac bifurcation
D. Growth of >1 cm over the past year
E. Multiple prior abdominal surgeries
F. 8 mm common femoral artery

5. A 93-year-old female is admitted to the hospital after experiencing transient weakness of her left arm and left leg, left facial droop, right visual loss, and slurred speech of less than 24 hours. Workup is significant for atrial fibrillation, an INR of 1.0, ultrasound demonstration of 70% bilateral carotid artery stenosis, and an echocardiogram showing no signs of clots or cardiac valve vegetations. CTA confirms the above ultrasound findings. Following cardiopulmonary risk assessment and appropriate optimization, what should be advised?

A. Coumadin anticoagulation alone
B. Aspirin and plavix medical management alone
C. Immediate bilateral carotid endarterectomy
D. No further management is necessary at this time
E. Right CEA only with close follow-up

6. A 72-year-old right-handed man presents with progressively worsening chronic kidney disease who is thought to require hemodialysis within 2 months. Which of the following is the correct order of preference for placement of angioaccess?

A. Left radial-cephalic arteriovenous fistula/right radial-cephalic arteriovenous fistula/left brachial-cephalic fistula
B. Left radial-cephalic arteriovenous fistula/left brachial-cephalic fistula/left upper arm e-PTFE brachial axillary graft
C. Left forearm brachial-brachial graft/left brachial-cephalic fistula/right radial-cephalic fistula
D. Right internal jugular tunneled dialysis catheter/left radial-cephalic fistula/left upper arm e-PTFE brachial axillary graft
E. Continue to monitor until hemodialysis is necessary

7. A 65-year-old female is admitted with chest pain and undergoes a diagnostic cardiac catheterization, which excluded a cardiac etiology of her chest pain. She is diagnosed with biliary colic and discharged. At follow-up visit in your office, she complains of fullness and a pulsatile mass in her groin. Ultrasound duplex shows a 3-cm pseudoaneurysm with a long, narrow neck. What is a pseudoaneurysm and what is the first-line treatment?
   A. The sac is completely surrounded by a vessel wall and treated with duplex-directed thrombin injection
   B. The sac is not completely bordered by the vessel wall and treated with duplex-directed thrombin injection
   C. The sac is completely surrounded by vessel wall and treated with duplex-directed compression
   D. The sac is not completely bordered by the vessel wall and treated with duplex-directed compression
   E. The sac is not completely bordered by the vessel wall and treated with surgical repair

8. A 73-year-old male presents 2 years after aortobifemoral bypass with a swollen, tender mass in his groin. CT scan shows air and fluid around the left femoral anastomosis that tracts into the abdomen. The correct management of this condition is:
   A. Culture-directed antibiotic treatment and close observation
   B. Endovascular repair
   C. Removal of aortobifemoral bypass and replacement with Rifampin soaked Dacron
   D. Removal of aortobifemoral bypass followed by axillary-bifemoral bypass the following day
   E. Axillary bifemoral bypass followed by excision of aortobifemoral bypass

9. A 53-year-old male presents to the emergency department with chest pain radiating to his back. His BP is 210/130 and his heart rate is 94. His labs are: Amylase-31, Hgb-13.1, Cr-1.0. He has no abdominal pain and he has palpable pulses in his lower extremities. CT shows a type B aortic dissection without any evidence of malperfusion. The next step in management is:
   A. Urgent open operative repair
   B. Urgent endovascular repair
   C. Admit to ICU, BP control with Nitroprusside
   D. Admit to ICU, BP control with Esmolol
   E. Admit to floor, BP control with PRN medication

10. A 34-year-old male presents with dry gangrene of his fingers that has progressed to autoamputation. He does not complaint of any symptoms of lower extremity arterial insufficiency. What is the most beneficial intervention for this pathology?
    A. Smoking cessation
    B. Amputation proximal to the gangrene
    C. Angiogram with possible intervention
    D. Gangrene biopsy
    E. Statin therapy

ANSWERS

1. **Answer: C.** This patient has acute arterial ischemia, likely secondary to embolization of cardiac etiology. Prompt heparin anticoagulation and surgical thromboembolectomy are key to management. Immediate arteriogram with possible lysis could also be considered, but treatment should not generally be delayed until the following day. Because you are evaluating this patient at least 6 hours after the embolic event, fasciotomy should be included in this patient's management.

2. **Answer: B.** The examination findings described in the question are consistent with venous ulcers having a typically nontender, moist, broad base over the medial malleolus associated with severe edema (can be pitting or nonpitting depending on chronicity of disease). Initial treatment recommendations should include limb elevation above heart level, compression garments, and weight loss with dietary and activity lifestyle changes. Given this patient's palpable pulses, arterial bypass is not currently indicated. The patient should be advised to follow up with a vascular or wound care specialist for ongoing care, and antibiotics should be considered for associated cellulitis.

3. **Answer: D.** The most important initial management for this patient is to control her bleeding with application of direct pressure over the vessel puncture site (not necessarily over the skin wound). An intact neurovascular examination with sensation intact, full range of motion, and no numbness, tingling, pain, or skin color changes does not support a diagnosis of compartment syndrome, but serial neurovascular examinations are absolutely essential to early identification and treatment should it develop.

4. **Answer: B.** Endovascular repair of abdominal aortic aneurysms has made aneurysm repair less invasive and often safer for many people with this disease, including those who may not have previously been candidates for repair before EVAR became available. Although this technology continues to evolve, specific requirements must still be met. Rupture is not a contraindication to endovascular repair. To the contrary, EVAR has become the preferred means of repair for ruptured AAAs with suitable anatomy. Growth of >1 cm/y is an indication for repair, whether endovascular or open, and an endovascular approach is preferred for a patient with multiple prior abdominal surgeries. Finally, femoral access vessels must be >7 mm, and a 15 mm normal diameter infrarenal aortic neck is required for currently available grafts. Although aneurysmal disease at the iliac bifurcation does not preclude endovascular repair, internal iliac embolization may be required to prevent a type II endoleak.

5. **Answer: E.** This patient's presentation is complicated by multiple potential reasons for her transient ischemic attack (<24 hours of symptoms), including bilateral carotid artery stenosis as well as atrial fibrillation either subtherapeutic or not on anticoagulation. However, her unilaterally symptomatic 70% carotid artery stenosis in the absence of echocardiogram-proven cardiac thrombus or valvular disease should be treated with carotid endarterectomy of the symptomatic side and close ultrasound follow-up of the asymptomatic contralateral 70% stenosis. Whether to anticoagulate this patient must be considered in the context of her risk for stroke due to atrial fibrillation and her risk of falling due to dementia, gait instability, or other common elderly risk factors. Antiplatelet drugs (aspirin, plavix) alone are not the preferred management for severe and symptomatic carotid artery stenosis, as demonstrated by the NASCET trial.

6. **Answer: B.** This patient is expected to require hemodialysis within 6 months, and is therefore a candidate for placement of permanent angioaccess. Autologous is preferred to prothetic, nondominant upper extremity is preferred to dominant upper extremity, and distal is preferred to proximal in creating access. A fistula usually takes 4 to 6 weeks to mature enough to be cannulated. This patient is not expected to need hemodialysis for 2 months; therefore, there is sufficient time for a fistula to mature, and therefore he would not require a catheter.

7. **Answer: B.** A pseudoaneurysm, or false aneurysm, is a complication after percutaneous femoral access that occurs at a rate of 0.6%. It is defined as extravascular blood flow that communicates with the vessel lumen and contained by the surrounding tissues. It often has a connective tissue wall and a pseudocapsule. In contrast, a true aneurysm is one that involves all 3 layers of the wall of an artery. Duplex-directed thrombin injection is now considered first-line therapy due to increase success rate, decreased time to perform, and decreased discomfort over ultrasound-guided compression. Surgical repair can be considered for patients who are on antiplatelet or anticoagulation therapy, pseudoaneurysms that have a short, wide neck or failure of minimally invasive therapy.

8. **Answer: E.** Infected prosthetic material is a devastating compilation of vascular surgery. Often an infection will present as a pseudoaneurysm that may or may not be symptomatic. This patient is presumed to have an infection based on the CT findings of air and fluid, which should not be present 2 years after surgery. The infected graft must be excised; antibiotics will not sterilize the graft material. Axillary-bifemoral bypass places prosthetic within a clean field and must be performed prior to removal of the indwelling bypass. The other options have a high rate of recurrent infection or ischemia.

9. **Answer: D.** This patient has an uncomplicated descending aortic dissection. Indications for operative repair of aortic dissection are rupture, ascending aortic dissection, rapid enlargement, intractable pain, or branch obstruction. This patient has no evidence of any complicating factors and treatment centers around anti-impulse control. The drug of choice to reduce aortic impulse is Esmolol (quick-acting beta-blocker). Nitroprusside reduces afterload and is indicated after beta blockade has been maximized. These patients need to be monitored in the ICU for medication infusion and monitoring for progression of disease.

10. **Answer: A.** This patient has Buerger disease (thromboangiitis obliterans), which most commonly affects young males. The most significant risk factor is smoking. Buerger disease is an acute inflammation and thrombosis of arteries and veins that affects the hands and sometimes the feet. Angiogram can show a "corkscrew" appearance of arteries that result from vascular damage, but only assists in diagnosis and not treatment. Dry gangrene does not require urgent amputation. A biopsy would not be helpful and would likely result in a chronic wound due to poor blood supply.

CHAPTER 25
Pediatrics

Doug Lehman, Jarom Gilstrap, and Anthony Georges

Test Taking Tips

- Remember typical ages at presentation for various congenital disorders that may manifest in similar fashion (eg, duodenal atresia vs malrotation). The age of a neonate can clue you in to the probably diagnosis.
- Many pediatric surgical disorders can be observed for possible resolution. Do not rush to the operative intervention. Examples include umbilical hernias, hernias, and MEN syndromes, where surgery is delayed until a certain age.

Is bilious vomiting a surgical emergency in the newborn and why?
Must rule out malrotation with mid-gut volvulus in a patient with proximal obstruction because the gut can be strangulated (time = bowel).
Differential diagnosis—(memorize this list—the ABSITE will point you toward one of these!) annular pancreas, malrotation, jejunoileal atresia, meconium ileus, meconium plug syndrome, duodenal web/atresia, Hirschsprung, hypoplastic left colon. Always remember 1 anomaly begets additional associated anomalies.

Meconium ileus is associated with what anomaly?
Cystic fibrosis

Duodenal atresia and malrotation are associated with what anomaly?
Down syndrome

What other abnormalities are associated with malrotation?
Diaphragmatic hernia, jejunoileal atresia, abdominal wall defects

Which abdominal wall defects are associated with malrotation?
Both omphalocele and gastroschisis

What is the diagnostic study of first choice to rule in malrotation with midgut volvulus?
Upper gastrointestinal

Surgical procedure for malrotation:
Ladd procedure
Counterclockwise rotation, divide peritoneal bands crossing the duodenum, position SB to right and colon to the left
Look for other abnormalities (see above)
Appendectomy (cecum is now on the left side of the abdomen, perhaps delaying the diagnosis of acute appendicitis.)

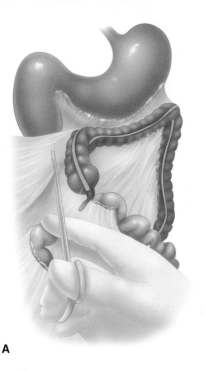

A

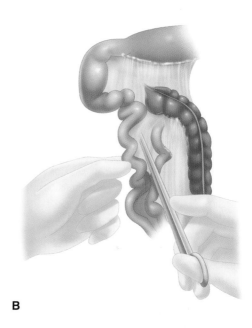

B

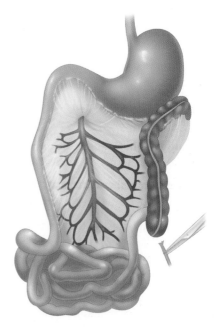

C

FIGURE 25-1. Ladd procedure for malrotation. (**A**) Lysis of cecal and duodenal bands. (**B**) Broadening of the mesentery. (**C**) Appendectomy. *(Reproduced from Brunicardi FC, Andersen DK, Billiar TR, et al. Schwartz's Principles of Surgery. 9th ed. http://www.accessmedicine.com. Copyright © The McGraw-Hill Companies, Inc. All rights reserved.)*

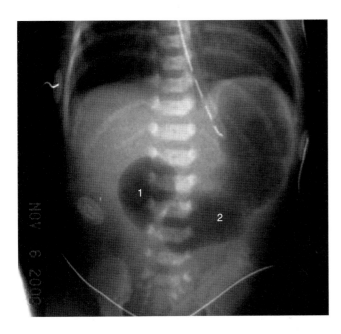

FIGURE 25-2. Abdominal radiograph showing the "double bubble" sign in a newborn infant with duodenal atresia. The 2 bubbles are numbered. *(Reproduced from Brunicardi FC, Andersen DK, Billiar TR, et al. Schwartz's Principles of Surgery. 9th ed. http://www.accessmedicine.com. Copyright © The McGraw-Hill Companies, Inc. All rights reserved.)*

Why do patients with malrotation have bilous vomiting?
Ladd bands cross the duodenum
Remember that BILIOUS vomiting in newborn is malrotation until proven otherwise. (most common presentation)

Why is blood flow to the bowel compromised in malrotation?
SMA twisted on its axis—detorsion counterclockwise will relieve this problem. (Malrotation results from failure of normal counterclockwise rotation in utero.)

Duodenal atresia—diagnosis and treatment (Rx):
"Double bubble sign"
Associated anomalies? Prematurity, polyhydramnios (most common), malrotation, annular pancreas, biliary atresia
Resuscitation and then duodenojejunostomy

Rx of duodenal atresia:
Decompression and resuscitation first and then duodenoduodenostomy or duodenojejunostomy

Rx of jeunoileal atresia:
Decompression and resuscitation first then resect atretic portion.
(Run the bowel [common ORALS mistake])!

Patient fails to pass meconium in first 24 hours, bilious vomiting, perforate anus, abdominal distention. "Babygram" shows terminal ileum is dilated; bowel contents have ground glass/soap bubble appearance without air/fluid levels. What is the diagnosis and Rx?
Simple meconium ileus
Rx is gastrograffin enema, pancreatic enzymes, and mucomyst
Get a chloride sweat test post-op
If patient is toxic → (Complicated meconium ileus) resuscitate and go to the OR (Don't mess with mucomyst when a patient is toxic!).

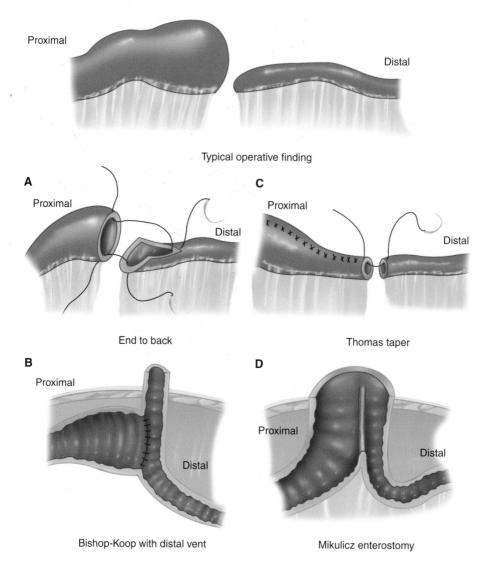

FIGURE 25-3. Techniques of intestinal anastomosis for infants with small-bowel obstruction. (**A**) End-to-back anastomosis. The distal limb has been incised to create a "fish mouth" to enlarge the lumen. (**B**) Bishop-Koop anastomosis. The proximal distended limb is joined to the side of the distal small bowel, which is vented by "chimney" to the abdominal wall. (**C**) Tapering anastomosis. A portion of the antimesenteric wall of the proximal bowel is excised, with longitudinal closure to minimize disparity in the limbs. (**D**) A Mikulicz double-barreled enterostomy is constructed by suturing the 2 limbs together and then exteriorizing the double stoma. The common wall can be crushed with a special clamp to create 1 large stoma. The stoma can be closed in an extraperitoneal manner. *(Reproduced from Brunicardi FC, Andersen DK, Billiar TR, et al. Schwartz's Principles of Surgery. 9th ed. http://www.accessmedicine.com. Copyright © The McGraw-Hill Companies, Inc. All rights reserved.)*

What is the difference between "meconium plug" and "meconium ileus?"
Meconium ileus is a misnomer. It is actually a distal obstruction. Meconium plug may be secondary to maternal condition, Hirschsprung or cystic fibrosis. It is also a distal obstruction. With passage of the meconium, the obstruction may be relieved.

Called to see a newborn, 27 weeks' gestation, acidotic, fever, free air on AXR, first stool was bloody. Diagnosis and Rx:
Necrotizing enterocolitis (NEC)!
Make the ABSITE push you to the OR on this one.

Absolute indication for OR:
Free air
Relative indications for OR. Clinical deterioration, worsening acidosis, persistent fixed loop on abdominal x-ray (AXR), thrombocytosis, portal venous air, abdominal wall erythema/cellulitis, positive paracentesis cultures. Portal venous gas and pneumatosis alone are not absolute indications for OR.
Nonoperative management is NPO, IVF, nasogastric tube (NGT), broad-spectrum IV antibiotics, correct coagulopathy, correct electrolytes, appropriate resuscitation, serial AXR, and bedside evaluations.

Operative management options:
In the neonatal intensive care unit: On high-frequency jet ventilator and can't be moved to OR ± extreme prematurity (<1000 g). Peritoneal drain at the bedside.
In the OR: Exploratory laparotomy, resection of dead bowel, bring up ostomies

Before establishing continuity, what study is needed and why?
A distal limb study because of the high incidence of associated strictures.

What is the expected urine output in this patient with NEC?
2 cc/kg

Called to L&D to see a patient with bowels outside the abdomen from defect to right of umbilical cord. Diagnosis and Rx:
Gastroschisis
The first step is always resuscitation.
Cover bowel with moist Kerlix, bowel bag.
"Bad bowel, good baby"—only 10% with associated anomalies. The bowel was exposed to amniotic fluid and looks bad.
Remember they will all have malrotation.
Place bowel in silo and slowly cinch the silo bag over time. The bowel may look congested/ purplish in the silo.
Do not try to reduce all viscera into the abdomen at the first operation—will result in respiratory distress and possibly abdominal compartment syndrome

Associated anomalies with omphalocele and gastroschisis:
Gastroschisis—intestinal atresia, malrotation
Omphalocele—skeleton, gastrointestinal (GI) tract, nervous system, genitourinary, GI tract. The most common and worrisome is cardiac, so get a STAT echo before going to the OR.

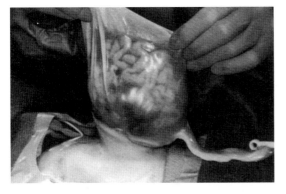

FIGURE 25-4. Neonate with omphalocele. The liver and bowel herniated through a midline abdominal wall defect and are surrounded by a sac of amnion and chorion from which the umbilical cord emanates. *(Reproduced with permission from Woo RK, Albanese CT. Pediatric surgery. In: Norton JA, ed. Surgery. 2nd ed. Copyright © 2008 Springer Science+Business Media, LLC. With permission of Springer Science+Business Media.)*

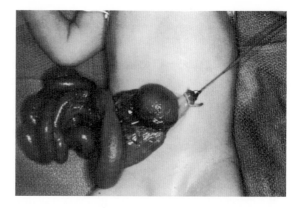

FIGURE 25-5. Neonate with a gastroschisis. The defect is to the right of the umbilical cord, and the bowel has no investing sac. Note edema of the bowel wall and the dilated stomach adjacent to the umbilical cord. *(Reproduced with permission from Woo RK, Albanese CT. Pediatric surgery. In: Norton JA, ed. Surgery. 2nd ed. Copyright © 2008 Springer Science+Business Media, LLC. With permission of Springer Science+Business Media.)*

Which condition is always associated with a sac, gastroschisis, or omphalocele?
Omphalocele always has a sac (may be ruptured); gastroschisis never has a sac

Where can the umbilical cord be found in gastroschisis compared to omphalocele?
In gastroschisis the umbilical cord if found to the left of the defect; in omphalocele the umbilical cord is attached to the sac

Infant with poor PO intake, life-threatening episodes of apnea (near miss SIDS), chronic cough, arching, recurrent pneumonia, asthma, hoarseness. Most likely diagnosis:
Gastroesophageal reflux disease (GERD)

Preoperative evaluation for GERD:
UGI—exclude other causes of vomiting
Gold standard is pH monitoring.
Endoscopy of esophagus, larynx, and trachea

Management of GERD:
Nonoperative: Thicken formulas, small feeds, acid suppression, modify posture
Operative: Nissen fundoplication
Indication for operative management: Failure of medical management, multiple aspiration, near miss SIDS, esophageal stricture, FTT

TRACHEOESOPHAGEAL FISTULA AND DIAPHRAGMATIC HERNIA

Most common TEF:
Gross type C (Type C—90%, Type A—7%, Type E—3%)

Describe Type C TEF:
Proximal EA (blind pouch)—distal tracheoesophageal fistula (TEF)

What is the 2nd most common TEF?
Type A

Describe Type A TEF:
Pure EA—no TEF

What is the common presentation of Type A TEF?
Newborn spits up feeds, excessive drooling, respiratory symptoms with feeds. NGT won't pass.

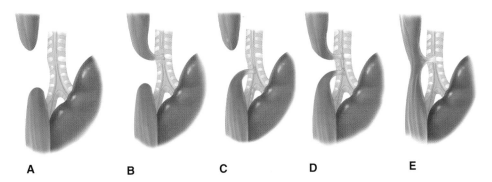

A   **B**   **C**   **D**   **E**

FIGURE 25-6. The 5 varieties of esophageal atresia (EA) and tracheoesophageal fistula (TEF). (**A**) Isolated EA. (**B**) EA with TEF between the proximal segment of the esophagus and the trachea. (**C**) EA with TEF between the distal esophagus and the trachea (**D**) EA with fistula between both the proximal and distal ends of the esophagus and the trachea. (**E**) TEF without EA (H-type fistula). *(Reproduced from Brunicardi FC, Andersen DK, Billiar TR, et al. Schwartz's Principles of Surgery. 9th ed. http://www.accessmedicine.com. Copyright © The McGraw-Hill Companies, Inc. All rights reserved.)*

AXR finding with Type A TEF:
Gasless abdomen, possibly with a scaphoid abdomen

Describe Type E TEF:
Normal esophagus—distal TEF

Most likely TEF to present in adulthood:
Type E

TEF is part of the VACTERL group of anomalies. Describe VACTERL:
Vertebral (ultrasound), Anorectal (rectal examination, imperforate anus), Cardiac (ECHO), TE Fistula, Renal (check renal ultrasound), Limb anomalies

Surgical management of TEF:
Rigid bronchoscopy, right extrapleural thoracotomy, divide fistula, close trachea, primary repair of esophagus, azygous often divided, ± G-tube. Prior to OR—Sump (NGT) for oral secretions, elevated head of bed, antibiotics, resuscitate, H2 blockers, NPO. Esophagogram to identify length of pouch

Patient with diaphragmatic hernia on the left. Do you expect both lungs to be dysfunctional or just the left?
Both are usually dysfunctional secondary to primary pulmonary hypertension

What percent of diaphragmatic hernia present on the left?
85%

Percent of diaphragmatic hernias associated with other congenital defects?
80%. Again, get an ECHO for associated cardiac defects before going to the OR!

Most common diaphragmatic hernia—located posterior-lateral:
Bochdalek

Rare diaphragmatic hernia—located anteriormedially, posterior to sternum:
Morgagni

When are most diaphragmatic hernias identified?
On prenatal ultrasound (typical presentation—no gastric bubble, bowel in chest, polyhydramnios)

NGT placed in child with Bochdalek hernia. CXR shows:
NGT in chest. Bowels in chest.

Failure of the diaphragm to fuse is called:
Eventration

PEDIATRIC NECK

What branchial cleft cyst is anterior to sternocleidomastoid muscle?
2nd branchial cleft cyst

Where does a 2nd branchial cleft cyst usually pass?
Fistula usually passed through carotid bifurcation and into tonsillar pillar.

Most common branchial cleft cyst?
2nd

Lateral neck, lymphatic malformation:
Cystic hygroma (75% present in posterior neck, 20% in the axilla)

Which branchial cleft cyst presents clinically as a firm mass in suprasternal notch or clavicular region?
3rd

The 1st branchial cleft cyst is often associated with which nerve?
1st branchial cleft cyst found at angle of mandible is often associated with facial nerve.

Midline neck mass draining pus:
Infected thyroglossal duct cyst. Give antibiotics to clear infection then Sistrunk procedure (excise tract and central portion of hyoid bone)

Patient presents with cervical lymphadenopathy suspected to be from URI who subsequently fails to respond to 10 days of antibiotics. Possible etiology:
Lymphoma (if it persists). Always check the scalp for a hidden infection.

Patient presents with head persistently rotated. Head noted to be rotated in the opposite direction of the affected muscle. Diagnosis and Rx:
Torticollis. ROM exercises (physical therapy)

TRAUMA

What size airway?
Uncuffed endotracheal tube if less than 8 to 10 years of age. Size is (4 + pt age)/4. Or can use the size of their pinkie as a clue! Remember, no cricothyroidotomy less than 12 years of age

IVF bolus? How much?
20 mL/kg. Blood if no response to 2 IVF boluses

Number 1 cause of death for children ages 1 to 20 years of age:
Trauma

Patient's mother gives a history of a fall that does not match the developmental stage of the child:
Suspect child abuse

Patient presents with history of fall from 15 feet, hypotensive, distended abdomen, open long bone fracture, blood draining from both ears, and an EMS report of decreased breathe sounds on the right. Next step in management:
Airway (ABC's)

Best indicator of shock:
Capillary refill/tachycardia. Pediatric trauma—children will look OK and then suddenly become very unstable.

PYLORIC STENOSIS

Ultrasound findings:
Pyloric wall thickness
Greater than 3 mm thick
Pyloric channel—greater than 15 mm long. All bilious vomiting does not equal pyloric stenosis. (For example, 20% of duodenal atresia occurs before the ampulla.)

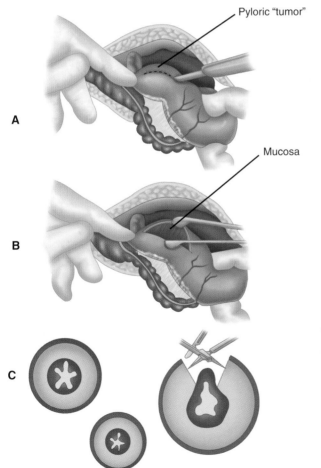

Pyloric "tumor"

A

Mucosa

B

C

FIGURE 25-7. Fredet-Ramstedt pyloromyotomy. (**A**) Pylorus delivered into wound and seromuscular layer incised. (**B**) Seromuscular layer separated down to the submucosal base to permit herniation of mucosa through the pyloric incision. (**C**) Cross-section demonstrating the hypertrophied pylorus, depth of incision, and spreading of muscle to permit mucosa to be herniated through the incision. (*Reproduced from Brunicardi FC, Andersen DK, Billiar TR, et al. Schwartz's Principles of Surgery. 9th ed. http://www.accessmedicine.com. Copyright © The McGraw-Hill Companies, Inc. All rights reserved.*)

Paradoxical aciduria:
Know the mechanism. Remember that they are volume-contracted and have lost H^+ in their vomit. The metabolic alkalosis and dehydration are the first things you need to treat. Use 0.9% NaCl boluses. When the baby is urinating, start 0.5% NaCl at 1.5 maintenance. Then replace the K^+. Again, we talk about the importance of K^+ levels in these patients, but you need a normal HCO_3^- before going to the OR. This is a semielective procedure.

Electrolyte findings:
Hypokalemic, hypochloremic, metabolic alkalosis

INTUSSUSCEPTION

3-year-old presents with a history of inconsolable crying from abdominal pain followed by periods in which they are happily playing. What is the diagnosis?
Intussusception

How to make diagnosis?
Start with plain AXR, then ultrasound

What are you looking for on ultrasound?
Target sign

Etiology:
Lead point is usually Peyer patches (classically secondary to viral gastroenteritis, URI, or administration of rotavirus vaccine).

When to operate?
Again, if the patient is toxic, resuscitate then go to the OR. Failure of nonoperative management with hydrostatic reduction/contrast or air enema. Bloody stool is not an indication for OR but ominous sign.

Success rate with nonoperative reduction:
80%

Push or pull?
Always push bowel out. Never pull bowel out. Recurrence after surgical reduction is low.

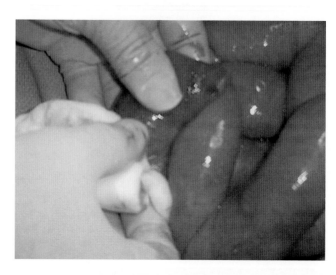

FIGURE 25-8. Open reduction of intussusception. The bowel is milked backward to relieve the obstruction. *(Reproduced from Brunicardi FC, Andersen DK, Billiar TR, et al. Schwartz's Principles of Surgery. 9th ed. http://www.accessmedicine. com. Copyright © The McGraw-Hill Companies, Inc. All rights reserved.)*

Incidental finding of Meckel:
Resect

What is intussusception?
Telescoping/invagination of a proximal segment of bowel into an adjacent distal segment of bowel

What is the most common cause of intestinal obstruction in infants/children ages 9 months to 4 years?
Intussusception

Where does intussusception most commonly occur?
At or near the ileocecal valve (ileocolic intussusception)

What percentage of pediatric intussusception cases are considered idiopathic?
95%

How many attempts at reduction of intussusception are usually tried before stopping?
3 attempts at reduction, may attempt more if progress being made

How long should each attempt at reduction of intussusception be in duration?
No longer than 3 minutes

When should a patient with intussusception undergo surgical exploration?
Presence of peritonitis and small bowel obstruction; incomplete reduction with retrograde enema; bowel perforation during diagnostic/therapeutic enema

What other structure is often routinely removed when operating on a patient with intussusception?
The appendix

What percentage of infants experience recurrent intussusception after either nonoperative or operative reduction?
~5% of infants

When trying to reduce an intussusception, what is the maximum barium column height or maximum air pressure that should be used?
Maximum column height of barium: 1 m
Maximum air pressure: 120 mm Hg

NUTRITION AND PHYSIOLOGY

Caloric intake for 0 to 1 year of age?
90 to 120 kcal/kg/d
Breast milk and formula is 20 kcal/ounce = 20 kcal/30 cc = 0.68 kcal/cc.
Infants should gain 30 g/d or about 1% of their body weight per day. For example, a 2-week-old, 1-kg, 34-week-gestation infant should gain about 10 g/d.
Weight gain is an important indicator of sufficient caloric intake.
Requirements for protein and calories are much higher for infants.

Other ages (not high-yield):
1 to 7 years: 75 to 90 kcal/kg/d
7 to 12 years: 60 to 75 kcal/kg/d
12 to 18 years: 30 to 60 kcal/kg/d

Temperature? Higher risk for hypothermia—large BSA.
Respond by nonshivering thermogenesis and mobilization of brown fat

Immune system:
Relatively immunodeficient, IgA from mother's breast milk. IgG is the only immunoglobulin to cross the placenta.

Woman in trauma bay, 30 weeks pregnant, with strong, regular contractions, cervical dilation without vaginal bleeding on speculum examination. Diagnosis and management? Patient is in labor-strong, regular contractions with cervical dilatation:
General considerations: Check ultrasound (fetal position, previa, abruption, etc), give steroids to help if premature lungs, tocolytics, hydration (number one cause of preterm labor is dehydration/hypovolemia!), antibiotics for GBS, check ratio of lecithin to sphingomyelin (L/S), check Rh, speculum examination before bimanual. Give mom oxygen and put the LEFT SIDE DOWN—insisting on putting the left side down to get the baby off the IVC. This alone will dramatically improve outcomes.

Insensible losses in an infant:
Higher! Notice the difference below (don't memorize)
Premature infant (<1500 g)—45 to 60 mL/kg/d
Term infant—30 to 35 mL/kg/d
Adult—15 mL/kg/d

Best indicator of adequate fluid intake:
Urine output: 1 to 2 mL/kg/d
Weigh diapers and weigh the baby
Urine osmolarity? Decreased. Max concentration for infant is 700 mOsm/kg
Know the 4, 2, 1 rule for maintenance fluids
No K^+ to any neonate/infant until making urine and potassium within normal serum levels

What structures are derived from the foregut?
Lungs, esophagus, stomach, pancreas, liver, gallbladder, bile duct, duodenum proximal to ampulla of Vater.

What structures are derived from the midgut?
Duodenum distal to ampulla, small intestine, colon to distal one-third of transverse colon.

What structures are derived from the hindgut?
Distal one-third of transverse colon to anal canal

What is the primary energy substrate for the fetus?
Glucose

What might you see with a linoleic acid deficiency?
Dryness/thickening of the skin, hair loss, and delayed wound healing

What is the most important carbohydrate source for infants?
Lactose

What is the most common cause of respiratory distress in neonates?
Respiratory distress syndrome (hyaline membrane disease)

What is the most common index of lung maturity?
The ratio of lecithin (phosphatidylcholine) to sphingomyelin in amniotic fluid (L/S ratio):
L/S ratio = 2.0, normal with extremely low risk of RDS
L/S ratio = 1.5 to 2.0 considered "immature" with low risk
L/S ratio <1.5 increased risk
L/S ratio <1.0 high risk

What drug inhibits prostaglandin synthetase and promotes closure of a patent ductus arteriosus if given within the first 2 weeks of life?
Indomethacin

Describe the fetal circulation:
Well-oxygenated blood from the placenta/umbilical cord passes through the hepatic ductus venosus→ IVC → Right atrium.
More oxygenated blood flows through foramen ovale into left atrium where it is pumped by the left ventricle into the aortic arch to supply the heart, brain, and upper body.
Less-oxygenated blood is pumped into pulmonary artery by right ventricle and shunted through ductus arteriosus into descending aorta, which then supplies the organs of the lower body and also gives blood back to the placenta through 2 umbilical arteries.

What is the most serious complication of neck masses in children?
Airway obstruction

What is the recurrence rate for thyroglossal duct cyst after the Sistrunk procedure?
<10%

What percentage of ectopic thyroid tissue is found to have thyroid neoplasia?
<1%

What is the most common presentation of a thyroglossal duct cyst?
A midline cystic neck mass versus a draining sinus

How might a thyroglossal duct cyst be differentiated from a branchial cleft cyst on physical examination?
A thyroglossal duct cyst often moves with protrusion of the tongue and swallowing because the cyst and tract are attached at the foramen cecum at the base of the tongue; branchial cleft cysts should not change position with tongue movement.

What is the most common deformity of the anterior chest wall?
Pectus excavatum

What is pectus excavatum?
A posterior curve in the body of the sternum from the manubrium to the xiphoid, resulting from abnormal regulation of costal cartilage growth

What do patients with pectus excavatum typically complain of clinically?
Chest pain or shortness of breath with exertion or both

What is the pectus index?
The ratio of the maximum internal transverse diameter of the thorax to the minimum sternovertebral distance

What is the optimal timing for repair of pectus excavatum?
Late childhood and early adolescence (ossification of key components of anterior chest wall not completed until late teenage years)

What procedure used to treat pectus excavatum utilizes a rigid U-shaped bar inserted transversely across the chest to push the deformity back into place?
The Lorenz bar/Nuss procedure

What chest wall defect features a protrusion of the sternum and ribs?
Pectus carinatum

What is included in Cantrell pentology?
Distal sternal cleft, omphalocele, (morgagni) diaphragmatic defect, pericardial defect, and intracardiac defect

What is a pulmonary sequestration?
Abnormal lung tissue that may or may not communicate with the trachea/bronchus

What is the usual vascular supply to an extralobar pulmonary sequestration?
Arterial blood supply: Systemic (frequently from aorta below diaphragm)
Venous drainage: Systemic

What is the usual Rx for a pulmonary sequestration?
Thoracotomy and lobectomy

What is the usual vascular supply to an intralobar pulmonary sequestration?
Arterial blood supply: thoracic or abdominal aorta
Venous drainage: pulmonary vein (can be systemic)

How may intralobar pulmonary sequestration present during childhood?
As recurrent localized pneumonia

What are the 3 stages of empyema?
Stage I: *Exudative:* Thin low cell count free-flowing fluid
Stage II: *Fibrinopurulent:* Encasement of lung parenchyma with thick purulent material with multiple loculations
Stage III: *Organizing:* A fibrotic peel from fibroblasts growing into the exudate

What are the 3 most common pathogens in pediatric pneumonia?
Haemophilus influenzae, Streptococcus pneumoniae, Staphylococcus aureus

What pleural fluid cell count differential makes the diagnosis of chylothorax in patients who are not being fed?
>90% lymphocytes

What may be administered to a patient prior to the OR that will make identification of the thoracic duct and an associated leak more obvious?
Cream

Are inguinal hernias more common in males or females?
Males (6:1)

How might acute, noncommunicating hydrocele be distinguished from incarcerated inguinal hernia?
Absence of symptoms of bowel obstruction; can usually palpate normal cord structures above the scrotal mass and transilluminate the hydrocele

When might you perform operative exploration of the contralateral asymptomatic groin in a pediatric patient with an inguinal hernia?
Controversial, but consider in males younger than 2 years (60%–70% incidence of a contralateral patent processus vaginalis) or female up to age 4.

What complications may follow repair of a pediatric inguinal hernia?
Complications from general anesthesia; wound infection; recurrence; injury to vas deferens/testicular vessels

What is a hydrocele?
A fluid collection in the processus vaginalis in the inguinal canal or the tunica vaginalis in the scrotum

What is the difference between a communicating versus a noncommunicating hydrocele?
A communicating hydrocele features a direct patency between the hydrocele and the peritoneal cavity, whereas a noncommunicating hydrocele does not increase or decrease in size over time.

How might a communicating hydrocele be distinguished from a noncommunicating hydrocele by history?
The communicating hydrocele will generally have a history of fluctuating size.

When should a communicating hydrocele be repaired?
Shortly after they are diagnosed (like an inguinal hernia)

When is operative management of a noncommunicating hydrocele indicated?
Acutely enlarging hydrocele; lesions that persist after age 12 months (usually spontaneously resolve before this time); question of communication of the hydrocele

What causes of neonatal intestinal obstruction have a higher incidence in infants with trisomy 21 compared to the general population?
Duodenal atresia/stenosis; Hirschsprung disease

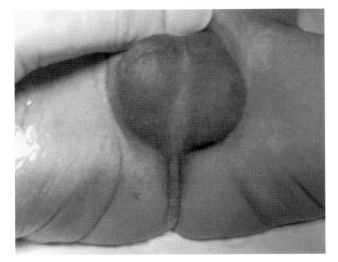

FIGURE 25-9. Low imperforate anus in a male. Note the well-developed buttocks. The perineal fistula was found at the midline raphe. (*Reproduced from Brunicardi FC, Andersen DK, Billiar TR, et al. Schwartz's Principles of Surgery. 9th ed. http://www. accessmedicine.com. Copyright © The McGraw-Hill Companies, Inc. All rights reserved.*)

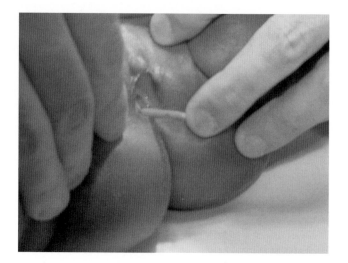

FIGURE 25-10. Imperforate anus in a female. A catheter has been placed into the fistula, which is in the vestibule of the vagina. *(Reproduced from Brunicardi FC, Andersen DK, Billiar TR, et al. Schwartz's Principles of Surgery. 9th ed. http://www.accessmedicine.com. Copyright © The McGraw-Hill Companies, Inc. All rights reserved.)*

What are the 2 most common anorectal malformations observed in males?
Low imperforate anus with perineal fistula; high anorectal agenesis with rectoprostatic urethral fistula

What is the most common anorectal malformation observed in females?
Low imperforate anus with fistula from rectum to either perineal body or vaginal vestibule

Which anorectal malformation has a more favorable prognosis for fecal continence: low, intermediate, or high anorectal lesion?
Low has a more favorable prognosis for fecal continence

What structure is used to delineate a low from high anorectal malformation?
Pubococcygeal line

What is the most common associated abnormality with anorectal malformation?
Renal anomaly (including both upper and lower tract)

What types of anorectal malformations are considered high lesions in females?
Anorectal agenesis with/without rectovaginal fistula; rectal atresia

What types of anorectal malformations are considered intermediate lesions in females?
Rectovestibular fistula, rectovaginal fistula, anal agenesis without fistula

What types of anorectal malformations are considered low lesions in females?
Rectovestibular fistula, anal stenosis

What types of anorectal malformations are considered high lesions in males?
Anorectal agenesis with/without rectoprostatic urethral fistula, rectal atresia

What types of anorectal malformations are considered intermediate lesions in males?
Rectobulbar urethral fistula, anal agenesis without fistula

What types of anorectal malformations are considered low lesions in males?
Anocutaneous fistula, anal stenosis

What do infants with an intermediate, high, or indeterminate anorectal malformation generally require as initial surgical management?
Divided diverting proximal sigmoidostomy, mucous fistula to study distally

When is anorectoplasty generally performed in an infant with an intermediate or high anorectal malformation?
8 to 12 months of age

What is the most widely used procedure for repair of high and intermediate anorectal malformations in the United States?
Posterior sagittal anorectoplasty

What complications may follow a repair of an anorectal malformation?
Infection, leak, anastomotic stricture, recurrent fistula

What is the most frequently encountered neonatal surgical emergency?
NEC

What percentage of NEC cases occur after the initiation of feeding?
>90%

What are the most common sites of involvement of necrotizing enterocolitis?
Terminal ileum, right colon

What causes of neonatal intestinal obstruction have a higher incidence in infants with trisomy 21 compared to the general population?
Duodenal atresia/stenosis Hirschsprung disease

What is the most common cause of colon obstruction in a pediatric patient?
Hirschsprung disease (vs constipation)

Which portion of the GI tract is most commonly involved in the aganglionosis of Hirschsprung disease?
Distal rectosigmoid colon (75%–80% of affected infants)

What is the characteristic lesion in the distal bowel seen with Hirschsprung disease?
Aganglionosis of the intermuscular and submucosal plexuses

What finding on rectal biopsy excludes a diagnosis of Hirschsprung disease?
The finding of ganglion cells on a rectal biopsy performed 1 to 1.5 cm above the dentate line

How do patients with Hirschsprung disease present?
Failure to pass meconium within the first 24 to 48 hours of life. Infants can have abdominal distension, feeding intolerance, bilious emesis, malnutrition, and failure to thrive. They can have enterocolitis with forceful expulsion of foul-smelling, liquid stool on rectal examination progressing to sepsis, transmural necrosis, and perforation; can have chronic constipation if older children/adults

When would you perform a full-thickness rectal biopsy under general anesthesia rather than a bedside suction biopsy for the diagnosis of Hirschsprung disease?
Inadequate suction biopsy in infants, older children

How would you treat a patient with Hirschsprung disease with enterocolitis or multiple associated anomalies/medical problems?
Resuscitation and broad-spectrum IV antibiotics
Diverting colostomy versus rectal irrigation and decompression followed by proximal diversion after stabilization

What is the most frequently encountered congenital anomaly of the GI tract?
Meckel diverticulum

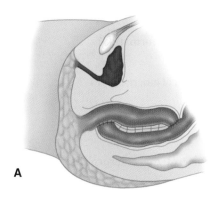
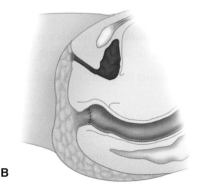

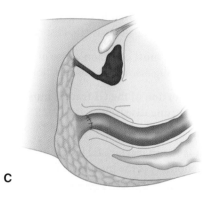

FIGURE 25-11. Three operations for surgical correction of Hirschsprung disease. **(A)** The Duhamel procedure leaves the rectum in place and brings ganglionic bowel into the retrorectal space. **(B)** Swenson procedure is a resection with end-to-end anastomosis performed by exteriorizing bowel ends through the anus. **(C)** In the Soave operation, endorectal dissection is performed and mucosa is removed from the aganglionic distal segment. The ganglionic bowel is then brought down to the anus within the seromuscular tunnel. *(Reproduced from Brunicardi FC, Andersen DK, Billiar TR, et al. Schwartz's Principles of Surgery. 9th ed. http://www.accessmedicine. com. Copyright © The McGraw-Hill Companies, Inc. All rights reserved.)*

What is a Meckel diverticulum?
A malformation resulting from persistence of the omphalomesenteric duct (vitelline duct)

Regarding Meckel diverticulum, what is the rule of 2's?
Found 2 ft from the ileocecal valve; In 2% of the population; 2% are symptomatic; 2 tissue types (gastric—most common and likely to be symptomatic, pancreatic); 2 presentations (bleeding, diverticulitis)

What is the #1 cause of painless lower GI bleeding in children?
Meckel diverticulum

Is a Meckel diverticulum a true diverticulum?
Yes, a Meckel diverticulum is a true diverticulum

What is the arterial blood supply to a Meckel diverticulum?
Persistent vitelline vessels (from SMA)

What is the test of choice to diagnose GI bleeding secondary to a Meckel diverticulum?
^{99m}Tc-pertechnetate radioisotope scan (Meckel scan)

What is the Rx of choice for a symptomatic Meckel diverticulum?
Antimesenteric wedge excision or segmental bowel resection with primary closure versus anastomosis

How does a patient with pyogenic liver abscess present?
Fever; jaundice; leukocytosis; may find tender liver/hepatosplenomegaly on physical examination

What is the Rx for a pyogenic liver abscess?
Broad-spectrum antibiotics and percutaneous drainage; rarely, may require open operative drainage

What parasite is responsible for amebic abscess of the liver?
Entamoeba histolytica

What is the most common cause of chronic cholestasis in infants?
Biliary atresia

What is the most frequent indication for pediatric liver transplantation?
Biliary atresia

What is biliary atresia?
Replacement of the extrahepatic/intrahepatic/both biliary tract ± gallbladder with dense, fibrous inflammatory tissue secondary to an inflammatory process

What is the cardinal sign of biliary atresia?
Progressive neonatal jaundice during the first few weeks of life

What degree of conjugated hyperbilirubinemia in an infant requires investigation?
Direct fraction of bilirubin >50%; direct bilirubin >2 mg/dL

What drug is given to infants orally to improve the sensitivity of a hepatobiliary scan in a patient with suspected biliary atresia?
Phenobarbital (5 mg/kg daily); increases hepatocyte processing ^{99m}Tc-IDA and induces hepatic microsomal enzymes. Workup is ultrasound, laboratories, HIDA

What is the most common ultrasonographic finding in biliary atresia?
A diminutive/absent gallbladder without associated intrahepatic duct dilatation

What will you see on liver biopsy in a patient with biliary atresia?
Periportal fibrosis; bile plugging; eventual cirrhosis

What medical condition should be ruled out before operative exploration in all patients with suspected biliary atresia?
α1-antitrypsin deficiency (difficult to differentiate from biliary atresia); check plasma α1-antitrypsin levels

What is the recommended initial procedure for the Rx of biliary atresia?
Portoenterostomy (Kasai procedure)

What fraction of patients undergoing the Kasai procedure for biliary atresia get better?
One-third

What fraction of patients undergoing the Kasai procedure for biliary atresia go on to liver transplant?
One-third

What fraction of patients undergoing the Kasai procedure for biliary atresia die?
One-third

What are indications for liver transplantation in a patient with biliary atresia?
Progressive hepatic failure despite portoenterostomy, growth retardation, complications of portal HTN

What condition is characterized by 2 separate pancreatic ducts resulting from the failure of the dorsal and ventral ducts to fuse normally?
Pancreas divisum

What is the most common exocrine pancreatic anomaly secondary to defective development during embryogenesis?
Annular pancreas (circumferential pancreatic tissue around duodenum)

What is the most common disorder of the pancreas in infants/children?
Acute pancreatitis

How is the definitive diagnosis of pancreas divisum made?
The demonstration of 2 separate, parallel ductal systems (magnetic resonance cholangiopancreatography)

If indicated, what would be the surgical management for pancreas divisum?
Sphincterotomy of the accessory duct (open dorsal duct sphincterotomy, endoscopic sphincterotomy)

In what percentage of hypospadias cases is the defect distal to the midshaft?
>85%

What are the principles of hypospadias repair?
To advance the urethral meatus to a normal position in the glans; correct penile chordee

When performing resection of a Wilm tumor, what is the consequence of intraoperative spillage of tumor?
Lesion is upstaged; will need whole-abdomen radiation

By what factor does intraoperative tumor spillage of Wilm tumor increase local abdominal recurrence?
6X

Which patients with resectable Wilm tumor should receive postoperative chemotherapy?
All patients with resectable Wilm tumor receive postoperative chemotherapy.

What is the surgical Rx of testicular torsion?
For torsed testis: orchiopexy if viable; orchiectomy if necrotic
For contralateral testis: orchiopexy

If suspect a torsed testes, don't waste time with Doppler's → go to OR!

MULTIPLE CHOICE QUESTIONS

1. A 6-week-old boy has a 6-day history of vomiting, intermittent fussiness, periods of inconsolability, and a 0.3-kg weight loss. On examination his anterior fontanelle is flattened and his mucous membranes are dry. Abdominal examination is unremarkable. Laboratory data are as follows: Na, 130; Ch, 87; CO_2, 30. An ultrasound of the abdomen reveals a 3.5 mm × 12 mm pylorus. The next most appropriate step in management of this child would be:
   A. Pyloromyotomy
   B. Esopahgeal pH monitoring
   C. Initiate proton pump inhibitor therapy
   D. Order an immediate small bowel follow-through study
   E. Begin IV fluid resuscitation

2. A 32-week gestational male presents with persistent cough when feeding and spits up after every feed. An abdominal radiograph reveals gasless stomach. Tracheoesophageal fistula is suspected. Appropriate workup should include:
   A. Ultrasound of the back
   B. Ultrasound of the kidneys
   C. Echocardiogram
   D. Rectal biopsy
   E. Chromosomal analysis

3. A two-day-old 34-week gestational female with Down syndrome presents with feeding intolerance and forceful bilious vomiting. A 'babygram' demonstrates two large gas-filled structures in the upper abdomen (presumed stomach and duodenum). What is the most appropriate surgical option?
   A. Duodenojejunostomy
   B. Duodenoduodenostomy
   C. Gastrojejunostomy
   D. Roux-en Y enterostomy
   E. Pyloromyotomy

4. What is the most common childhood malgnancy?
   A. Neuroblastoma
   B. Wilm tumor
   C. Leukemia
   D. Lymphoma
   E. Hepatoblastoma

5. A 4-day-old 28-week gestational male develops increasing abdominal distention and feeding intolerance. His nurse notes scant blood with the patient's last bowel movement. An abdominal radiograph reveals portal venous gas and pneumatosis intestinalis. An orogastric tube is placed and IV antibiotic therapy is initiated. All of the following are indications for immediate operation except:
   A. Worsening pneumatosis intestinalis and portal venous gas
   B. Worsening acidosis
   C. Abdominal wall erythema
   D. Positive paracentesis cultures
   E. None of the above

6. You see a 4-year-old boy regarding an abdominal mass. His parents have noted that he has been increasingly lethargic over the past several weeks. They think he is pale, and he has recently started to take long afternoon naps. His appetite has been poor, and he has lost 4 pounds in the last 2 months.

Upon physical examination, the child is thin and pale. His lungs are clear with equal breath sounds. His heart tones are normal. His abdomen is quite full. You feel a large mass under the left costal margin that is firm and immobile.

The most likely diagnosis is:

A. Wilm tumor
B. Hodgkin disease
C. Non-Hodgkin disease
D. Neuroblastoma
E. Rhabdomyosarcoma

7. Which of the following factors influence this patient's prognosis?

A. Age
B. Stage of the tumor
C. Histologic appearance
D. Cytogenetic analysis
E. All of above

8. Which of the following are associated with an increased incidence of neuroblastoma?

A. Maternal phenytoin use
B. Fetal alcohol syndrome
C. Hirschprung disease
D. Beckwith-Weidermann syndrome
E. All of the above

9. Which of the following should be included in the initial evaluation of patients with neuroblastoma?

A. A CT scan of the head
B. Bone marrow biopsy
C. Lumbar puncture
D. MIBG scan
E. All of the above

10. If bone marrow did not reveal small round blue cells consistent with neuroblastoma. Which of the following is the most appropriate Rx for this 4-year-old boy?

A. Fine-needle aspiration cytology under local anesthesia
B. Wide resection of the mass with resection of all contiguous structures
C. Laparotomy and tumor biopsy followed by chemotherapy
D. Limited resection with preservation of all vital structures followed by chemotherapy
E. Chemotherapy without biopsy

ANSWERS

1. **Answer: E.** The age of this child's presentation should exclude diagonoses of duodenal atresia (which typically present earlier) and the clinical presentation, as well as age, may exclude later presenting pathologies, such as intussusception. GERD may be suspected. However, in light of weight loss, dehydration, and electrolyte derangement, other diagnosis must be excluded. This child presents with metabolic alkalosis and subclinical findings on ultrasound of pyloric stenosis (typically 4 mm × 14 mm pylorus effectively clenches the diagnosis). The first goal should be correction of the electrolytes and close monitoring.

2. **Answer: E.** TEF can be seen in the VACTERL association and additional anomalies should be ruled out.

   Vertebral anomalies: Defects of the spinal column usually consist of hypoplastic vertebrae or hemivertebra. 70% of patients with VACTERL association will have vertebral anomalies.

   Imperforate **A**nus: Anal atresia or imperforate anus is seen in about 55% of patients with VACTERL association.

   Cardiac defects: Up to 75% of patients with VACTERL association have been reported to have congenital heart disease. The most common heart defects seen with VACTERL association are ventricular septal defect, atrial septal defects, and tetralogy of Fallot.

   Tracheo-**E**sophageal fistula: EA with TEF is seen in about 70% of patients with VACTERL association, although it can frequently occur as an isolated defect.

   Renal anomalies: Renal defects are seen in approximately 50% of patients with VACTERL association. In addition, up to 35% of patients with VACTERL association have a single umbilical artery. These defects can be severe with incomplete formation of one or both kidneys or urologic abnormalities such as obstruction of outflow of urine from the kidneys or severe reflux of urine into the kidneys from the bladder. These problems can cause kidney failure early in life and may require kidney transplant. Many of these problems can be corrected surgically before any damage can occur.

   Limb anomalies: Limb defects occur in up to 70% of babies with VACTERL association and include a displaced or hypoplastic thumb, polydactyly, syndactyly, and forearm defects such as radial aplasia.

3. **Answer: B.** Approximately 20% to 40% of all infants with duodenal atresia have Down syndrome and approximately 8% all infants with Down syndrome have duodenal atresia. Forceful bilious vomiting is commonly seen and the diagnosis of duodenal atresia is usually confirmed by radiography. A duodenodeuodenostomy is the surgical Rx of choice in these cases because it provides physiologic continuity of the GI tract.

4. **Answer: C.** The most common solid tumor in children is neuroblastoma. However, the most common overall malignancy is leukemia (40% of all childhood malignancies).

5. **Answer: A.** Initial therapy for NEC is medical; however, the pathologic process may progress to frank peritonitis and systemic sepsis. Close monitoring of children with NEC is required.

6. **Answer: D.** The most common solid abdominal tumors of childhood are Wilm tumor and neuroblastoma. Patients with Wilm tumor are typically asymptomatic and present when they are found to have a large abdominal mass on routine examination. Children with neuroblastoma, on the other hand, typically present with a variety of constitutional symptoms.

7. **Answer: A.** The age of the patient at the time of diagnosis has a profound influence on outcome for neuroblastoma. Survival rates for children with neuroblastoma under 1 year of age are between 70% and 90%, whereas survival rates for children older than 1 year are 20% to 30%. Much of this discrepancy is explained by the unusual maturation seen in neuroblastoma in infancy.

8. **Answer: E.** Hirschsprung disease is a disorder of ganglion cell migration in the large intestine. These ganglion cells are thought to be neural crest in origin. Beckwith-Weidermann syndrome results in an increased incidence of a number of abdominal tumors, including Wilm tumor, neuroblastoma, hepatoblastoma, and adrenocortical carcinoma. Fetal alcohol syndrome and maternal Dilantin use have been found to correlate with neuroblastoma by unknown mechanisms.

9. **Answer: B.** Bone marrow biopsy should be obtained in order to rule out any metastatic disease in the case of neuroblastoma.

10. **Answer: C.** Neuroblastoma is commonly metastatic to the bone marrow. In fact, the diagnosis can often be made by means of bone marrow examination without biopsy of the primary tumor. In this particular case, the best procedure would be small laparotomy with tumor biopsy for histologic and cytogenetic analysis. This information would then be used to guide most appropriate course of chemotherapy.

CHAPTER 26
Plastic and Reconstructive Surgery

Ramon Garza III

SKIN

What type of UV radiation is linked with skin cancer?
UVB

What is the most common skin malignancy in the United States?
Basal cell carcinoma

What are the classic physical findings of basal cell carcinoma?
Pearly appearance with rolled edges, +/− telangiectasia

What type of basal cell carcinoma is the most aggressive?
Morpheaform type (produces collagenase)

What margins are appropriate for basal cell?
3 mm margins are acceptable and frozen section can be used intraoperatively.

What is the most common physical finding of squamous cell carcinoma?
Scaly appearance, papulonodular, ulceration

What is the name of the cancer associated with a previous burn injury?
Marjolin ulcer; can also develop in areas of chronic inflammation, that is, enteric fistula.

What are appropriate margins for squamous cell carcinoma?
0.5 to 1.0 cm margins

What are risk factors for the development of squamous cell carcinoma?
Actinic keratosis, arsenics, atrophic dermatitis, Bowen disease, chlorophenols, fair skin, HPV, immunosuppression, nitrates, previous skin cancer, radiation exposure, sun exposure, xeroderma pigmentosum

What is the natural history of squamous cell carcinoma?
Actinic keratosis, Bowen disease (squamous cell carcinoma in situ), squamous cell carcinoma

Aside from sun exposure, what is classically a risk factor for squamous cell carcinoma?
History of organ transplantation, or any other immunocompromised state

Can squamous cell carcinoma metastasize?
Yes, it is uncommon, but it can metastasize to lymph nodes. Regional adenectomy should be performed.

When can Mohs surgery be used for basal cell or squamous cell carcinoma?
Delicate areas that include perioral, perioccular, perinasal, ears, hands, and genitalia

What is the most common melanoma site on the skin in men? In women?
Men—back
Women—legs

What is the most common location for distant melanoma metastasis?
The lung (surgery can help relieve pain caused by metastatic melanoma to the lung, but is not a cure)

What is the most common metastasis to the small bowel?
Melanoma

What margins are recommended for a melanoma skin lesion with thickness of 1 mm?
1 cm margins are recommended; for lesions greater than 2 mm a 2 cm margin is recommended. 0.5 cm margins are acceptable for thin lentigo maligna melanomas or melanoma in situ.

Can electrocautery be used for excisional biopsy of melanoma?
No, cold knife excision should be used so as to not disturb the deep margin with burn artifact.

What types of melanoma are there?
Superficial spreading, lentigo maligna, acral lentiginous, nodular

What is the most common type of melanoma?
Superficial spreading

Clark level	Breslow (mm)	AJCC T
I		
II	≤0.75	T1
III	0.76–1.50	T2
IV	1.51–4.00	T3
V	≥4.00	T4

FIGURE 26-1. Although Breslow thickness has traditionally been used to anticipate clinical outcomes based on the depth of melanoma invasion, more recent staging criteria advanced by the American Joint Committee on Cancer (AJCC) are today's standard of care. *(Reproduced from Brunicardi FC, Andersen DK, Billiar TR, et al. Schwartz's Principles of Surgery. 9th ed. http://www.accessmedicine.com. Copyright © The McGraw-Hill Companies, Inc. All rights reserved.)*

What is the least aggressive type of melanoma?
Lentigo maligna

What is the most aggressive type of melanoma?
Nodular, but acral lentiginous is also aggressive and presents late because of location on feet/hands.

If a melanoma lesion is less than 1 mm thickness and no lymphadenopathy is palpated, does any additional workup need to be performed?
No. Optional CXR, liver function test (LFT's), and sentinel lymph node biopsy (SNLB) can be performed for lesions greater than 1 mm thickness. If SNLB is positive, then all the above workup and an MRI of brain and CXR should be performed. If there are palpable nodes present, a formal lymph node dissection should be performed.

Can Mohs surgery be used for melanoma?
No, never!

Can frozen sections be used to determine if margins are negative for melanoma?
No, frozen sections have no role in the management of melanoma (permanent section only).

What is the difference between a keloid and hypertrophic scar?
A hypertrophic scar does not extend beyond the borders of the original scar.

What is the treatment for a keloid?
First-line therapy for most keloids is intralesional corticosteroids. They can also be treated with radiation, silicone sheets, surgery with interferon or triamcinolone injections, and pressure garments.

What is the treatment for a hypertrophic scar?
Intralesional corticosteroids, silicone sheets, pressure garments

What is the treatment for hidradenitis?
Improve hygiene, antibiotics, surgery to remove infected tissue and apocrine sweat glands

WOUND HEALING

What is the reconstructive ladder?
It is a way of organizing approaches to reconstruction and wound healing. The first step of the reconstructive ladder is the simplest and least invasive method progressing to the most complex method at the top of the ladder.

What are the general categories in the steps of the reconstructive ladder in order from simple to complex?
Healing by secondary intention
Healing by primary intention/tertiary (delayed primary) intention
Split-thickness/full-thickness skin graft (STSG/FTSG)
Local flap
Regional flap
Distant flap
Free flap

What patient factors are important when evaluating a wound?
Immune deficiency/suppression
Nutritional status/obesity
Diabetes
Smoking
Healing disorders
Age

How can you diagnose a skin infection in a burn patient?
Biopsy the skin; if bacteria are present on deep dermis, then the patient likely has an infection.

How do you obtain a sample of bone for biopsy to evaluate for osteomyelitis?
A separate incision is made, away from open wound, and bone biopsy is performed through this incision.

What is the utility of imaging in evaluating osteomyelitis?
MRI is a good modality to evaluate extent of osteomyelitis, plain film will not show osteomyelitis changes for 2 weeks, and bone scan is not specific in the face of an open wound or a fracture.

True or false: A moist environment is key for a clean wound to heal.
True. Clean wounds heal faster and with less scarring if the wound is kept moist.

What adverse side effect is associated with silver nitrate? Silvadene? Sulfamylon?
Silver nitrate = hypo-(calcium, sodium, potassium, chloride)
Sulfamylon = metabolic acidosis
Silvadene = neutropenia and thrombocytopenia

What is the strength layer in closing an incision?
Dermis

RECONSTRUCTION

How does a Z-plasty work?
It increases length by rearranging the tissues and borrowing from the width.

What are the angles of a Z-plasty that would give you a theoretical increase in length of 75%?
60 degrees

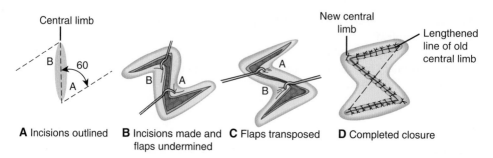

A Incisions outlined **B** Incisions made and **C** Flaps transposed **D** Completed closure
flaps undermined

FIGURE 26-2. Z-plasty. *(Reproduced from Doherty GM. Current Diagnosis and Treatment: Surgery. 13th ed. http://www.accessmedicine.com. Copyright © The McGraw-Hill Companies, Inc. All rights reserved.)*

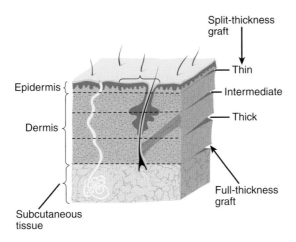

FIGURE 26-3. Depths of full-thickness and split-thickness grafts. *(Reproduced from Doherty GM. Current Diagnosis and Treatment: Surgery. 13th ed. http://www.accessmedicine.com. Copyright © The McGraw-Hill Companies, Inc. All rights reserved.)*

How do you design a Z-plasty?
The common limb of the Z-plasty is in the direction to be lengthened. All the limbs should be the same length.

What is a STSG?
Its components include all of the epidermis and a portion of the dermis. STSG vary in thickness depending on how much dermis is included.

What is a FTSG?
Its components include all of the epidermis and all of the underlying dermis.

How do skin grafts survive?
Within the first 24 to 48 hours, skin grafts survive on nutrients that diffuse from the surrounding tissue to the dermis of the skin graft (plasmatic imbibition). After this occurs, revascularization of the skin graft occurs (inosculation).

Can a skin graft survive on exposed tendon or bone?
Yes, as long as the peritenon and periosteum are in place, respectively.

What is the difference between a flap and a graft?
A flap has its own inherent blood supply. A graft receives its nutrition from the recipient tissue until revascularization occurs.

What is a random skin flap?
It is a flap that does not have a large-bore artery as its arterial supply (axial blood supply). It receives its blood supply from a random subdermal arterial plexus.

What is a pedicle?
It is the vascular supply to a flap that is left intact when mobilizing a flap.

What is surgical delay with regard to skin flaps?
It is the process in which there is a partial interruption of the skin flap's blood supply to build a more robust arterial supply from the other feeding vessels (likely the future pedicle).

What is the safe (flap length):(base width) for a random skin flap? For the face?
1:1; 1:1.5 for face

What is an axial skin flap?
It is a skin flap that is fed by a named or clearly identifiable artery.

What is the (flap length):(base width) for an axial skin flap? For the face?
3:1; 6:1

What is a fasciocutaneous flap?
Fascia + skin; can be used as a pedicled flap or as a free flap.

What is a myocutaneous flap?
Muscle + skin; can be used as a pedicled flap or as a free flap.

What is meant by major vascular pedicle in the Mathes and Nahai muscle classification system?
It is a vascular pedicle able to maintain adequate perfusion to the entire muscle if its other arterial supplies were interrupted.

What is the blood supply to pectoralis major?
Major blood supply from pectoral artery from thoracoacromial vessel and minor blood supply from segmental branches from internal mammary

What is the blood supply to Latissimus Dorsi?
Major blood supply from thoracodorsal artery, minor contributions from intercostal and lumbar arteries

What is the blood supply to gracilis?
Ascending branch from medial circumflex femoral artery

What is the blood supply to the rectus abdominis?
The inferior epigastric and superior epigastric arteries

What is the success rate of a free flap surviving?
Greater than 90%

What is the most common reason for free flap failure?
Venous thrombosis

What is the most sensitive way to determine pedicle/free flap viability?
Clinical monitoring

What are signs of a viable flap?
Warm flap, pink in color, cap refill <2 to 3 seconds

BREAST RECONSTRUCTION

What are the various methods for postmastectomy breast reconstruction?
Tissue expander with subsequent breast implant, pedicled autologous tissue (TRAM/latissimus dorsi), free flap (free TRAM, DIEP, SIEA, SGAP)

What do TRAM, DIEP, SIEA, and SGAP stand for?
TransRectus abdominis myocutaneous flap, deep inferior epigastric artery perforator flap, superficial inferior epigastric artery flap, superior gluteal artery perforator flap

What is a perforator?
It is an arterial branch from a larger artery that travels through a muscle ("perforates") to supply the overlying fascia and skin with blood.

What is the first stage of a tissue expander breast reconstruction?
Placement of the expanders in a subpectoral pocket with minimal inflation of the expander.
The expander will be slowly filled over the next several weeks/months until the tissue has expanded enough to accept the final implant at a second stage procedure.

What is the blood supply to a pedicled TRAM flap?
Superior epigastric artery

Where does the superior epigastric artery come from?
It is the distal extent of the internal mammary.

What is the blood supply for a DIEP flap?
It is a perforator from the deep inferior epigastric artery that travels through the rectus abdominis muscle to supply the overlying fascia, fat, and skin

HAND

How many phalanges are located in the digits of one hand?
14; all of the digits have 3 phalanges (proximal, middle, and distal) with the exception of the thumb, which has 2 (proximal and distal).

What is a quick way to assess function of the median nerve in an injured hand/ forearm?
Ask the patient to make an "Ok" sign.

What muscles are innervated by the ulnar nerve in the hand?
Palmar and dorsal interossei, opponens digiti minimi, flexor digiti minimi, abductor digiti minimi, palmaris brevis, deep portion of flexor pollicis brevis, adductor pollicis, lumbricals to ring and small finger

What is Allen test?
It is a way to assess the patency of the ulnar and radial artery to the hand.

What are the indications for replantation?
Thumb replantation, multiple finger amputations, single digit distal to flexor digitorum superficialis (FDS) insertion (zone I), hand amputation through palm, hand amputation through distal wrist, any part in a child, distal forearm

What are the structures in the carpal tunnel?
There are 9 tendons and one nerve (median nerve). Tendons from FDS and flexor digitorum profundus plus the flexor pollicis longus

How do you diagnose carpal tunnel syndrome?
Nerve conduction tests that show motor latency greater than 4.5 msec and sensory latency greater than 3.5 msec

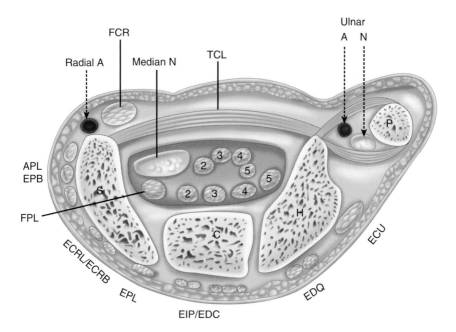

FIGURE 26-4. Cross-section of the wrist at the midcarpal level. The relative geography of the neurologic and tendinous structures can be seen. The transverse carpal ligament (TCL) is the roof of the carpal tunnel, passing volar to the median nerve and long flexor tendons. The TCL is also the floor of the ulnar tunnel, or Guyon canal, passing dorsal to the ulnar artery and nerve. The wrist and digital extensor tendons are also seen, distal to their compartments on the distal radius and ulna. Bones: C, capitate; H, hamate; P, pisiform; S, scaphoid. Tendons (flexor digitorum superficialis is volar to flexor digitorum profundus within the carpal tunnel): 2, index finger; 3, middle finger; 4, ring finger; 5, small finger. A, artery; APL, abductor pollicis longus; ECRB, extensor carpi radialis brevis; ECRL, extensor carpi radialis longus; ECU, extensor carpi ulnaris; EDC, extensor digitorum communis; EDQ, extensor digiti quinti; EIP, extensor indices proprius; EPB, extensor pollicis brevis; EPL, extensor pollicis longus; FCR, flexor carpi radialis; FPL, flexor pollicis longus; N, nerve. *(Reproduced from Brunicardi FC, Andersen DK, Billiar TR, et al. Schwartz's Principles of Surgery. 9th ed. http://www.accessmedicine.com. Copyright © The McGraw-Hill Companies, Inc. All rights reserved.)*

How do you surgically treat carpal tunnel?
Complete release of transverse carpal ligament with care to avoid median recurrent motor branch of median nerve.

Which 2 nonthumb fingers are needed for grip strength?
Little and ring fingers

MULTIPLE CHOICE QUESTIONS

1. **How does a skin graft survive within the first 24 hours?**
    A. Capillary network neovascularization
    B. Neovascularization
    C. Imbibition
    D. Oxygen diffusion from open air

2. **What is the most common reason for free flap failure?**
    A. Arterial thrombosis
    B. Venous thrombosis
    C. Capillary thrombosis
    D. Arterial embolus

3. **What is the perfusion pressure of the capillary network of skin?**

   A. 10 mm Hg
   B. 15 mm Hg
   C. 30 mm Hg
   D. 50 mm Hg

4. **What is the third layer of the epidermis called?**

   A. Stratum basalis
   B. Stratum spinosum
   C. Stratum lucidum
   D. Stratum granulosum

5. **What is a local anesthetic that has both anesthetic and vasoconstrictive properties?**

   A. Lidocaine
   B. Bupivacaine
   C. Cocaine
   D. Novacaine

6. **Which topical antimicrobial has the adverse side effect of metabolic acidosis?**

   A. Silvadene
   B. Sulfamylon
   C. Silver nitrate
   D. Bacitracin

7. **Which nerve supplies the pectoralis minor muscle?**

   A. Medial pectoral nerve
   B. Lateral pectoral nerve
   C. Nerve to pectoralis
   D. Medial and lateral pectoral nerves

8. **Which artery supplies the latissimus dorsi muscle?**

   A. Long thoracic artery
   B. Intercostal muscle perforator artery branches
   C. Thoracoacromial artery
   D. Thoracodorsal artery

9. **Which muscle flap is most affected in a patient that has undergone coronary artery bypass graft with the left internal mammary artery?**

   A. Pectoralis major
   B. Pectoralis minor
   C. Serratus
   D. Rectus abdominis

10. **In a 100 kg man, what is the safe dose of bupivicaine that can be administered for local anesthesia?**

    A. 1 to 2 mg/kg
    B. 2.5 to 3 mg/kg
    C. 5 to 7 mg/kg
    D. 7 to 10 mg/kg

ANSWERS

1. **Answer: C.** Plasmotic imbibition is how the skin graft survives for the first 24 hours; capillary inosculation occurs in the next 48 hours followed by neovascularization.

2. **Answer: B.** Venous thrombosis is the most common reason for free flap failure; clinical signs of venous thrombosis include congested blue appearing flap, cap refill <2 seconds, eventual loss of Doppler signals, and arterial insufficiency.

3. **Answer: B.** Once tissue compression exceeds perfusion pressure, tissue necrosis can occur. Generally tissues can tolerate ischemia for short periods of time as long as compression is relieved every 1 to 2 hours for 5 to 10 minutes, hence the reason debilitated patients are turned Q2 hours to prevent pressure sores.

4. **Answer: D.** Starting from outside to in, the skin layers are stratum corneum, stratum lucidum (not always present), stratum granulosum, stratum spinosum, and stratum basalis. When measuring depth of extension for melanoma, the stratum granulosum is used as the starting point of the lesion for Breslow thickness.

5. **Answer: C.** Cocaine is the only topical anesthetic that provides both an anesthetic and vasoconstrictive effect. It is often used in nasal surgery because of the added bonus of vasoconstriction in an extremely vascular area.

6. **Answer: B.** Sulfamylon is a carbonic anhydrase inhibitor that has the known side effect of metabolic acidosis. This can be especially problematic in burn patients during their initial hospital course because of lactic acidosis or respiratory acidosis from inhalation injury.

7. **Answer: A.** The pectoralis minor muscle is innervated by the medial pectoral nerve. Pectoralis major is innervated by both medial and lateral pectoral nerves.

8. **Answer: D.** The thoracodorsal artery supplies the latissimus dorsi muscle.

9. **Answer: D.** Rectus abdominis has a dual blood supply from the deep inferior epigastric artery and the superior epigastric artery (distal extension of the internal mammary). For sternal wound infections in a patient that is post CABG, the rectus muscle flap may not be of use if the ipsilateral internal mammary has been used in the CABG.

10. **Answer: B.** 2.5 to 3 mg/kg of bupivicaine can be administered to a patient. Bupivicaine has a tendency to cause more systemic side effects than other local anesthetics.

CHAPTER 27
Thoracic Surgery

Timothy Misselbeck

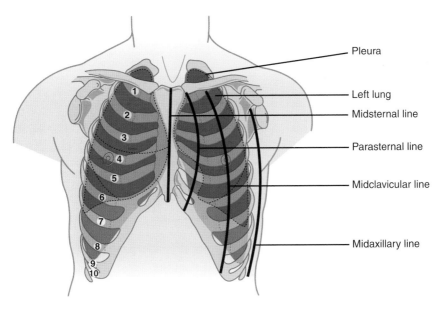

FIGURE 27-1. The thorax, showing rib cage, pleura, and lung fields. *(Reproduced from Doherty GM. Current Diagnosis and Treatment: Surgery. 13th ed. http://www.accessmedicine.com. Copyright © The McGraw-Hill Companies, Inc. All rights reserved.)*

ANATOMY/PHYSIOLOGY

Which ribs are true ribs (directly articulate with the sternum by means of cartilages)?
The upper 7 ribs (numbered 1–7)

Which ribs are false ribs (no direct connection with sternum anteriorly; usually connect with the costocartilage above)?
The lower 5 ribs (numbered 8–10)

Which ribs are floating ribs (articulate only with thoracic spine)?
Ribs 11 and 12

What structure perforates and connects the alveoli?
The pores of Kohn

What type of epithelium lines the larger upper airways as a single layer?
Ciliated tall columnar epithelium

What are type I pneumocytes?
Gas exchange; constitute ~40% of the number of cells lining the alveoli and cover >90% of the alveolar lining

What are type II pneumocytes?
Granular pneumocytes that contain lipid inclusion bodies and manufacture surfactant, a lipoprotein (dipalmitoyl-lecithin) that decreases surface tension.

What are the lobes and fissures of the right lung?
The right lung is composed of 3 lobes: the upper, middle, and lower.
The major (oblique) fissure separates the right lower lobe from the right upper and middle lobes.
The minor (horizontal) fissure separates the right upper lobe from the right middle lobe.

Right lung and bronchi

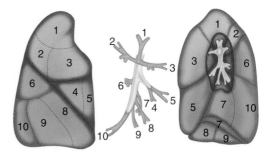

Segments	
1. Apical	6. Superior
2. Posterior	7. Medial Basal*
3. Anterior	8. Anterior Basal
4. Lateral	9. Lateral Basal
5. Medial	10. Posterior Basal

*Medial basal (7) not present in left lung

Left lung and bronchi

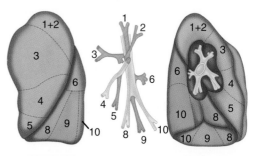

FIGURE 27-2. Segmental anatomy of the lungs and bronchi. *(Reproduced from Brunicardi FC, Andersen DK, Billiar TR, et al. Schwartz's Principles of Surgery. 9th ed. http://www.accessmedicine.com. Copyright © The McGraw-Hill Companies, Inc. All rights reserved.)*

What are the lobes and fissures of the left lung?
The left lung has 2 lobes—the left upper lobe and the left lower lobe.
The lingula is a portion of the left upper lobe and corresponds embryologically to the right middle lobe.
A single oblique fissure separates the left upper lobe from the left lower lobe.

What is the blood supply to the lung?
Unoxygenated blood is pumped to the lung from the right ventricle through the pulmonary artery.
Oxygenated blood is returned to the left atrium through the pulmonary veins.
Blood supply to the bronchi is from the systemic circulation by bronchial arteries arising from the superior thoracic aorta or the aortic arch (discrete branches or in combination with intercostal arteries).
In most individuals, there are 2 left and 1 right main bronchial artery but ~25% of patients have the bronchial arteries arise as a common trunk.

What lobe of the lung is more commonly affected by pulmonary arterial branching variation?
Left upper lobe

What is actually associated with increased surgical risk when performing lung surgery: hypercarbia or hypoxia?
Elevated pCO_2 is actually associated with increased surgical risk more significantly than hypoxia.
pCO_2 >43 to 45 mm Hg suggests severe disease (50% functional loss of the lung) and may be associated with underlying pulmonary hypertension (relative contraindication to surgical resection).

What is the most commonly used predictor of postoperative pulmonary reserve?
The predicted postoperative forced expiratory volume in 1 second (FEV_1)

What percentage of predicted FEV_1 should most patients exceed to tolerate an anatomic lobectomy?
FEV_1 in excess of 60% of predicted

What carbon monoxide diffusing capacity (DLCO) levels are associated with increased perioperative risk following lung surgery?
DLCO levels <40% to 50% are associated with increased perioperative risk.

CHEST WALL CONDITIONS

What is the most common chest wall deformity?
Pectus excavatum (also called funnel chest)

How does pectus excavatum arise?
Pectus excavatum results from an imbalance/excessive growth of the lower costal cartilages leading to posterior sternal depression.

What is pectus excavatum associated with?
Other musculoskeletal abnormalities (~20%) such as scoliosis (15%) and Marfan syndrome and congenital heart disease (1.5% of patients)

Name the defect characterized by an anterior protrusion deformity of the sternum and costal cartilages:
Pectus carinatum (also called pigeon breast)

Which is more common pectus carinatum or pectus excavatum?
Pectus excavatum is more common than pectus carinatum (5:1)

What is Poland syndrome?
The absence of the pectoralis major muscle, absence or hypoplasia of the pectoralis minor muscle, absence of costal cartilages, hypoplasia of breast and subcutaneous tissue (including the nipple complex), and a variety of hand anomalies.

Is Poland syndrome more common on the right side or left side?
Poland syndrome in 2X more common on the right side of the body than on the left

Where do most bony chest wall tumors arise?
In the ribs (85%)

What is the most common malignant chest wall tumor?
Metastatic disease to the ribs

Primary bone tumors account for what percentage of all chest wall malignancies?
7% to 8% of all chest wall malignancies

What is the preferred method to obtain pathologic confirmation of a chest wall tumor?
Excisional biopsy with a minimum of a 1 to 2 cm margin (incisional biopsy may be appropriate for a large tumor)

Fibrous dysplasia of bone accounts for what percentage of benign chest wall tumors?
>30% of benign chest wall tumors

How does fibrous dysplasia most commonly present?
As an asymptomatic mass in the lateral or posterior aspect of the rib

What does fibrous dysplasia look like on chest radiography?
A fusiform expansion in the posterior aspect of the rib with a characteristic soap bubble, or ground glass appearance

When is excision of fibrous dysplasia indicated?
For relief of symptoms (pain) and for confirmation of the diagnosis

What syndrome might you suspect in a patient with multiple areas of fibrous dysplasia, precocious puberty, and skin pigmentation?
Albright syndrome

Chondromas account for what percentage of benign chest wall tumors?
15% to 20% of benign chest wall tumors

How does chondroma usually present?
As an asymptomatic, slowly growing tumor at the anterior costochondral junction

From where do chondromas arise?
Chondromas can arise from the medulla (enchondroma) or the periosteum (periosteal chondroma).

How do chondromas appear on chest radiography?
Chondromas appear as lytic lesions with sclerotic margins.

What is the treatment for chondroma?
Although benign, wide excision to rule out malignancy (chondrosarcoma)

What kind of benign chest wall tumor presents as a mass originating from the cortex of the rib?
Osteochondroma

What of patients are most commonly affected by osteochondromas?
Young males

What is the characteristic finding on chest radiography for osteochondroma?
A pedunculated bony mass capped with viable cartilage

What might you suspect if multiple osteochondromas are found in the same patient?
Familial osteochondromatosis

What is the treatment for osteochondroma?
Treatment of choice is complete excision

What is the term for the benign component of malignant fibrous histiocytosis?
Eosinophilic granuloma

What is the most common malignant tumor of the chest wall?
Chondrosarcoma (20% of all bone tumors)

What is the appearance on chest radiography of chondrosarcoma?
A poorly defined tumor mass that destroys cortical bone

What site is most frequently involved by chondrosarcoma?
The anterior costochondral junctions of the sternum

What is the treatment of choice for chondrosarcoma?
Resection with wide margins

What is the reported 5-year survival rate after complete excision of a chondrosarcoma?
70% 5-year survival rate

What tumor arises most frequently in the long bones of adolescents and young adults, accounts for 10% to 15% of malignant tumors in the chest, and typically presents as a rapidly enlarging mass with a characteristic sunburst pattern on chest radiography?
Osteosarcoma (osteogenic sarcoma)

What is the 5-year survival for osteosarcoma with complete excision and adjuvant chemotherapy?
The 5-year survival approaches 60%

What is the third most common chest wall malignant chest wall tumor?
Ewing sarcoma (10%–15%)

What bones are commonly affected by Ewing sarcoma?
Pelvis, humerus, femur

What is the characteristic appearance of Ewing sarcoma on chest x-ray?
Onion peel appearance (caused by periosteal elevation and bony remodeling)

What is the 5-year survival in a patient with Ewing sarcoma treated with multimodality therapy (chemotherapy, radiotherapy, and surgery)?
~50%

How does multiple myeloma appear on chest x-ray?
A diffuse, punched-out appearance of the bone (caused by myelogenous deposits)

How does multiple myeloma commonly present?
Multiple myeloma commonly presents as pain without a mass

What is the primary mode of therapy for multiple myeloma?
Radiotherapy

What syndrome is characterized by a benign inflammation of one or more of the costal cartilages?
Tietze syndrome

What is the difference between Tietze syndrome and costochondritis?
Tietze syndrome is characterized by swelling of the costal cartilages.
Costochondritis is characterized by the absence of swelling of the costal cartilages.

THORACIC OUTLET SYNDROME (TOS)

What syndrome is characterized by compression of the subclavian vessels and nerves of the brachial plexus in the region of the thoracic inlet?
Thoracic outlet syndrome

Name the various anatomic structures that may compress the neurovascular structures of the upper extremity:
Bone (cervical rib, long transverse process of C7, abnormal first rib, osteoarthritis)
Muscles (scalenes)
Trauma (neck hematoma, bone dislocation)
Fibrous bands (congenital and acquired)
Neoplasm

What type of symptoms commonly develop in patients with TOS?
Neurologic

What patient population is most commonly affected by TOS?
Middle-aged women

Name the borders of the scalene triangle:
Scalenus anticus anteriorly, scalenus medius posteriorly, first rib inferiorly

What might you expect with ulnar nerve (C8–T1) involvement by TOS?
Motor weakness and atrophy of the hypothenar and interosseous muscles, pain and paresthesia along medial aspect of arm and hand, fifth finger, and medial aspect of fourth finger

Where might you expect symptoms with median nerve (C5–8, T1) involvement by TOS?
Symptoms in the index and middle fingers and the flexor compartment of the forearm

What symptoms might be seen with subclavian artery compression from TOS?
Fatigue, weakness, coldness, ischemic pain, paresthesia

What syndrome is characterized by effort-induced thrombosis of the axillary or subclavian vein secondary to unusual, repetitive, or excessive arm exertion or exercise?
Paget-Schroetter syndrome

How is the Adson (scalene) test performed?
The patient inspires maximally and hold his/her breath with the neck fully extended and the head turned toward the affected side.
A decrease or loss of the ipsilateral radial pulse suggests compression from narrowing of the space between the scalenus anticus and medius with resultant compression of the subclavian artery and the brachial plexus.

What should the initial management of TOS be?
Nonsurgical: improvements in postural sitting, standing, and sleeping positions, behavior modification at work, muscle stretching and strengthening exercises as instructed by physiotherapists.

What percentage of patients with TOS can be successfully treated with nonsurgical methods and patient education?
50% to 90%

What are indications for operation for TOS?
Failure of conservative management, progression of sensory or motor symptoms, presence of excessively prolonged ulnar or median nerve conduction velocities, narrowing or occlusion of the subclavian artery, thrombosis of the axillary or subclavian vein

What should the initial operation for TOS include?
Complete removal of the first rib, division of the scalenus anticus and medius

Name some complications that can arise from a first rib removal:
Brachial plexus injuries, vascular injuries, pleural effusion, winged scapula, infection

What is the treatment for subclavian vein thrombosis from TOS?
Anticoagulant therapy and simultaneous surgical decompression

CHEST TRAUMA

What might you suspect in a patient with palpable subcutaneous emphysema on the chest wall?
Injury to the airway or lung parenchyma leading to a pneumothorax, esophageal perforation

What does a patient with a circumferential burn to the chest require?
Escharotomy: to allow for adequate chest wall expansion

What ribs are most likely to be injured?
Thoracic ribs 5 to 10 are most likely to be injured.
Upper thoracic rib fractures (T1–T4) are uncommon because of their relatively protected position below the upper extremity girdle musculature and fractures of the lower thoracic ribs (T11–T12) are uncommon because the ribs are short and less exposed.

What patient population is commonly affected by spontaneous pneumothorax?
Tall, thin men, 25 to 40 years of age

At what rate does an uncomplicated pneumothorax reabsorb?
~1% per day

What is the treatment for a first-time asymptomatic small spontaneous pneumothorax (<20%) in a stable patient?
Monitor the patient, follow up the pneumothorax with a chest radiograph within 24 to 48 hours, smoking cessation in patients who are smokers; indications for intervention include progressive pneumothorax, delayed pulmonary expansion, or development of symptoms

Where do you place the 18-gauge needle or angiocatheter for emergent needle decompression for tension pneumothorax?
At the midclavicular line in the second anterior intercostal space on the affected side; relieves the tension created within the thorax but does not treat the pneumothorax and requires subsequent chest tube insertion.

What is the preferred approach for chest tube placement?
Through the fourth, fifth, or sixth intercostal space in the mid to anterior axillary line

Name a unidirectional valve that can be placed at the end of a chest tube to function as a one-way valve that lets air escape from the hemithorax:
Heimlich valve

List some complications that may occur with chest tube placement:
Laceration of an intercostal vessel, laceration of the lung, intrapulmonary or extrathoracic placement of the chest tube, infection

What is the risk for first-time recurrence in a patient with a spontaneous pneumothorax?
~25% to 30%

When is surgery recommended for a patient with an uncomplicated unilateral spontaneous pneumothorax?
Recurrence or the development of a contralateral pneumothorax

When is surgical intervention recommended for a first-time pneumothorax?
Bilateral simultaneous pneumothoraces, complete (100%) pneumothorax, pneumothorax associated with tension or borderline cardiopulmonary reserve, patients in high-risk professions or activities involving significant variations in atmospheric pressure (pilots, scuba divers), patients with complications of pneumothorax (empyema, hemothorax, or chronic pneumothorax)

PLEURAL DISEASE

What are the 3 histologic subtypes of mesothelioma that have been identified?
Epithelial, sarcomatous, mixed histology

What histologic subtype of mesothelioma has a more favorable prognosis than the other 2 subtypes?
Epithelial

What is the best method to obtain a tumor sample sufficient to distinguish mesothelioma from other tumors (adenocarcinoma) and to determine the specific subtype of malignant pleural mesothelioma?
Open or video-assisted thoracoscopic surgery (VATS) biopsy

What is the survival for mesothelioma with supportive care?
4 to 12 months

Name the 2 surgical cytoreductive procedures used in the treatment of malignant pleural mesothelioma?
Extrapleural pneumonectomy and radical pleurectomy with decortication

What is the term for a pyogenic or suppurative infection of the pleural space?
Empyema

What are the 3 categories of an empyema based on the chronicity of the disease process?
The acute phase: characterized by pleural effusion of low viscosity and cell count.
The transitional, exudative, or fibrinopurulent phase: begins after 48 hours and is characterized by an increase in white blood cells (WBCs) in the pleural effusion; the effusion begins to loculate, and is associated with fibrin deposition on visceral and parietal pleurae leading to progressive lung entrapment.
The organizing or chronic phase: occurs after as little as 1 to 2 weeks and is associated with an ingrowth of capillaries and fibroblasts into the pleural rind and nonexpansile lung.

What is the usual cause of an empyema?
Empyemas are usually the result of a primary infectious process in the lung

What are the basic principles that apply to all successful interventions in the treatment of empyema?
Early detection of empyema, rapid and effective pleural drainage, complete lung re-expansion

Name the procedure associated with open drainage of a chronic empyema:
Eloesser flap

DISEASES OF THE MEDIASTINUM

What are the borders of the mediastinum?
1. Thoracic inlet—superiorly
2. Diaphragm—inferiorly
3. Sternum—anteriorly
4. Vertebral column—posteriorly
5. Parietal pleura—laterally

What are the 3 subcompartments that the mediastinum is divided into?
Anterosuperior, middle, posterior

What are the most common mediastinal masses?
Neurogenic tumors (23%), thymomas (21%), lymphomas (13%), germ cell tumors (12%)

In which subcompartment of the mediastinum are mediastinal masses most frequently located?
Anterosuperior mediastinum (54%), followed by the posterior (26%) and middle mediastinum (20%)

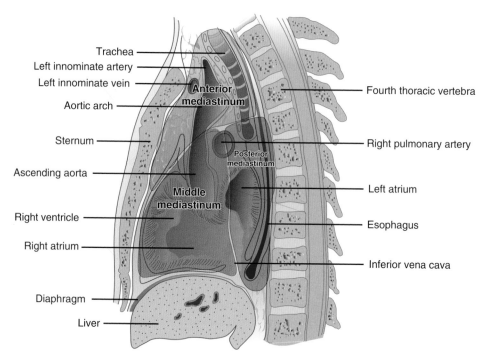

FIGURE 27-3. Divisions of the mediastinum (Burkell classification). Light screening: anterior mediastinum; lower dark screening: middle mediastinum; dotted area at right: posterior mediastinum. *(Reproduced from Doherty GM. Current Diagnosis and Treatment: Surgery. 13th ed. http://www.accessmedicine.com. Copyright © The McGraw-Hill Companies, Inc. All rights reserved.)*

95% of tumors in the anterosuperior compartment of the mediastinum are made up by the 4 Ts? What are the 4 "Ts"?
Thymoma
Teratoma (germ cell tumors)
Thyroid goiter
Terrible lymphoma

What is the term for a neurogenic tumor with extension into the spinal column?
Dumbbell tumor: has a characteristic shape from the relatively large paraspinal and intraspinal portions connected by a narrow isthmus of tissue traversing the intervertebral foramen.

What is the recommended surgical approach to dumbbell tumors?
A one-stage excision of the intraspinal component before resecting the thoracic component (to minimize any spinal column hematoma)

What pattern are the small, round, immature cells of a neuroblastoma arranged?
A rosette pattern

What is the usual location of a ganglioneuroma?
The paravertebral region

What is the most common neurogenic tumor?
Neurilemoma (schwannoma)

What are the 2 morphologic patterns seen with neurilemoma (schwannoma)?
Antoni type A—organized architecture with a cellular palisading pattern of growth
Antoni type B—loose reticular pattern of growth

What is the peak incidence of neurilemoma (schwannoma)?
3rd to 5th decades of life

What is the most common neoplasm of the anterosuperior mediastinum?
Thymoma

What is the second most common mediastinal mass?
Thymoma

What systemic syndrome is associated with thymoma?
Myasthenia gravis

What is the peak incidence of thymoma?
3rd to 5th decades, but may occur throughout adulthood

How is the differentiation between benign and malignant thymoma determined?
By the presence of gross invasion of adjacent structures, metastasis, microscopic evidence of capsular invasion

What approach is used to obtain the best operative exposure when excising a thymoma?
A median sternotomy

THYMOMA STAGING

Table 27-1	Staging and Treatment for Thymoma	
Stage	Description	Treatment
I	Macroscopically, completely encapsulated, microscopically, no capsular invasion	Complete surgical resection
IIa	Macroscopic invasion into surrounding fatty tissues or mediastinal pleura (without microscopic invasion)	Surgical resection with adjunctive radiation
IIb	Microscopic evidence of capsular invasion or microscopic invasion of surrounding fatty tissues or mediastinal pleura	Surgical resection with adjunctive radiation
III	Macroscopic invasion into a neighboring organ (pericardium, great vessels, or lung)	Surgical resection with adjunctive radiation
IVa	Pleural or pericardial dissemination	Chemotherapy, followed by surgical exploration with the goal of complete resection, and postoperative radiation therapy
IVb	Lymphatic or hematogenous distant metastases	Chemotherapy, followed by surgical exploration with the goal of complete resection, and postoperative radiation therapy

Modified from Doherty GM, ed. *Current Diagnosis & Treatment: Surgery.* 13th ed. http://www.accessmedicine.com. Copyright © The McGraw-Hill Companies, Inc. All rights reserved.

What is the most common mediastinal germ cell tumor?
Teratoma

What is the peak incidence for a germ cell tumor?
2nd to 3rd decade of life

What is the most common extragonadal primary site of germ cell tumors?
The anterosuperior mediastinum

What are the current recommendations for evaluating the testes of a patient with mediastinal germ cell tumor?
Careful physical examination and ultrasonography with biopsy reserved for positive findings; blind biopsy/orchiectomy is contraindicated.

Why are serologic measurements of α-fetoprotein and β-HCG useful in the treatment of germ cell tumors?
Can differentiate seminomas from nonseminomas, can quantitatively assess response to therapy in hormonally active tumors, can diagnose relapse or failure of therapy before changes that can be observed in gross disease

What is the relationship of seminomas and nonseminomas to α-fetoprotein and β-HCG?
Seminomas rarely produce β-HCG and never produce α-fetoprotein; >90% of nonseminomas secrete one or both of these hormones.

What is the histologic appearance of a seminoma?
Large cells with round nuclei, scant cytoplasm, and abundant glycogen

How do nonseminomas differ from seminomas?
Nonseminomas are more aggressive tumors that are frequently disseminated at the time of diagnosis, nonseminomas are rarely radiosensitive, and >90% of nonseminomas produce either β-HCG or α-fetoprotein.

What is the treatment of choice for seminoma?
Cisplatin-based chemotherapy is the treatment of choice; treatment usually consists of chemotherapy with or without secondary surgery or combination chemotherapy and radiation therapy.

What is the treatment for a nonseminomatous tumor?
Cisplatin- and etoposide-based chemotherapy
If a complete serologic and radiologic response—observe closely
If disease progresses—initiate salvage chemotherapy
If serologic response but a radiographic abnormality remains, surgery to remove as much remaining tumor as possible

What is the most common type of Hodgkin lymphoma seen in the mediastinum?
Nodular sclerosing

What are the neoplastic cells in Hodgkin lymphoma called?
The neoplastic cells in Hodgkin disease are Reed-Sternberg cells

What is the treatment for non-Hodgkin lymphoma?
Anthracycline containing chemotherapeutic regimens with or without consolidation-involved field radiotherapy in lymphoblastic lymphoma; central nervous system prophylaxis is given in conjunction with the standard chemotherapeutic regimen (intrathecal chemotherapy, with or without cranial irradiation).

What is giant lymph node hyperplasia otherwise known as?
Castleman disease

What associations have been made to multicentric Castleman disease?
HIV infection; human herpes virus 8

LUNG CANCER

ALGORITHM FOR SINGLE PULMONARY NODULE

What cancer remains the leading cause of cancer-related death in the United States?
Lung cancer

What is the best predictor of survival for patients with lung cancer?
Tumor stage

Approximate percentage of all patients diagnosed with lung cancer that are considered resectable (stages I–IIIA):
~20%

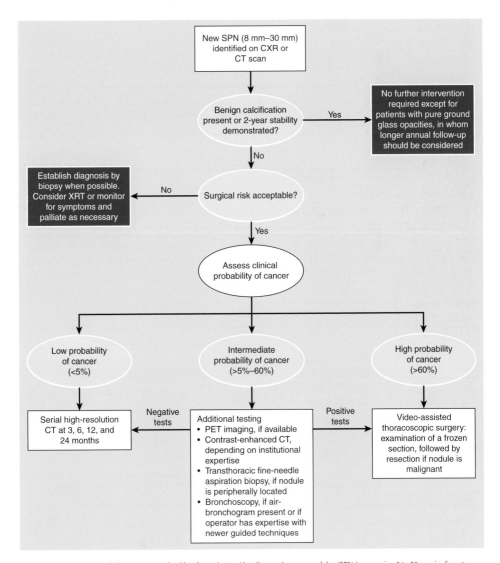

FIGURE 27-4. Recommended management algorithm for patients with solitary pulmonary nodules (SPNs) measuring 8 to 30 mm in diameter. CT, computed tomography; CXR, chest radiograph; PET, positron emission tomography; XRT, radiotherapy. *(Reproduced with permission from Gould MK, Fletcher J, Iannettoni MD, et al. Evaluation of patients with pulmonary nodules: when is it lung cancer? ACCP evidence-based clinical practice guidelines (2nd edition). Chest. 2007;132(3 suppl):108S. Reproduced with permission from the American College of Chest Physicians.)*

Table 27-2	American Joint Committee on Cancer Staging System for Lung Cancer
Stage TNM	
IA T1 N0 M0	
IB T2 N0 M0	
IIA T1 N1 M0	
IIB T2 N1 M0	
T3 N0 M0	
IIIA T3 N1 M0	
T1–3 N2 M0	
IIIB T4 Any N M0	
Any T N3 M0	
IV Any T Any N M1	

TNM Definitions

T TX Positive malignant cell, but primary tumor not visualized by imaging or bronchoscopy

T0 No evidence of primary tumor

Tis Carcinoma in situ

T1 Tumor ≤3 cm, surrounded by lung or visceral pleura, without bronchoscopic evidence of invasion more proximal than the lobar bronchus

T2 Tumor with any of the following features of size or extent:

>3 cm in greatest dimension

Involves main bronchus, ≥2 cm distal to the carina

Invades the visceral pleura

Associated with atelectasis or obstructive pneumonitis that extends to the hilar region but does not involve the entire lung

T3 Tumor of any size that directly invades any of the following: chest wall (including superior sulcus tumors), diaphragm, mediastinal pleura, parietal pericardium; or tumor in the main bronchus <2 cm distal to the carina, but without involvement of the carina; or associated atelectasis or obstructive pneumonitis of the entire lung

T4 Tumor of any size that invades any of the following: mediastinum, heart, great vessels, trachea, esophagus, vertebral body, carina; or tumor with a malignant pleural or pericardial effusion, or with satellite tumor nodule(s) within the ipsilateral primary-tumor lobe of the lung

N NX Regional lymph nodes cannot be assessed

N0 No regional lymph node metastasis

N1 Metastasis to ipsilateral peribronchial and/or ipsilateral hilar lymph nodes, and intrapulmonary nodes involved by direct extension of the primary tumor

N2 Metastasis to ipsilateral mediastinal and/or subcarinal lymph node(s)

N3 Metastasis to contralateral mediastinal, contralateral hilar, ipsilateral or contralateral scalene, or supraclavicular lymph node(s)

M MX Presence of distant metastasis cannot be assessed

M0 No distant metastasis

M1 Distant metastasis present [including metastatic tumor nodule(s) in the ipsilateral nonprimary tumor lobe(s) of the lung]

(*continued*)

Table 27-2	American Joint Committee on Cancer Staging System for Lung Cancer (*Continued*)
Summary of Staging Definitions	
Occult stage	Microscopically identified cancer cells in lung secretions on multiple occasions (or multiple daily collections); no discernible primary cancer in the lung
Stage 0	Carcinoma in situ
Stage IA	Tumor surrounded by lung or visceral pleura ≤3 cm arising more than 2 cm distal to the carina (T1 N0)
Stage IB	Tumor surrounded by lung >3 cm, or tumor of any size with visceral pleura involved arising more than 2 cm distal to the carina (T2 N0)
Stage IIA	Tumor ≤3 cm not extended to adjacent organs, with ipsilateral peribronchial and hilar lymph node involvement (T1 N1)
Stage IIB	Tumor >3 cm not extended to adjacent organs, with ipsilateral peribronchial and hilar lymph node involvement (T2 N1)
	Tumor invading chest wall, pleura, or pericardium but not involving carina, nodes negative (T3 N0)
Stage IIIA	Tumor invading chest wall, pleura, or pericardium and nodes in hilum or ipsilateral mediastinum (T3, N1–2) or tumor of any size invading ipsilateral mediastinal or subcarinal nodes (T1–3, N2)
Stage IIIB	Direct extension to adjacent organs (esophagus, aorta, heart, cava, diaphragm, or spine); satellite nodule same lobe, or any tumor associated with contralateral mediastinal or supraclavicular lymph node involvement (T4 or N3)
Stage IV	Separate nodule in different lobes or any tumor with distant metastases (M1)

Data from the American Joint Committee on Cancer (AJCC). *AJCC Cancer Staging Manual.* 7th ed. Chicago, Illinois: Springer Science and Business Media LLC; 2010.

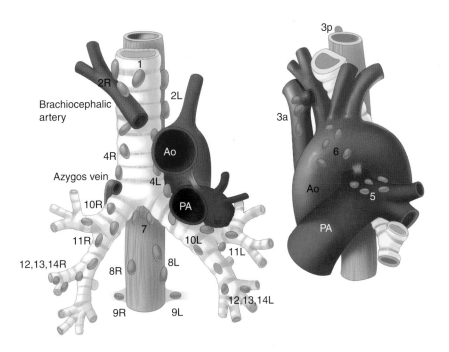

FIGURE 27-5. The location of regional lymph node stations for lung cancer staging. Station, Description: 1, highest mediastinal lymph nodes; 2, upper paratracheal nodes; 3, prevascular, precarinal, and retrotracheal nodes; 4, lower paratracheal nodes; 5, aortopulmonary nodes; 6, preaortic nodes; 7, subcarinal nodes; 8, paraesophageal nodes; 9, pulmonary ligament nodes; 10, tracheobronchial nodes; 11, interlobular nodes; 12, lobar bronchial nodes; 13, segmental nodes; 14, subsegmental nodes. Note: Stations 12, 13, and 14 are not shown in their entirety. *(This article was published in Ferguson MK. Thoracic Surgery Atlas. Philadelphia: W.B. Saunders, Inc. Copyright © Elsevier 2007.)*

MULTIPLE CHOICE QUESTIONS

1. A 65-year-old woman presents to your office with an incidental chest radiograph (CXR) finding of a 2-cm nodule in the periphery of her right upper lobe. This was confirmed by a CT scan and there are no other nodules or adenopathy noted. She has a heavy smoking history and you suspect this could be a lung cancer. Of the following choices, which represents the best first test to order?

   A. Fiberoptic bronchoscopy
   B. Positron emission tomography (PET) scan
   C. Percutaneous image-guided biopsy
   D. VATS
   E. Mediastinoscopy

2. A 24-year-old man was involved in a high-speed car accident. The patient has right- and left-sided rib fractures and pneumothoraces. Bilateral chest tubes are inserted and there is a large airleak. You suspect an airway injury and perform a bronchoscopy. Indeed, there is a nearly circumferential tear of the distal trachea, which extends past the carina into the proximal left main bronchus. What is the optimal operative approach to surgically repair this injury?

   A. Median sternotomy
   B. Right posterolateral thoracotomy
   C. Left posterolateral thoracotomy
   D. Clamshell thoracotomy
   E. Anterior thoracotomy

3. You are asked to evaluate a patient who has a history of colon cancer treated by primary resection and adjuvant chemotherapy several years ago. The patient now has pulmonary metastatic nodules that have been biopsy proven. When considering a patient for pulmonary metastectomy, what is the most important concept to keep in mind?

   A. The histology of the primary tumor
   B. Overall time of disease-free interval
   C. The total number of metastasis
   D. Control of the primary tumor
   E. Ability to completely resect the disease

4. The trauma service asks you to evaluate a 75-year-old lady who fell at home. On admission, a chest x-ray showed several rib fractures and a hemothorax. She takes coumadin for atrial fibrillation. A chest tube placed in the emergency center drained about 1000 mL of dark blood and stopped. The patient remains hemodynamically stable, but there is still evidence of a retained hemothorax on the follow-up chest x-ray. What is the next best course of action?

   A. Place another chest tube
   B. Evacuation via thoracotomy
   C. Evacuation via VATS
   D. Instillation of intrapleural thrombolytic drugs (tPA)
   E. Observation

5. A 56-year-old man underwent an uneventful right middle lobe resection and mediastinal lymph node dissection for a pulmonary carcinoid tumor. He is discharged but returns in 3 days with complaints of shortness of breath, and x-ray shows a pleural effusion. A chest tube is placed to drain the effusion and it then drains about 1200 mL of milky fluid the next 24 hours. You suspect a chylothorax and send off the fluid for a cell count. What is the best way to initially treat this problem?

A. Immediate operation and ligation of the thoracic duct
B. Make the patient NPO and provide total parenteral nutrition (TPN)
C. Lymphatic mapping and embolization of the thoracic duct
D. Octreotide
E. Observation

6. A 25-year-old man presents to the emergency center with complaints of vague chest discomfort. Acute coronary syndromes have been ruled out and the patient is noted to have a large anterior mediastinal mass. The α-fetoprotein levels are markedly elevated. What is the likely diagnosis?

A. Nonseminomatous germ cell tumor
B. Seminoma
C. Thymoma
D. Lymphoma
E. Ectopic thyroid goiter

7. You are asked to evaluate a 56-year-old lady with widely metastatic breast cancer and a new unilateral pleural effusion. She underwent a thoracentesis, which removed about 1500 mL of fluid and had relief of her symptoms. The fluid was positive for malignancy. She still has a residual effusion. She has a reasonable performance status and is undergoing chemotherapy. What is the best way to palliate the patient?

A. Repeat thoracentesis as needed
B. Thoracotomy and manual pleurodesis
C. Tube thoracostomy with bedside chemical pleurodesis
D. VATS pleurodesis
E. Observation

8. A 65-year-old man comes to your office with a newly diagnosed right upper lobe lung cancer. He underwent a complete staging workup and the disease appears localized with no evidence of metastasis and is otherwise healthy. His FEV_1 is 2.5 L, 98% predicted. You are considering him for resection with curative intent but the mass is abutting the bronchus intermedius. In the operating room, you are able to resect the right upper lobe, but the bronchial margin is positive for cancer. What is the best option?

A. Right pneumonectomy
B. Right upper lobe sleeve resection
C. Resect the staple line and attempt to get a negative margin
D. Place clips on the bronchus and send the patient for radiation postop

9. A 60-year-old lady was being evaluated for persistent bronchitis and was sent for a chest x-ray. This x-ray revealed a mass and a follow-up CT scan showed this to be a 10-cm anterior mediastinal mass, which was applying a mass effect on the heart and lungs. She is currently asymptomatic and in good general health. What is the best option?

   A. PET scan
   B. Tumor markers
   C. Needle biopsy
   D. Operative resection
   E. Observation

10. You are consulted to see a 43-year-old homeless man. He is well known to the house staff from his numerous admissions. He has been treated intermittently for pneumonia for the past few weeks and has been noncompliant with his treatment, signing out of the hospital only to be readmitted a few days later. In order to better characterize his lung infiltrates, a CT scan was performed and shows the entire left lung encased in a thick rind with multiple pockets of loculated fluid. The patient has a WBC of 11 and a T_{max} of 101. What is the best option?

   A. Thoracotomy and decortication
   B. VATS decortication
   C. Tube thoracostomy drainage
   D. Instillation of pleural streptokinase (lytics)

ANSWERS

1. **Answer: C.** It is unlikely you can biopsy a nodule in the periphery of the lung with a standard fiberoptic bronchoscopy. A mediastinoscopy is not indicated at this point, since there are no enlarged lymph nodes. A PET scan will not give you a diagnosis. VATS resection could be a reasonable answer, but you should never go to the operating room without a diagnosis. Image-guided biopsy of a peripheral nodule can be done quickly and safely with a sensitivity >90% for malignancy.

2. **Answer: B.** A right posterolateral thoracotomy will give access to the entire trachea, carina, and proximal left-sided bronchial tree.

3. **Answer: E.** All of these issues play a role in cure; however, the ability to completely resect the disease is the most important factor in deciding if this patient should have surgery.

4. **Answer: A.** Retained hemothorax needs to be drained. Usually, if you can see it on a CXR, there is too much blood to leave in the chest and observation is not really a good option since this may lead to loss of lung volume and infection. Placing a second chest tube is a good first step and may avoid more invasive options. If unable to drain with tube thoracostomies, then the patient may need operative drainage via VATS or formal thoracotomy. Instilling thrombolytics into the pleural space has also had good success in some centers and is an option to consider.

5. **Answer: B.** Chylothorax is more frequently seen after esophageal surgery, but can also occur after pulmonary surgery or coronary artery bypass graft. The diagnosis is confirmed by cell count of the pleural fluid showing >300 lymphocytes or triglycerides higher than the plasma levels. A trial of conservative therapy should be tried first and

consists of making the patient NPO and nourishment with TPN. Greater than 50% of the chylous leaks will stop within a few days. If conservative therapy fails, then ligation of the thoracic duct via surgery is often necessary. Octreotide has shown some success as an adjunct to conservative therapy but should not be used alone. Embolization of the thoracic duct is also a good option, but its success is limited to highly specialized centers and the techniques are not reproducible.

6. **Answer: A.** An anterior mediastinal mass in a young male patient with markedly elevated α-fetoprotein levels is pathognomonic for a nonseminomatous germ cell tumor. He should also undergo a testicular examination and ultrasound as part of the staging workup. Usually the mass is easily amenable to percutaneous core needle biopsy and the role of the surgeon is only to obtain tissue for diagnosis, although this should not delay treatment. This is one of the few scenarios where chemotherapy can be initiated while the tissue diagnosis is being confirmed.

7. **Answer: D.** VATS pleurodesis is the best option to reduce the risk of the pleural effusion recurring. This does involve general anesthesia but allows for complete evacuation of the pleural space and allows the surgeon to apply the pleural sclerosant under direct vision. In patients who are sicker and at higher risk for anesthesia, then a bedside pleurodesis may be a better option. There is no role for a formal thoracotomy in a patient with widely metastatic disease. Observation and serial thoracentesis may be options for selected patients but this would be a suboptimal treatment strategy.

8. **Answer: B.** The best option would be to completely resect the bronchial stump and perform a sleeve resection, creating an anastomosis between the right main bronchus and the bronchus intermedius. It is always better to preserve functional lung tissue if it can be done while maintaining the oncologic integrity of the operation. A pneumonectomy can be considered if clear bronchial margins cannot be obtained. Simply resecting the staple line is suboptimal since it will lead to a close margin and potentially narrows the native bronchus. Leaving a patient with positive margins and sending them for postop radiation should only be considered in high-risk patients with no pulmonary reserve.

9. **Answer: D.** A 10-cm anterior mediastinal mass is too large to observe. In an asymptomatic patient, PET scans or needle biopsies will not change the management of choice, which is complete excision.

10. **Answer: A.** This patient has an empyema and needs operative complete decortication. In a patient with this type of chronicity of symptoms, this is best accomplished safely via a standard thoracotomy approach. VATS approaches to decortication are better suited to earlier stages of empyema and less extensive disease. Tube thoracostomy and lytic therapy are unlikely to be successful in advanced empyema.

CHAPTER 28
Orthopedics

Joshua Gish and Scott Sexton

Test Taking Tip

Orthopedics is not usually a high-yield topic for the ABSITE, although they will occasionally ask a question related to trauma. Look over injury patterns and know which fractures are associated with each other (eg, calcaneal fractures and spinal compression fractures).

TYPES OF FRACTURES

Which type of fracture is characterized by sharp fragments?
Acute fractures

Which type of fracture is characterized by rounded fragments with callous formation?
Chronic fractures; callous indicates an attempt at healing.

What are "greenstick" fractures?
Incomplete disruptions of all aspects of the bony cortex in children; bone can be bent but not displaced with greenstick fractures.

Which type of fracture occurs through diseased bone (eg, a tumor or osteopenic bone)?
Pathologic fractures

What are fractures called that have a communication to the skin?
Open fractures (sometimes called "compound fractures")

What type of fracture is caused by rotational forces?
A spiral fracture

What term is given to a fracture that breaks in multiple places?
A comminuted fracture

What is a "butterfly fragment?"
A smaller portion of bone that is separated from the larger portions by comminution; implies greater force and a bending mechanism; must be at least 3 fragments

Define a Monteggia fracture:
Fracture of the proximal one-third of the ulna with associated dislocation of the radial head

Define a Galeazzi fracture:
Fracture of the mid radius with associated dislocation of the distal radial-ulnar joint

Define a Lisfranc injury:
A disruption of the Lisfranc ligament—the ligament binding the first metatarsal to the second

Scaphoid fractures most commonly occur as a result of:
Fall on an outstretched hand

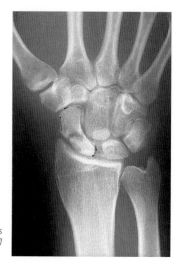

FIGURE 28-1. Scaphoid fracture: nonunion. *(Reproduced from Doherty GM. Current Diagnosis and Treatment: Surgery. 13th ed. http://www.accessmedicine.com. Copyright © The McGraw-Hill Companies, Inc. All rights reserved.)*

Where does a scaphoid (navicular) fracture of the wrist classically produce tenderness?
Pain on the radial aspect of the wrist with tenderness over the anatomic snuffbox

Define a Chance fracture:
A distraction-type injury of the spine where the anterior ligament fails under tension; often caused by a seatbelt injury. There is a high likelihood of associated abdominal injury (~60%).

Define a Jefferson fracture:
Burst fracture of C1, the atlas—actually widens the spinal canal; therefore, spinal cord injury is uncommon.

Define a Hangman fracture:
Fracture of the pars interarticularis of C2, the axis, with dissociation of the C2-C3 articulation—has a high incidence of neurologic injury.

Define a clay shoveller fracture:
Avulsion of the lower cervical spinous process—no association with the spinal canal, therefore has no association with neurologic injury

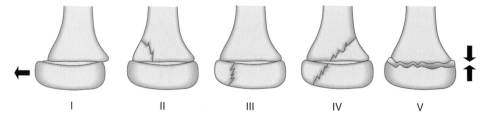

I   II   III   IV   V

FIGURE 28-2. Salter-Harris classification of physeal injuries occurring at the zone of provisional calcification of the growth plate. *(Reproduced from Doherty GM. Current Diagnosis and Treatment: Surgery. 13th ed. http://www.accessmedicine.com. Copyright © The McGraw-Hill Companies, Inc. All rights reserved.)*

What is the "Salter Harris" classification?
It is a classification of physeal fractures in children
    Grade 1: Transphyseal parallel to the joint
    Grade 2: Fracture extends away from the joint
    Grade 3: Fracture extends toward the joint
    Grade 4: Fracture crosses the physis from joint to metaphysis
    Grade 5: Crush injury to the physis

What is a Holstein-Lewis fracture?
Fracture of the distal third of the humerus resulting in radial nerve entrapment

MECHANISM/TYPES OF INJURIES

What associated injury must be ruled out in posterior knee dislocations?
Popliteal artery injury

What test is indicated in posterior knee dislocations in order to rule out intimal injury?
Arteriography

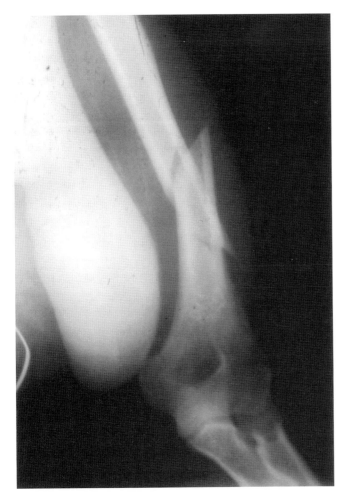

FIGURE 28-3. An anteroposterior x-ray of a spiral fracture of the distal third of the humerus. This fracture is called a Holstein-Lewis fracture. It is frequently associated with radial nerve palsy. *(Reproduced from Felliciano DV, Mattox KL, Moore EE. Trauma. 6th ed. http://www.accesssurgery.com. Copyright © The McGraw-Hill Companies, Inc. All rights reserved.)*

What injuries can be associated with supracondylar humerus fractures?
Brachial artery, radial nerve, and/or median nerve (most common nerve is the anterior interosseus nerve, which is a branch of the median nerve)

What injury must you worry about with a midshaft humerus fracture?
Radial nerve injury

What injury must you worry about with an elbow dislocation?
Brachial artery injury

What injury must you worry about with a distal radius fracture?
Median nerve injury

What injury must you worry about with a anterior shoulder dislocation?
Axillary nerve injury

What injury must you worry about with a posterior shoulder dislocation?
Axillary artery injury

What injury must you worry about with a posterior hip dislocation?
Sciatic nerve injury (peroneal division)

What injury must you worry about with a fibula neck fracture?
Common peroneal nerve injury

What is the typical mechanism of action of a calcaneal fracture?
Fall from a height unto outstretched legs

What injuries are associated with calcaneal fractures?
Contralateral foot fractures, pelvic fractures (vertical shear), spinal compression fractures

Name the 3 broad types of pelvic fracture mechanisms:
Anterior-posterior compression, lateral compression, vertical shear

Which is the most common mechanism of pelvic fracture?
Lateral compression

What is the Gustilo-Anderson classification of open fractures?

Table 28-1	Classification of Open Fractures According to Gustilo and Anderson
Type	
I	Skin opening <1 cm, clean; most likely inside-to-outside lesion; minimal muscle contusion; simple transverse or oblique fracture
II	Laceration >1 cm with extensive soft tissue damage, flaps, or avulsion; minimal-to-moderate crushing; simple transverse or short oblique fracture with minimal comminution
III	Extensive soft tissue damage, including muscle, skin, and neurovascular structures; often a high-velocity injury with a severe crushing component
IIIA	Extensive laceration, adequate bone coverage; segmental fracture; gunshot injuries
IIIB	Extensive soft tissue damage with periosteal stripping and bone exposure; usually associated with massive contamination
IIIC	Vascular injury requiring repair

What is the usual surgical treatment for type I, II, and IIIA open fractures of the tibia?
Intramedullary nailing

What is the usual surgical treatment for type IIIB and IIIC open fractures of the tibia?
Some form of external fixation with conversion to a reamed, locked nail within 2 weeks of injury

MANGLED EXTREMITY SEVERITY SCORE

What mangled extremity severity score (MESS) consistently predicts the need for amputation?
MESS >7

How many points do you get on the MESS with low-energy (stab, simple fracture, "civilian" gunshot wound) skeletal and soft tissue injury?
1

How many points do you get on the MESS with medium-energy (open or multiplex fractures, dislocation) skeletal and soft tissue injury?
2

How many points do you get on the MESS with high-energy (close-range shotgun or "military" gunshot wound; crush injury) skeletal and soft tissue injury?
3

How many points do you get on the MESS with very high-energy (same as above plus gross contamination, soft tissue avulsion) skeletal and soft tissue injury?
4

How many points do you get on the MESS with a reduced or absent pulse with normal perfusion?
1 (doubled if limb ischemia >6 hours)

How many points do you get on the MESS with pulselessness, paresthesias, and diminished capillary refill?
2 (doubled if limb ischemia >6 hours)

How many points do you get on the MESS with a cool, paralyzed, insensate, numb limb?
3 (doubled if limb ischemia >6 hours)

How many points do you get on the MESS with a systolic blood pressure always >90 mm Hg?
0

How many points do you get on the MESS with transient hypotension?
1

How many points do you get on the MESS with persistent hypotension?
2

How many points do you get on the MESS with age <30 years?
0

How many points do you get on the MESS with age 30 to 50 years?
1

How many points do you get on the MESS with age >50 years?
2

LOWER EXTREMITY AND COMPARTMENT SYNDROME

What are the 6 "P's" of an acute compartment syndrome?
1. Pain out of proportion to exam or on passive stretch (most important)
2. Pallor
3. Pulselessness
4. Paraesthesia
5. Paralysis
6. Poikiliothermia

Which is the last of the "P's" to occur?
Pulselessness—usually does not occur unless there is concomitant vascular injury

What diagnostic test can be helpful in the diagnosis of compartment syndrome of the extremities?
Measurement of compartment pressures—requires a special device and in general, should not be used to rule out compartment syndrome, only to rule in

What 5 methods have been described for evaluation of compartment pressure?
Stic (Stryker) catheter, wick catheter, slit catheter, Whitesides' infusion technique; near-infrared spectroscopy

What intracompartmental pressure is generally regarded as indicative of compartment syndrome in the extremities?
30 mm Hg. A better measurement is the compartment perfusion pressure, measured by CPP = diastolic pressure – intracompartmental pressure. If the CPP <30, then this indicates poor perfusion.

What is the order in which compartment syndrome causes vascular compromise?
1. Capillary perfusion
2. Venous outflow
3. Arterial inflow (pressure must be extremely elevated)

What are the compartments of the leg?
Anterior, lateral, deep posterior, and superficial posterior

To perform an adequate fasciotomy of the leg, which compartments must be opened?
All of them

What test is indicated in posterior knee dislocations in order to rule out intimal injury?
Arteriography

What must be documented before and after all attempts at reduction?
A neurovascular examination

What is the most common cause of compartment syndrome in an orthopedic patient?
Muscle edema from direct trauma to the extremity or reperfusion after vascular injury

What level of compartment pressure is needed before surgical intervention is required?
Controversial; compartment pressure approaching 20 mm Hg below diastolic pressure in the presence of worsening general condition, documented rising tissue pressure, significant tissue injury, or a history of 6 hours of total ischemia time of an extremity versus absolute tissue pressure of 30 mm Hg versus critical compartment pressure = 45 mm Hg

How long can peripheral nerves and muscles survive under ischemic conditions without irreversible damage?
Up to 4 hours

Place the following in order of decreasing frequency of compartment syndrome in the lower extremity: anterior compartment; deep posterior compartment; lateral compartment; superficial posterior compartment?
Anterior compartment; lateral compartment; deep posterior compartment; superficial posterior compartment

Most frequent compartment in the thigh to develop compartment syndrome:
Anterior quadriceps compartment

What might the first neurologic finding be in a patient with compartment syndrome of the calf?
Numbness of the great toe web space (anterior compartment most commonly affected (pressure on deep peroneal nerve)

Describe how to do a 2-incision, 4-compartment fasciotomy?
Make a longitudinal incision just posterior to the tibia; carry incision through the fascia into the superficial posterior space; incise the soleus muscle longitudinally near its tibial insertion; incise the deep fascia longitudinally to decompress the deep posterior compartment; make a second longitudinal anterolateral calf incision; carry incision down through the fascia into the anterior compartment; make another longitudinal fascial incision over the lateral compartment to decompress the peroneus muscles

What is the most common iatrogenic injury during an anterior fasciotomy?
Injury to the superficial peroneal nerve in the superior aspect of the incision

What muscles are contained in the anterior compartment of the leg?
Tibialis anterior; extensor hallucis longus; extensor digitorum communis

What vessels are contained in the anterior compartment of the leg?
Anterior tibial vessels

What nerve is contained in the anterior compartment of the leg?
Deep peroneal nerve

What muscles are contained in the deep posterior compartment of the leg?
Tibialis posterior; flexor hallucis longus; flexor digitorum longus

What vessels are contained in the deep posterior compartment of the leg?
Posterior tibial and peroneal vessels

What nerve is contained in the deep posterior compartment of the leg?
Tibial nerve

What muscles are contained in the superficial posterior compartment of the leg?
Gastrocnemius, soleus, plantaris

What muscles are contained in the lateral compartment of the leg?
Peroneals

What nerve is contained in the lateral compartment of the leg?
Superficial peroneal

MISCELLANEOUS

What is the technical term for the growth plate?
Physis

What is the term for the part of the bone that is between the physis and the articular surface?
Epiphysis

What is the term for the section of bone between the epiphysis and the bony shaft (the diaphysis)?
The metaphysis (This includes the physis.)

What term is given to a ligamentous injury in which the ligament remains in continuity?
Sprain

What term describes a tendinous or muscular injury?
Strain

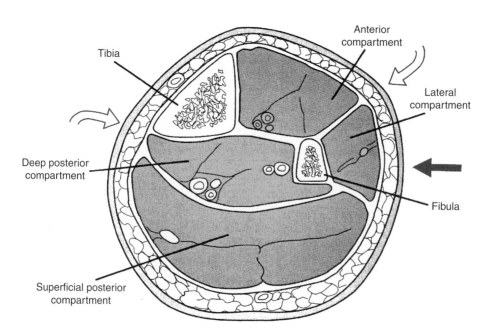

FIGURE 28-4. Cross-section of mid-calf showing the 4 fascial compartments and their contents. Open arrows show sites of double-incision fasciotomy; closed arrow shows site of single-incision fasciotomy. *(This article was published in Cooper C, Scalea TM. Abdominal compartment syndrome. In: Cameron JL, ed. Current Surgical Therapy. 5th ed. Mosby-Year Book; 1995:850. Copyright © Elsevier 1995.)*

Early reduction should be performed in hip dislocations and femoral neck fractures in order to prevent what complication?
Avascular necrosis of the femoral head—the blood vessels travel in the femoral neck

What is the recommended time period that all open fractures should be treated?
Within the first 8 hours after injury

What is external fixation?
Stabilization of an injured limb segment with pins or wires connected to the rods of a rigid construct external to the body via clamps or rings

In what situations is external fixation used?
Complex fractures where open reduction plus internal fixation (ORIF) is not indicated; fractures with associated vascular injuries requiring stabilization and urgent vascular repair; fractures in unstable patients unable to tolerate significant blood loss or anesthesia time; treatment of open fractures; specialized limb reconstruction surgery

What is open reduction and internal fixation?
An incision is made at or near the site of injury and the fracture is reduced under direct vision (open reduction) and subsequently rigidly stabilized with plates, screws, wires, or a combination (internal fixation).

What is the incidence of fat emboli syndrome?
1% to 17%

Fat emboli syndrome is characterized by:
Respiratory distress, altered mental status, skin petechiae

MULTIPLE CHOICE QUESTIONS

1. **Which of the following is most closely associated with calcaneal fractures?**
   A. Spiral fracture of the tibia
   B. Compression fractures of the lumbar spine
   C. Lateral compression fractures of the pelvis
   D. Calvarial fractures
   E. Clavicular fractures

2. **What is described by the term Monteggia fracture?**
   A. Fracture of the proximal one-third of the ulna with associated dislocation of the radial head
   B. Fracture of the mid radius with associated dislocation of the distal radial-ulnar joint
   C. A distraction-type injury of the spine where the anterior ligament fails under tension
   D. Burst fracture of C1
   E. Disruption of the ligament binding the first metatarsal to the second

3. **What must be done in all posterior knee dislocations if there is no other sign of trauma?**

   A. Application of a long leg splint
   B. Application of a long leg cast
   C. Determination of compartment pressures above and below the knee
   D. Arteriogram
   E. Amputation

4. **Which artery can be injured in a humeral shaft fracture and, if compromised, indicates operative repair of the humerus?**

   A. Radial artery
   B. Ulnar artery
   C. Brachial artery
   D. Subclavian artery
   E. Aorta

5. **Which of the following indicates nonaccidental trauma?**

   A. Multiple fractures in various stages of healing
   B. Spiral fracture of the femur
   C. Conjunctival hemorrhage
   D. Alleged mechanism that does not fit the injury
   E. All of the above indicate nonaccidental trauma

6. **Which Salter-Harris class is defined as a fracture that crosses the growth plate from the articular surface to the metaphysis?**

   A. Salter-Harris I
   B. Salter-Harris II
   C. Salter-Harris III
   D. Salter-Harris IV
   E. Salter-Harris V

7. **Which of the following is an incomplete fracture?**

   A. Compound fracture
   B. Greenstick fracture
   C. Comminuted fracture
   D. Spiral fracture
   E. None of the above

8. **Which of the following fractures is most closely associated with intra-abdominal injuries?**

   A. Calcaneal fractures
   B. Distal radius fractures
   C. Chance fractures
   D. Jefferson fracture
   E. Femoral neck fractures

9. **Which of the following is an early sign of compartment syndrome?**

    A. Paresthesias
    B. Paralysis
    C. Pulselessness
    D. Piloerection
    E. Putrifaction

10. **Which of the following pelvic fracture injury patterns would be most likely following a side-impact motor vehicle accident?**

    A. Anterior-posterior compression (APC)
    B. Lateral compression
    C. Vertical shear
    D. Greenstick
    E. Open book

ANSWERS

1. **Answer: B.** A calcaneal fracture is classically caused by a fall from height onto outstretched legs, such as a parachute jump or a fall from a ladder. Thus, someone who sustains this type of fracture is likely to have other fractures that are caused by an axial load. The choice that is most likely to be caused by an axial load is a compression fracture of the lumbar spine.

2. **Answer: A.** The other choices describe a Galeazzi fracture, Chance fracture, Jefferson fracture, and a Lisfranc injury, respectively.

3. **Answer: D.** An evaluation of the popliteal artery is essential for all patients who suffer from a posterior knee dislocation to rule out occult injury to the artery. The other modalities may be helpful in selected instances, but not necessarily in every circumstance.

4. **Answer: C.** The radial and ulnar arteries are in the forearm and are not associated with a humeral fracture. Similarly, the subclavian artery and the aorta are not in the proximity of the humeral shaft; only the brachial artery incurs risk with a humeral shaft fracture.

5. **Answer: E.** All of these findings can indicate a nonaccidental mechanism of injury. A high index of suspicion is necessary to correctly diagnose these injuries since misdiagnosis can have devastating effects on a child. Collaboration with child protection services is mandated by law.

6. **Answer: D.** A Salter-Harris I is a fracture through the growth plate, parallel to the joint. Salter-Harris II extends away from the joint. Salter-Harris III extends toward the joint. A type V fracture is a crush injury to the growth plate.

7. **Answer: B.** A greenstick fracture is seen in children due to the increased pliability of their bones. One cortex of the bone fails under tension, but the other one remains intact.

8. **Answer: C.** A Chance fracture is a failure of the anterior spinal ligament under tension. It is often caused by a seatbelt injury and there is approximately a 60% chance of an associated abdominal injury.

9. **Answer: A.** Paresthesia occurs early due to ischemic dysfunction of sensory nerves. Motor nerve dysfunction occurs much later. Pulselessness is a very late and very ominous sign. Piloerection is not associated with compartment syndrome.

10. **Answer: B.** Lateral compression, which is the most common injury pattern type for pelvic fractures, occurs when a force vector is applied laterally as in this case. Open book or APC-type fractures occur with anterior to posterior vectors, whereas vertical shear injuries occur with falls onto the outstretched lower extremities. A greenstick fracture is an incomplete fracture that occurs in children.

CHAPTER 29
Neurosurgery

Joshua Gish

Make sure that you are familiar with the Glasgow Coma Score prior to the test.

Review the neurosurgery section in the trauma chapter.

What components are present in the cranium?
Brain tissue, cerebrospinal fluid (CSF), blood vessels and blood volume, pathological volume (eg, neoplasm, hematoma, abscess, etc)

What may cause an increase in the brain tissue component (not including neoplasms)?
Edema, inflammatory, perineoplastic, vasogenic

What can be given to decrease swelling due to edema?
Mannitol, hypertonic saline

What can be given to decrease the brain tissue component if swelling is caused by inflammation or perineoplastic syndrome?
Steroids

What can be done to decrease the blood volume component?
Hyperventilation, diuretics, head elevation, remove venous obstruction

What can be done to decrease the CSF component?
Drainage (either external or internal such as a VP shunt), acetazolamide (temporary), steroids (temporary)

What can be done to decrease volume due to a mass lesion?
Evacuation or removal of the cause of the mass lesion

What is the Monro-Kelly doctrine?
The total volume of the cranial vault is fixed and thus an increase in one component must be offset by a decrease in another component.

True or false: CSF production rate is affected by intracranial pressure (ICP)?
False. CSF production rate is constant and is not affected by "back pressure."

What is the site of CSF production?
The arachnoid granulations

What is the name of the process that maintains cerebral blood flow at a constant rate despite changes in systemic blood pressure?
Autoregulation

Define cerebral perfusion pressure:
Mean arterial pressure (MAP) – ICP

Why do older people tend to be more tolerant of mass lesions?
They tend to have larger ventricles, which are more tolerant of compression than brain tissue

What is a raised ICP with no mass lesion termed?
Pseudotumor cerebri or idiopathic intracranial hypertension

What is increased ventricular volume without increased intracranial pressure called?
Normal pressure hydrocephalus

What is a failure of proper capillary formation termed?
Arteriovenous malformation (AVM)

What is the risk of hemorrhage associated with an AVM?
4% per year

What percentage of AVM-associated hemorrhages is classified as severe?
25%

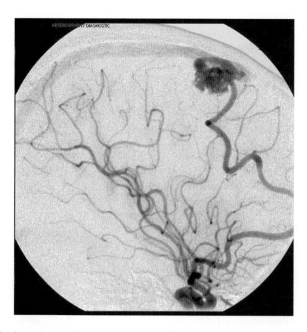

FIGURE 29-1. Cerebral angiogram demonstrating a frontal arteriovenous malformation filling from the left anterior cerebral artery. *(Reproduced from Doherty GM. Current Diagnosis and Treatment: Surgery. 13th ed. http://www.accessmedicine.com. Copyright © The McGraw-Hill Companies, Inc. All rights reserved.)*

This process is caused by defects in the arterial media and is increased in patients with connective tissue disorders such as Ehlers-Danlos or Marfan syndromes:
Berry aneurysms

What is the risk of hemorrhage with an aneurysm measuring less than 1 cm?
0.05% to 0.5% per year

What is the risk of hemorrhage with an aneurysm measuring more than 1 cm?
1% to 2% per year

If not treated, what is the risk of rebleed within 2 weeks from an aneurysm that has ruptured?
20%

Which cerebrovascular moniker derives from the Japanese term for "puff of smoke?"
Moyamoya—it is characterized by idiopathic narrowing of the major intracrainial vessels with formation of a compensatory collateral circulation.

Which medication is prescribed to reduce swelling related to brain tumors?
Dexamethasone

Which class of tumors accounts for half of all primary brain tumors?
Astrocytomas

What is the term for grade IV astrocytomas?
Glioblastoma multiforme

What is the most common Schwannoma?
Vestibular schwannoma

What brain tumor will tend to cause bitemporal hemianopsia?
Pituitary adenomas

What dopamine agonist is useful in 75% of prolactinomas?
Bromocriptine

What is the most common primary lesion for metastatic tumors of the brain?
Lung (~50%)

What is the second most common primary lesion for metastatic tumors of the brain?
Breast (15%–20%)

Chemotherapy is useful for brain metastatic tumors for which 2 primary lesions?
Small cell lung cancer and seminomas

Up to how many lesions can surgery be indicated for metastatic disease in the brain?
Up to 3 (provided they are accessible)

What is the most common cause of subarachnoid hemorrhage?
Trauma

What is the term for rotational acceleration and deceleration injuries that disrupt the white matter tracts of the brain?
Diffuse axonal injury

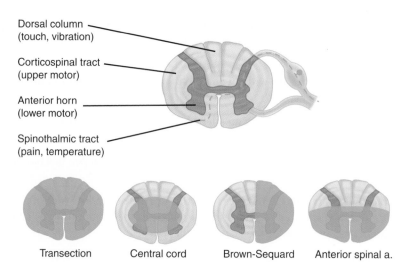

Dorsal column
(touch, vibration)

Corticospinal tract
(upper motor)

Anterior horn
(lower motor)

Spinothalmic tract
(pain, temperature)

Transection   Central cord   Brown-Sequard   Anterior spinal a.

FIGURE 29-2. Spinal cord injury patterns. a., artery. *(Adapted with permission from Hoff J, Boland M. Neurosurgery. In: Principles of Surgery. 7th ed. New York: McGraw-Hill; 1999:1837.)*

Which imaging test is paramount in assessing for brain injury following a trauma?
Head computed tomography (CT)

What Glasgow coma score (GCS) is considered the "cutoff" as an indication for ICP monitoring?
8

How can one differentiate between CSF and mucus secretions in cases of suspected ethmoid plate disruptions?
CSF will contain glucose

What syndrome results in weakness of the upper extremities with relative sparing of the lower extremities?
Central cord syndrome

Which syndrome results in ipsilateral paralysis and contralateral loss of sensation?
Brown-Sequard or hemitransection of the spinal cord

Which syndrome is characterized by paralysis and sensory loss but preservation of deep sensation and proprioception?
Anterior cord syndrome

What is the most common CNS infection in patients with acquired immunodeficiency syndrome?
Toxoplasma gondii

What are considered the symptoms of a carotid stenosis?
Ipsilateral amaurosis fugax (temporary blindness often described as a window shade caused by ophthalmic artery emboli), ipsilateral transient ischemic attack, or stroke

Table 29-1 Spinal Tumor Characteristics				
Compartment	Tumor	Predilection	Treatment Options	Comments
Extradural	Vertebral hemangioma	Thoracic	Preoperative embolization + resection (+ XRT) for progressive symptoms	Honeycomb radiographic appearance
	Giant cell tumor	Sacral	Resection (+ XRT)	Aggressive spread, often biopsy for diagnosis before treating
	Plasmacytoma	Thoracic	(XRT + steroids + surgical stabilization)	Precursor to multiple myeloma
	Osteoid osteoma	Lumbar	Resection of nidus (+ fusion)	Peak incidence in adolescence
	Osteoblastoma	Lumbar	En bloc resection (+ XRT)	Similar to osteoid osteoma but >1.5 cm
	Osteochondroma	Cervical	Resection (+ fusion) to treat symptoms	Often causes spinal deformity
(nonneoplastic)	Eosinophilic granuloma	Cervical	Spine stabilization	Classic vertebra plana in children
(nonneoplastic)	Aneurysmal bone cyst	Thoracic and lumbar	GTR (+ fusion)	Aggressively expansile, peak incidence in adolescence
(nonneoplastic)	Angiolipoma	Thoracic	Resection to treat symptoms	Onset of symptoms often during pregnancy
	Metastasis		XRT + steroids	
Extradural	Chordoma	Sacral, cervical	En bloc resection (+ XRT)	Most common primary bone malignancy of the spine
	Ewing sarcoma	Sacral	Resection + XRT + chemotherapy	Usually metastatic from another site, HBA-71 Ag
	Multiple myeloma		Chemotherapy + XRT (+ steroids + surgical stabilization)	Pathological fractures seen in 50% at presentation
	Lymphoma		Chemotherapy	Hodgkin and non-Hodgkin
	Chondrosarcoma	Thoracic	En bloc resection	Second-most common primary bone malignancy
	Osteosarcoma		Chemotherapy + en bloc resection (+ XRT)	Bimodal age distribution, potentially curable
	Paravertebral sarcomas		En bloc resection + XRT + chemotherapy	Often painless, presents with neurological deficits
Intradural-extramedullary	Schwannoma	Thoracic	GTR	Associated with dorsal root origin
	Neurofibroma	Thoracic	Resection	Associated with ventral root origin
	Meningioma	Thoracic	GTR (+ XRT for recurrence)	Extension common

(continued)

Table 29-1   Spinal Tumor Characteristics (*Continued*)

Compartment	Tumor	Predilection	Treatment Options	Comments
	Metastasis		XRT + steroids	Drop metastases from GBM, AA, ependymoma, and MB
	Myxopapillary ependymoma	Conus	Resection + XRT	Dissemination common
	Lymphoma		Chemotherapy	
	Lipoma	Lumbosacral	Resection	Congenital, can cause tethered cord
	Paraganglioma	Conus	GTR	Can secrete hyperadrenergic state
	Neuroganglioma			Rare nerve sheath tumor
	Dermoid and epidermoid		GTR (+ steroids for chemical meningitis)	Commonly in children
	Teratoma	Sacral	GTR	Can be in any compartment
Intramedullary	Ependymoma	Cervical	GTR	Strongly enhancing, well-circumscribed
	Astrocytoma	Cervical	Biopsy ± resection + XRT	Infiltrative, common in children
	Lipoma	Cervical and thoracic	Debulking	
	Hemangioblastoma	Thoracic and cervical	GTR	Cystic with mural nodule, associated with von Hippel-Lindau syndrome
	Metastasis	Cervical and conus	XRT + steroids	Most commonly small-cell lung cancer
	Ganglioglioma	Thoracic	GTR + XRT	Commonly in children
	Oligodendroglioma	Thoracic	GTR + XRT	Spinal deformity, syrinx common
	Neuroblastoma	Cervical	GTR	

AA, anaplastic astrocytoma; GBM, glioblastoma multiforme; GTR, gross total resection; MB, medulloblastoma; XRT, radiation therapy.

MULTIPLE CHOICE QUESTIONS

1. **A patient is intubated in the ICU, but can follow commands with his right arm, extends with his lower extremities, and does not move his left arm. His eyes open to command. What is his GCS?**

   A. 14T

   B. 11T

   C. 10T

   D. 9T

   E. 5T

2. **A patient comes into the trauma bay with a large laceration of his scalp with a skull deformity after a motor vehicle collision. He seems to be moving all 4 extremities spontaneously, and he is tachycardic. He has a large pool of blood on the stretcher. He also has a large flail segment of his right chest. What should your first move be?**

A. Attempt to stop the bleeding with pressure or with suture repair of his scalp
B. Transfer the patient to CT scan to rule out intracranial trauma
C. Assess the patient's airway
D. Transfuse 2 units of uncross-matched blood
E. Obtain a chest x-ray

3. **You are seeing a patient in the ICU who has suffered a head injury. He has a ventricular monitor placed for measuring intracranial pressure, as well as an arterial catheter placed. His blood pressure is 120/80 with a mean of 90 and his ICP is 20. What is his cerebral perfusion pressure?**

A. 100
B. 90
C. 80
D. 70
E. 60

4. **Which intracranial component can be affected most rapidly to decrease intracranial pressure in an acute situation?**

A. Intravascular blood
B. Cerebral spinal fluid
C. A mass lesion
D. An extra-axial hematoma
E. Brain tissue

5. **Which of the following patients is most likely to require emergent surgical decompression?**

A. An 85-year-old female with advanced dementia who has a 1-cm left subdural hematoma following a fall at her nursing home
B. An 8-month-old baby with an intraparenchymal hemorrhage after a fall from her sister's arms
C. A 17-year-old male with a 2-cm frontal epidural hematoma with a GCS of 15
D. A 56-year-old male with bilateral subdural hematomas found after a CT scan for headache
E. An 18-year-old female with a small fracture of her skull following a gunshot wound, with no appreciable underlying hematoma.

6. **A patient presents with weakness of his upper extremities, but four-fifth strength of his lower extremities. Which syndrome is most likely to be the cause of his findings?**

A. Brown-Sequard
B. Central cord
C. Anterior cord
D. Monro-Kelly
E. Total cord disruption

7. **Which of the following therapies is useful in the majority of prolactinomas?**

   A. Octreotide
   B. Insulin
   C. Corticosteroids
   D. Prolactin
   E. Bromocriptine

ANSWERS

1. **Answer: C.** This patient would get 1 point out of 5 for verbal (the lowest that you can get in a single category is 1), but would get the designation T to indicate that he is intubated. He would get all 6 points for verbal because this follows the best result (the right arm). He would get 3 out of 4 points for eyes.

2. **Answer: C.** When in a trauma resuscitation, the first priority is to secure the patient's airway. All other choices may be necessary, but the airway is of prime importance.

3. **Answer: D.** Cerebral perfusion pressure is defined as MAP − ICP. In this case, 90 − 20 = 70.

4. **Answer: A.** The intravascular blood volume can be decreased rapidly, but transiently by methods such as hyperventilation and mannitol dieresis. This can provide the necessary time to affect a more permanent solution.

5. **Answer: C.** An epidural hematoma is caused by a disruption of the middle meningeal artery and thus is exposed to higher pressures than a subdural hematoma, which is caused by tearing of bridging veins. In addition, younger patients have more brain tissue that increases pressure by mass lesions proportionately more than in an older individual with significant atrophy. An epidural hematoma classically has a "lucid interval" in which the patient's GCS may be normal. This should not delay decompression, as the epidural hematoma can rapidly expand causing herniation.

6. **Answer: B.** Central cord syndrome results in weakness of the upper extremities with relative sparing of the lower extremities. Brown-Sequard is a hemitransaction that would cause ipsilateral paralysis and contralateral sensory deficit. Anterior cord leaves proprioception and deep sensation intact. Total cord disruption results in paralysis of both the upper and lower extremities distal to the lesion. Monro-Kelly is a doctrine that describes the contents of the calvarium.

7. **Answer: E.** Bromocriptine is a dopamine agonist that inhibits prolactin secretion from the anterior pituitary. The other options are not helpful in this condition.

CHAPTER 30
Obstetrics and Gynecology

Leon Plowright and Christine Chen

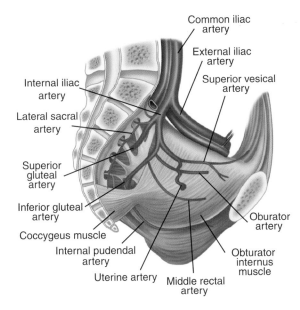

Common iliac artery

External iliac artery

Internal iliac artery

Superior vesical artery

Lateral sacral artery

Superior gluteal artery

Inferior gluteal artery

Coccygeus muscle

Internal pudendal artery

Uterine artery

Middle rectal artery

Oburator artery

Obturator internus muscle

FIGURE 30-1. The muscles and vasculature of the pelvis. *(Reproduced from Brunicardi FC, Andersen DK, Billiar TR, et al. Schwartz's Principles of Surgery. 9th ed. http://www.accessmedicine.com. Copyright © The McGraw-Hill Companies, Inc. All rights reserved.)*

ANATOMY

What are the branches of the internal iliac artery (hypogastric)?
Posterior division: Iliolumbar, lateral sacral, superior gluteal
Anterior division: Obturator, internal pudendal, inferior gluteal, umbilical, middle vesicle, inferior vesicle, middle hemorrhoidal, uterine, vaginal

Arterial supply to the uterus:
Uterine artery from the hypogastric and ovarian arteries directly from the aorta

Right ovarian vein originates from:
Inferior vena cava

Left ovarian vein originates from:
Left renal vein

Vaginal arterial supply
Upper: cervical branch of the uterine artery
Middle: inferior vesical
Lower: internal pudendal and middle hemorrhoidal

The major arterial supply to the cervix is located:
In the lateral cervical walls at the 3 and 9 o'clock positions

The external pudendal artery supply:
The rectum, labia, clitoris, perineum

Artery that supplies the round ligament:
Sampson

Inferior epigastric artery and vein originates from:
External iliac artery and external iliac vein, respectively

Levator ani complex:
Iliococcygeus, pubococcygeus, puborectalis

Boundaries of the femoral triangle:
Sartorius, adductor longus muscle, and inguinal ligament

Floor of the femoral triangle is formed by:
Iliopsoas, pectineus, and adductor longus

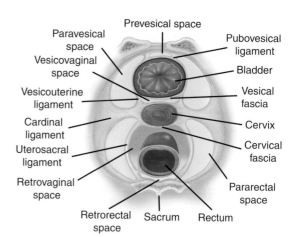

FIGURE 30-2. The avascular spaces of the female pelvis. *(Reproduced from Brunicardi FC, Andersen DK, Billiar TR, et al. Schwartz's Principles of Surgery. 9th ed. http://www.accessmedicine.com. Copyright © The McGraw-Hill Companies, Inc. All rights reserved.)*

Space of Retzius:
The area between the bladder and the symphysis pubis, bounded laterally by the obliterated hypogastric arteries

Cul-de-sac of Douglas:
Also known as the rectouterine pouch or fold and is located anterior to the rectum, separating the uterus from the large intestine

Boundaries of the paravesical space:
Anterior: pubic symphysis
Posterior: cardinal ligament
Medial: superior vesical artery
Lateral: obturator internus muscle

Boundaries of the pararectal space:
Anterior: cardinal ligament
Posterior: sacrum
Medial: rectum
Lateral: iliac vessels

Anatomic relationship between the uterine artery and the ureter:
At approximately 2 cm from the cervix, the uterine artery crosses above and in front of the ureter.

Support of the uterus:
The cardinal and uterosacral ligaments

Vaginal lymphatics:
Upper third: Iliac
Middle third: hypogastric
Lower third: inguinal

Aorta lies at this spinal level:
L4

Innervation to the uterus:
Hypogastric plexus by sympathetic merging at Frankenhauser plexus (uterovaginal plexus)
Pain sensory to T11 to 12

Sensory innervation of the vagina:
Pudendal nerve (S2–S4)

Obturator nerve:
Sensory and motor to the medial thigh

Sciatic nerve:
L4 to S2; passing through the greater sciatic foramen to supplying the muscles of lateral leg and foot

PHYSIOLOGY

Increases in pregnancy:
GFR by 50%: 90 mL/min prepregnancy versus 125 mL/min pregnancy
Total T4
Total T3
PTH
Prolactin
Plasma fibrinogen: 300 mg/dL prepregnancy versus 600 mg/dL pregnancy
ESR
TBG: thyroxine-binding globulin
Cholesterol
Heart rate: Increased 10 to 15 bpm
Cardiac output: 1.5 mL/min more than prepregnant average
Prostacyclin
Thromboxane
Plasma volume
Red cell volume
Alkaline phoshatase

Human placental lactogen
Progesterone
Estradiol

Decreases in pregnancy:
Total serum calcium
Albumin (decrease by 30%)
BUN and creatinine: due to increase in GFR
Hgb and Hct
Factor XI
Factor XIII
TSH
Systemic vascular resistance
pCO_2: 35 to 40 mm Hg prepregnant to 28 to 30 mm Hg pregnant
Respiratory volume
Antithrombin III (anti-factor Xa)
Anticoagulant protein S

Cross the placenta:
Propylthiouracil, TRH, iodine, magnesium sulfate, IgG, propanolol, warfarin

Does not cross the placenta:
T3, T4, TSH, insulin, glucagon, heparin, prednisone

hCG peaks at:
8 to 10 weeks gestation

Average weight gained in pregnancy:
25 lb

Average weight and volume of non-pregnant uterus:
40 to 70 g and 10 mL

Average weight and volume of pregnant uterus:
1100 to 1200 g and 5000 mL

What supports pregnancy during the first 14 weeks of pregnancy prior to the development of the placenta?
The corpus luteum, which secretes progesterone

Gestational age at which the uterus rises out of the pelvis:
12 weeks gestation

In late pregnancy blood flow rate to the uterus:
450 to 650 mL/min

Percentage of uterine blood flow direct to the placenta at term:
80% to 90%

Pulmonary function in pregnancy:
Increase: Tidal volume, inspiratory capacity, minute ventilation, minute oxygen uptake
Decrease: Functional residual capacity (by 15%), residual volume, expiratory reserve volume
Unchanged: Maximum breathing capacity, forced expiratory volume (FEV_1)

Physiologic hydronephrosis of pregnancy resolve in:
12 to 16 weeks postpartum

Gastric acid production and gastric emptying:
Increased and decreased, respectively, in pregnancy

Two GI disorders in third trimester pregnancy:
Acute fatty liver of pregnancy and cholestasis of pregnancy

OBSTETRICAL CONDITIONS AND COMPLICATIONS

Incidence of hypertensive disease in pregnancy:
12% to 22%

New onset hypertension and proteinuria after 20 weeks gestation in a previously normotensive woman:
Preeclampsia

Criteria for diagnosis of preeclampsia:
Mild: BP 140/90, 6 hours apart plus at least 1+ protein on urine dip or >300 mg of protein on 24-hour urine
Severe: BP 160/110 6 hours apart plus at least 3+ protein on urine dip or 5000 mg of protein on 24-hour urine protein

New-onset hypertension without proteinuria after 20 weeks gestation in a previously normotensive woman:
Gestational hypertension

New-onset grand mal seizure in woman with preeclampsia:
Eclampsia

Treatment of preecalmpsia:
Magnesium sulfate for seizure prophylaxis, labetalol and hydralazine for BP control and expedient delivery

HELLP syndrome is characterized by:
Hemolysis, elevated liver enzymes, and low platelets

Most common cause of serious blunt trauma during pregnancy:
Motor vehicle accidents

Frequency of placental abruption caused by trauma
1% to 6% of "minor" injuries and up to 50% of "major" injuries

Percent of uterine rupture because of blunt trauma:
Less than 1%

Minimal amount of time of fetal monitoring after maternal trauma:
At least 4 hours for minor trauma and 24 hours for major trauma

Best diagnostic imaging in pregnancy in order of preference:
Ultrasound, MRI, chest x-ray, CT scan

Estimated fetal exposure from common imaging modalities:
Chest x-ray (2 views): 0.02 to 0.07 mrad
Abdominal film (single view): 100 mrad
Intravenous pyelography: ≥1 rad
Hip film (single view): 200 mrad
Mammography: 7 to 20 mrad

Barium enema or small bowel series: 2 to 4 rads
CT scan of head or chest: <1 rad
CT scan of abdomen and lumbar spine: 250 mrad

X-ray exposure level thought to be safe during pregnancy:
Less than 5 rads has not been associated with an increase in fetal anomalies or
pregnancy loss

Test used to determine percentage of fetal red blood cells in maternal blood:
Kleihauer-Betke (KB)

Most common form of isoimmunization:
Rh (D) alloimmunization

Women who are Rh negative are given this to prevent alloimmunization:
Anti-D immune globulin (IgG anti-D), that is, RhoGAM

Rhogam is given in the setting of:
Rh negative women status posttrauma or invasive procedure with a high probability of
maternal fetal hemorrhage (despite a negative KB) and it should be administered within
72 hours of the event.

Painless vaginal bleeding:
Placenta previa: placental tissue overlying or proximal to the internal cervical os

Painful vaginal bleeding:
Placental abruption: decidual hemorrhage leading to the premature separation of the
placenta prior to delivery.

**Condition where the placenta attaches deep into the uterine wall but not through the
myometrium:**
Placenta accreta

**Condition where the placenta attaches into the uterine wall with penetration deep into
the myometrium but not to the uterine serosa:**
Placenta increta

**Placenta accreta with penetration of the entire myometrium to the uterine serosa and
sometimes even the bladder:**
Placenta percreta

Safest treatment for placenta accreta:
Cesarean with possible need for hysterectomy

Most common cause of postpartum hemorrhage:
Uterine atony

**The administration of what drugs can cause uterine contractions and aid in
postpartum hemorrhage:**
Oxytocin (pitocin): excess use may cause antidiuretic effect
Methylergonovine (methergine): contraindicated in those with hypertension or preeclampsia
15 Methylprostaglandin F2 α (hemabate): contraindicated in those with pulmonary or
renal disease
Misoprostol (Cytotec)

Surgical options for postpartum hemorrhage when pharmacologic measures have failed:
Embolization of uterine vessels
Ligation of uterine vessels
Ligation of utero-ovarian vessels
Ligation of hypogastric vessels
Uterine compression suture (ie, B-lynch)
Abdominal packing
Hysterectomy

Of the branches of the posterior division that is responsible for gluteal ischemia as a complication of hypogastric artery ligation:
Superior gluteal artery

Percentage of pregnant women who require surgery during pregnancy:
About 0.1% to 2.0%

The most common surgical procedure complicating pregnancy:
Appendectomy (1 per 500)

The second most common general surgical procedure encountered during pregnancy:
Cholecystectomy

Which side is pyelonephritis most likely?
Right

Leading cause of maternal death in the United States:
Pulmonary embolism

Pregnancy increases the risk factor for venous thrombosis by:
5 times

GYNECOLOGIC CONDITIONS AND COMPLICATIONS

Heavy or excessive menses (greater than 7 days duration or >80 mL)
Menorrhagia

Painful cyclical menses:
Dysmenorrhea

Absence of menses during the reproductive years for at least 6 months:
Amenorrhea

Differential diagnosis for adnexal masses:
Benign gyn: Functional cyst, leiomyomata, endometrioma, tubo-ovarian abscess, ectopic pregnancy, teratoma, mucin and serous cystadenoma, hydrosalpinx, paratubal cyst
Benign non-gyn: Diverticula abscess, appendicular abscess, pelvic kidney, bladder, diverticulum, urethral diverticulum, nerve sheath tumors
Malignant gyn: Epithelial carcinoma, sex cord or stroma tumor, germ cell tumor
Malignant non-gyn: Gastrointestinal cancers, retroperitoneal sarcomas, metastases colon, and breast

Presence of endometrial stroma and glands at extrauterine sites:
Endometriosis: Found in 15% of reproductive age women undergoing laparoscopy

Etiology of endometriosis:
Sampson: Retrograde menstruation
Halban: Lymphatic-vascular spreading
Meyer: Coelomic metaplasia
Dimowski: Decreased cellular immunity

Clinical features of endometriosis:
Chronic pelvic pain
Dysmenorrhea
Dyspareunia
Bowel and bladder symptoms
Subfertility
Abnormal menstrual bleeding
Chronic fatigue
Low back pain

Diagnosis of endometriosis:
By direct visualization with confirmed pathology

Endometrial glands and stroma within the myometrium:
Adenomyosis: Most common physical finding is diffusely enlarged uterus

Diagnostic criteria for pelvic inflammatory disease (PID):
History and presence of lower abdominal pain
Cervical motion tenderness
Adnexal tenderness

Pregnancy outside of the uterine cavity:
Ectopic: Annual rate in the United States 1.5 per 1000 women, age 15 to 44

Acute severe, unilateral, lower abdominal and pelvic pain, waxing and waning associated with nausea and vomiting:
Ovarian torsion: ovarian enlargement of 8 to 10 cm. Occurs most commonly in the reproductive years with average patient in their mid-20s.

Average age of menopause:
52

Differential for postmenopausal bleeding:
Atrophy: 59%
Polyps: 12%
Endometrial cancer: 10%
Endometrial hyperplasia: 9.8%
Hormonal effect: 7%
Cervical cancer: <1%
Other: 2%

Most common placental tumor:
Choriocarcinoma

Most common gynecologic malignancy:
Endometrial cancer

Most lethal gynecologic malignancy:
Ovarian cancer

Most common gynecologic malignancy in pregnancy:
Cervical cancer

Most infrequent gynecologic cancer encountered:
Tubal cancer

CA 125 tumor marker (a glycoprotein antigen) is elevated in the following conditions:
Endometriosis
Uterine leiomyoma
Adenomyosis
Functional ovarian cyst
Meigs syndrome
Pelvic inflammatory disease
Menstruation
Ovarian hyperstimulation
Benign ovarian neoplasm
Active hepatitis
Chronic liver disease
Cirrhosis
Acute pancreatitis
Diverticulitis
Malignancy of the ovary, endometrium, breast, lung, and pancreas
Congestive heart failure
Pneumonia
Mesothelioma
Renal disease
Systemic lupus erythematous
Diabetes (poorly controlled)

Staging for gynecologic cancers:
Endometrial: surgical
Ovarian: surgical
Cervical: clinical

BRCA **gene mutations have this associated risk of breast and ovarian cancer:**
BRAC1: 45% to 85% risk of breast cancer and 20% to 45% risk for ovarian cancer
BRAC2: 30% to 50 % risk of breast cancer and 10% to 20% risk of ovarian cancer

Family members with lynch syndrome type II are at risk for developing which cancers?
Colorectal
Endometrial
Ovarian

Surgical staging and therapy for ovarian cancer includes:
Peritoneal cytologic examination
Total abdominal hysterectomy
Bilateral salpingo-oophorectomy
Pelvic and periaortic lymph node dissection
Omentectomy
Biopsy of the diaphragm and peritoneal surfaces
Removal of all visible tumors possible

Hysterectomy types:

Supracervical: Uterus transected at the level of the internal cervical os.

Simple hysterectomy (type I): Also known as *extrafascial hysterectomy*, and entails removing the uterus and cervix without excision of the parametrium.

Modified radical hysterectomy (type II): Removes the cervix, proximal vagina, and parametrial and paracervical tissue.

Radical hysterectomy (type III): Requires greater resection of the parametria, and extension to the pelvic sidewalls. The ureters are completely dissected from their beds and the bladder and rectum mobilized.

Five **locations where ureteral injuries can occur at the time of gynecologic operations:**

The base of the broad ligament, where the ureter passes beneath the uterine vessels

Beyond the uterine vessels as the ureter passes through its tunnel in the cardinal ligament

The intramural portion of the ureter that traverses the bladder

At or below the infundibulopelvic ligament

Along the course of the ureter on the lateral pelvic sidewalls just above the uterosacral ligaments

Incisional approaches used to gain entry into the abdomen:

Pfannenstiel: Transverse incision 2 finger breaths above the pubic symphysis. Less infection, greater strength, greater comfort, increased blood loss, greater exposure of the lateral pelvis.

Vertical midline incision: Midline or paramedian incision made from the pubic symphysis to the level of the umbilicus and beyond. More dehiscence, weaker, more painful, less blood loss, increased exposure to abdomen, ability to extend.

Cherney incision: The rectus muscle is transected at least 0.5 cm above its insertion site at the posterior aspect of the pubic bone.

Maylard incision: The rectus muscle is transected more cephalad, at the level of the superior iliac spine.

MULTIPLE CHOICE QUESTIONS

1. **Which artery if transected during uterine artery ligation can result in gluteal ischemia?**

   A. Superior gluteal
   B. Inferior gluteal
   C. Lateral sacral
   D. Iliolumbar

2. **Describe the relationship of ureter in reference to the cervix.**

   A. The ureter can be found extremely lateral from the internal cervical os
   B. At approximately 2 cm from the cervix, the uterine artery crosses above and in front of the ureter
   C. At approximately 2 cm from the cervix, the uterine artery crosses below and in front of the ureter
   D. Supracervical hysterectomy is only performed to avoid ureteral injury

3. **What level of radiation exposure is thought to be safe in pregnancy?**

   A. 500 mrad
   B. 5 rad
   C. 50 mrad
   D. 100 mrad

4. **The incidence of hypertensive disease in pregnancy.**

   A. 7%
   B. 10%
   C. 12% to 22%
   D. 2%

5. **Tumor marker used to assess progression of disease in ovarian cancer:**

   A. CA-125
   B. CEA
   C. CA 19-9
   D. BHCG

6. **Which space is traversed by trocars during a retropubic midurethral sling procedure?**

   A. Inguinal canal
   B. Pouch of Douglas
   C. Space of Retzius
   D. Paravesical space

7. **How long is fetal monitoring required after the mother sustains major trauma?**

   A. Until the nonstress test is reactive
   B. 1 hour
   C. 4 hours
   D. 24 hours

8. **Which is NOT a symptom of pelvic inflammatory disease?**

   A. Abdominal pain
   B. Cervical motion tenderness
   C. Urinary frequency
   D. Nausea/vomiting

9. **Which is the most common gynecologic cancer?**

   A. Endometrial
   B. Cervical
   C. Ovarian
   D. Tubal

10. **The risk of endometrial and ovarian cancers is increased in which hereditary cancer syndrome?**

    A. Cowden syndrome
    B. Li-Fraumeni syndrome
    C. Lynch II syndrome
    D. Peutz-Jeghers syndrome

ANSWERS

1. **Answer: A.** Choice A is the major blood supply to gluteus maximus and minimus. Choice B provides branches to gluteus maximus and an anastomotic branch contributes to the cruciate anastomosis of the back of the thigh. Choice C supplies the sacrum and coccyx. Choice D supplies the bone and muscles of the iliac fossa.

2. **Answer: B.** The ureter runs under the uterine artery (remember, "water under the bridge") and they cross at a point approximately 2 cm from the cervix. This point is also called point A in radiation oncology (2 cm anterior and 2 cm lateral from the cervical os). A is incorrect because the ureter runs near the internal cervical os. C is incorrect because the uterine artery crosses above the ureter (the correct choice B). There are a number of reasons to opt to perform a supracervical hysterectomy but the sole reason is not to avoid ureteral injury.

3. **Answer: B.** Less than 5 rad has not been associated with an increase in fetal anomalies or pregnancy loss.

4. **Answer: C.** Depending on the study population, studies have shown that the incidence of hypertensive disease (gestational hypertension, preeclampsia, eclampsia) is 12% to 22%.

5. **Answer: A.** Elevated CA-125 can indicate ovarian cancer (as well as tubal and primary peritoneal cancer). Increasing CA-125 after treatment often indicates progression of disease. Choice B is associated with colon/GI cancer; choice C, pancreatic cancer; choice D, gestational trophoblastic disease/neoplasia.

6. **Answer: C.** The space of Retzius is located between the urinary bladder and the symphysis pubis. During a retropubic midurethral sling procedure, trocars are passed from the area of the midurethra up through the urogenital diaphragm, with the trocar hugging the posterior of symphysis pubis. The trocar should pass laterally to the bladder. Bladder perforation is a risk of this procedure.

7. **Answer: D.** Following major trauma, fetal monitoring is required for at least 24 hours. After minor trauma, a minimum of 4 hours is required. The risk of a placental event (eg, abruption) is highest during these time frames and may necessitate delivery.

8. **Answer: B.** Cervical motion tenderness is a sign not a symptom. The symptoms of clinically suspected pelvic inflammatory disease are abdominal pain, abnormal discharge, intermenstrual bleeding, postcoital bleeding, fever, urinary frequency, low back pain, and nausea/vomiting.

9. **Answer: A.** Endometrial cancer is the most common gynecologic cancer with approximately 40,000 new cases diagnosed each year. It is the fourth most common cancer in women after breast, lung, and colon cancers. Ovarian cancer is the most common cause of gynecologic cancer mortality.

10. **Answer: C.** Lynch II syndrome increases risk of colorectal, endometrial, ovarian, gastric, hepatobiliary, small bowel, and brain cancers; Cowden—thyroid, breast, mucocutaneous lesions, colonic neoplasms; Li-Fraumeni—soft tissue sarcoma, leukemia, breast, brain, adrenocortical, pancreatic, lung and possibly prostate cancer, melanoma, gonadal germ cell tumors; Peutz-Jeghers—abnormal melanin deposits, GI tract polyposis and cancer, sex cord tumors, breast cancer.

CHAPTER 31
Statistics

Lung Ching Lee and Dale A. Dangleben

1. Memorize the table below for easy calculation of sensitivity, specificity, and positive and negative predictive values.
2. Know the differences between different types of statistical tests.

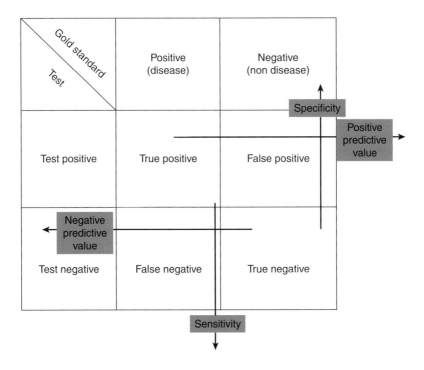

What is sensitivity?
Proportion of truly diseased persons in a screened population who are identified as being diseased by the test. It is a measure of the probability of correctly diagnosing a condition.

Sensitivity equation:
True positive/(true positive + false negative)

What is specificity?
The proportion of truly nondiseased persons who are so identified by the screening test

Specificity equation:
True negative/(false positive + true negative)

False-positive rate:
1 – specificity

False-negative rate
1 – sensitivity

What is positive predictive value?
The probability that a person with a positive test result has the disease

What is the positive predictive equation?
True positive/(true positive + false positive)

What is the negative predicted value?
The probability that a patient with a negative test result really is free of the disease

What is the negative predicted value equation?
True negative/(false negative + true negative)

Definition of prevalence:
The total number of cases of a given disease in a specified population at a designated time

Definition of incidence:
The number of new cases of a given disease during a given period in a specified population

What is the absolute risk reduction?
The absolute arithmetic difference in outcome rates between control and experimental patients in a trial

What is relative risk reduction?
The proportional reduction in outcome rates between control and experimental patients in a trial

A range of values that has a specified probability of containing the rate or trend:
Confidence intervals

A method of studying a drug or procedure in which both the subjects and investigators are kept unaware of who is actually getting which specific treatment:
Double-blind method

The number of patients who need to be treated to prevent one adverse outcome:
Number Needed To Treat

The probability that an event will occur:
Risk

The number of units in a population to be studied:
Sample size

The number of deaths during a specific time period:
Mortality

The proportion of patients alive at some point after the diagnosis:
Survival

What is the null hypothesis?
Denoted by H_o; it is a proposal that there is no difference in a comparison.

What is a Type I error?
Rejecting the null hypothesis tested when it is true (α)

What is a Type II error?
Failing to reject the null hypothesis when a given alternative hypothesis was true (β)

The probability that the test will reject the hypothesis tested when a specific alternative hypothesis is true:
Power $(1 - \beta)$

Sum of all results divided by the number of results:
Mean

The middle value that divides the distribution of data:
Median

The most common value in data set:
Mode

The extent to which a test measures what it claims to measure:
Validity

The consistency with which the data collection process measures whatever it measures:
Reliability

An estimate of the population mean is:
Sample mean

What is central limit theorem?
For a large enough sample size n, the distribution of the sample mean will approach a normal distribution

What is standard deviation (SD)?
It is a predictable measure of dispersion from the mean in a Gaussian normal distribution

What is the square root of the variance?
SD

What are case-control studies?
Observational retrospective study to study risk factors and causation for desired/predefined cases (outcome). Good for rare diseases.
For example, comparing smoking history of acute myocardial infarction (MI) (cases) patient versus smoking history of patient without MI (control)

What are prospective cohort studies?

Observational study of treatment outcome for patient groups that could not be randomized (cohorts) for ethical reasons.

For example, following long-term weight loss outcome of patients who received roux-en-y gastric bypass versus sleeve gastrectomy

What are retrospective cohort studies?

Differ from prospective cohort studies in that the exposure in question being studied are collected retrospectively

For example, studying if certain preprocedural comorbidities will affect the long-term weight loss outcome of patients who received roux-en-y gastric bypass versus sleeve gastrectomy

What are randomized controlled trials?

Randomly selecting subjects to be allocated into treatment versus control group. Best design, minimizes biases

What are the different levels of evidences?

Level I: Evidence from at least 1 randomized controlled trial

Level II-1: Evidence from well-designed controlled trial without randomization

Level II-2: Evidence from well-designed cohort or case control studies

Level II-3: Evidence from multiple time series with or without the treatment, or dramatic result in uncontrolled trials

Level III: Expert opinion, clinical experience

What are t tests used for?

To assess statistical difference between sample means of the testing group versus known population mean (1-sample t test) or sample means of 2 independent or dependent groups (2-sample t test) for continuous variables

What is a paired t test?

A specific t test to compare 2 sample groups that are not randomly selected.

For example, the second sample group is the first sample group after treatment.

What are Z tests?

Similar to t test, however, is used when sample size is greater than 30 (t test is for a limited sample size, ie, less than 30) and when SDs of the population are known

What is ANOVA?

Analysis of variance. It is used to determine whether there is a difference between the means of several different groups (as opposed to t tests, which only compare 2 groups).

What is χ^2 test?

It tests whether the distribution of multiple categorical variables in the experimented population differs from the control.

For example, proportion of surviving and nonsurviving cancer patients in 5 years after chemotherapy versus proportion of surviving and nonsurviving cancer patients without treatment.

What is Fisher exact test?

Similar to χ^2 test, but specifically only compares 2 categorical variables

MULTIPLE CHOICE QUESTIONS

1. What is the *mode* in the following data set:
   1, 1, 1, 1, 1, 1, 3, 4, 5, 5, 5, 5, 5, 7, 8, 8, 8?

   A. 1
   B. 3
   C. 4
   D. 5
   E. 8

2. What is the *median* in the following data set:
   1, 1, 1, 1, 1, 1, 3, 4, 5, 5, 5, 5, 5, 7, 8, 8, 8?

   A. 1
   B. 3
   C. 4
   D. 5
   E. 8

3. A university research student wishes to study possible risk factors for disease X and decides to collect and compare the medical histories of 200 disease X patients within his institution in the last 10 years and compare with 200 other patients with similar age group, demography, and ethnicity but disease X free. What type of study is this?

   A. Case series
   B. Case-control
   C. Prospective cohort
   D. Randomized control studies

4. What level of evidence would the above scenario (question 3) provide?

   A. Level I
   B. Level II-1
   C. Level II-2
   D. Level II-3
   E. Level III

5. A university researcher has developed a new screening test for disease X. When tested against 100 patients with known diagnosis of disease X, 89 were positive and the remaining tested negative. When tested against 100 patients without disease X, 50 were negative and the remaining tested positive. What is the specificity of the new screening test?

   A. 89%
   B. 82%
   C. 64%
   D. 50%

6. In the above scenario (question 5), what is the negative predictive value of the new screening test?

   A. 89%
   B. 82%
   C. 64%
   D. 50%

7. A university research group has devised a novel therapy for disease X. In their research protocol, 300 patients with disease X were randomly assigned to either novel therapy or placebo therapy. Which of the following test is best to analyze if the novel therapy affects the 5-year survival rate?

   A. 1-sample t test
   B. Paired t test
   C. ANOVA
   D. Fisher exact test

8. In the above scenario (question 7), which of the following test is best to analyze whether the novel therapy affects the survival time in disease X patients versus nontreated patients?

   A. 1-sample t test
   B. Paired t test
   C. ANOVA
   D. Fisher exact test

9. What level of evidence would above scenario (question 7) provide?

   A. Level I
   B. Level II-1
   C. Level II-2
   D. Level II-3
   E. Level III

10. In the above scenario (question 7), the research group showed that patients with disease X has an increase in 5-year survival rate after novel therapy with P value >0.002. A research student decided to randomly take only 5 patient's results and calculated that the P value between the 5-year survival rate is actually 0.9 and concludes that there is no difference in 5-year survival rate between novel and placebo therapy. What statistical error is demonstrated?

    A. Bias error
    B. Standard error
    C. Type I error
    D. Type II error
    E. Type III error

ANSWERS

1. **Answer: A.** Mode is the most common value in the data set; in the above case, there are 6 value 1's.

2. **Answer: D.** Median is the value that divides the distribution of the data set. There are 17 numbers in the above data set; the 9th number (the middle number that divides the data set in half) in the above data set is 5. In case of even numbers of values in a data set, the mean of the 2 values that divide the data set would be the median. For example, the median of the data set 1, 1, 3, 5 would be $(1 + 3)/2 = 2$.

3. **Answer: B.** This is a case-control study; the study is predefining disease X cases versus nondisease X case and trying to identify possible risk factors.

4. **Answer: C.** Evidence from case-control studies is considered Level II-2.

5. **Answer: D.** After constructing 2 × 2 table based on the question stem, Specificity = true negative/(false positive + true negative) = 50/(50 + 50) = 50%.

6. **Answer: B.** After constructing 2 × 2 table based on the question stem, negative predictive value = true negative/(false negative + true negative) = 50/(11 + 50) = 82%.

7. **Answer: D.** Fisher exact test tests, if there is a statistical difference between the percentage of disease X patient who survived 5 years or not after the novel therapy versus placebo therapy. All other tests listed analyze quantitative data instead of categorical data sets.

8. **Answer: A.** 1-sample *t* test tests whether there is a statistical difference between the mean survival time of disease X patient after novel therapy treatment versus survival time of disease X patient in control group. Paired *t* test is to test for differences before and after treatment. ANOVA is used when there are more than 2 groups to be compared. Fisher exact tests are used for categorical data sets.

9. **Answer: A.** Evidence from randomized control study is considered Level I.

10. **Answer: D.** Type II error is failing to reject null hypothesis when alternative hypothesis is true. The null hypothesis for the experiment is to assume there is no difference in 5-year survival between novel therapy group and placebo group. The alternative hypothesis is that there is a difference. Type II error can be minimized by increasing sample size, such as shown by the *P* value from calculating the result of the 300-patient data set in the original research.

CHAPTER 32
Ethics and Professionalism

Robert D. Barraco and Stephen E. Lammers

ETHICS

PRINCIPLES

What is respect for autonomy?
When the patient has the capacity to act intentionally, with understanding, and without controlling influences that would mitigate against a free and voluntary act, surgeons ought to respect patient decisions, even when those decisions are different from the surgeon's recommendations.

What is beneficence?
The duty of health care providers is to benefit the patient and to bring about good for the patient.

What is nonmaleficence?
Health care providers may not intentionally create a needless harm or injury to the patient, through acts of commission or omission. In addition, health care providers ought to take positive steps to remove harm from the patient.

What is justice?
In our context, it is defined as a form of fairness. This implies the fair distribution of goods and services in society, which are in short supply; thus, some fair means of allocating scarce resources must be determined.

DECISION MAKING—SFNO APPROACH

What is the SFNO approach?
So Far No Objections = Stakeholders, Facts, Norms, Options

What are the 3 major sources of uncertainty in medical ethics decisions?
1. Different people are involved who have competing interests.
2. Uncertainty or disagreement exists about relevant facts.
3. Uncertainty, conflict, or disagreement exists regarding ethical norms.

Who are the stakeholders?

Those who will be affected by the decision made. It helps to state why people are stakeholders or how they are affected.

What are the facts?

They are factual issues that might generate disagreement or are relevant to a solution. It may be helpful to refer to the experts or the literature.

What are the norms?

They are ethical principles (see above), norms, or values that are at stake. Some may be relevant and others only appear to be. For assistance, reference can be made to professional ethical codes or regulations. Advice of colleagues should be sought when it is not clear what ethical principle or principles apply.

What defines the options?

They are actions or policies as well as compromises that deserve consideration for potential solutions. They may be best arrived at by group brainstorming with others.

JUSTIFYING ETHICAL DECISIONS

How do I justify an ethical decision?

It depends on the source of the disagreement.

If the source of the disagreement involves the competing interests of stakeholders, 2 questions must be asked:

1. Do ethically justified reasons exist for giving priority to the interests of one party over another?
2. Who is invested with decision-making authority?

If the source of the disagreement involves the facts in the widest sense of the word (benefit and harms of procedures or research, worldview beliefs), the resolutions differ. It is easiest if concerning facts where irrefutable data exist. When the facts concern probabilities, experts in given areas as well as existing literature may help. Other considerations here include quality of life, autonomous wishes, etc.

If the source of the disagreement involves ethical norms and values, goals must be clarified first.

How many types of norms are there to consider?

2: moral absolutes and prima facie norms. An example of a moral absolute is "it is wrong to kill a human for personal gain." Professional codes and laws often contain such norms. If a worthy goal conflicts with a moral absolute, the absolute trumps the goal. Prima facie norms express commitment to a value that deserves respect and should always be taken into account. Examples include confidentiality, or informed consent. Although these values should always be considered, there are circumstances where a breach of the norm is appropriate. An example includes the Tarasoff case, where a viable threat to another human being warrants the potential victim being informed.

PROFESSIONALISM

What is a profession?

An occupational group with internal ethical standards related to the primary goals of the profession.

What is professionalism?
It is "something that resides in the interface between the possession of specialized knowledge and a commitment to use that knowledge for the betterment of others." (Goode, 1969)
It is "aspiring toward altruism, accountability, excellence, duty, service, honor, integrity, and respect for others." (American Board of Internal Medicine, 1995)

CONCEPTS

What are the ACGME Core Competencies of Professionalism?
Resident should demonstrate:
- Respect, compassion, integrity, and altruism in their relationships with patients, families, and colleagues
- The ability to serve as patient's advocate
- Willingness to provide needed care regardless of ability to pay
- Avoidance of conflicts of interest
- Avoidance of inappropriate gifts

Residents should demonstrate knowledge of:
- The proscription against sexual relationships with patients
- Issues of impairment, including substance abuse
- Health care resources available in the community
- Health care needs of the community

What defines a conflict of interest?
A conflict of interest exists whenever a duty of a physician to a patient is in tension with some interest or interests of the physician. This might possibly adversely influence a physician's decisions or actions.

Name 3 types of conflicts of interests:
Financial—These include investments, gifts, and interactions with third-party payers.
Professional—These include multiple roles, that is, research and patient care, and dealing with impaired or inappropriate colleagues.
Personal—These include family, social, and other personal issues.

Name types of communication issues:
Delivering bad news
Truth telling about complications and bad outcomes
Obtaining informed consent

List issues of palliative care, death, and dying
Do Not Resuscitate (DNR) in the operating room
Advance directives
Futility
Withdrawing and withholding treatment
Euthanasia and physician-assisted suicide

What is an advance directive?
A health care power of attorney, living will, a written combination of these, or other written expression of a patient's wishes for treatment or the person(s) they want to make decisions for them.

What is futile treatment?
Any clinical circumstance in which the doctor and his/her consultants, consistent with the available medical literature, conclude that further treatment (except comfort care) cannot, within reasonable possibility, cure, improve, or restore a quality of life that would be beneficial to the patient.

What is euthanasia?
Decisions or acts that end the life of a patient suffering from an illness. Active euthanasia involves the use of lethal substances. Withholding of life-sustaining treatments is accepted in modern medical practice under the right circumstances.

What is physician-assisted suicide?
When a physician helps another person voluntarily end their life

What is confidentiality?
The duty of the physician to not disclose protected health information or information obtained in the delivery of health care

Are there cases where a breach of confidentiality is warranted?
Yes. They can include threat to specific individuals, reporting of issues such as child abuse to the authorities and to individuals assisting the care of the patient.
There may also be cases where patient behavior has the possibility of harming others, and different jurisdictions might authorize or mandate reporting these cases.

Name 3 situations of inappropriate breaches of confidentiality:
Discussing confidential information in public
Giving information to a colleague not caring for the patient for personal reasons
Leaving a hospital computer without logging out

What is an impaired physician?
This is defined by the American Medical Association as a physician unable to fulfill professional or personal responsibilities due to psychiatric illness, alcoholism, or drug dependency.

What is the Hidden Curriculum in medical training?
Day-to-day experiences that challenge or diminish professionalism in trainees

MULTIPLE CHOICE QUESTIONS

1. **An attending surgeon asks a resident to look up medical information on the attending's family member since the resident is logged in and has his computer open. The norm most at risk in this scenario involves:**
   A. Beneficence
   B. Justice
   C. HIPAA/Privacy
   D. Autonomy

2. **In response to the request in question 1, the best course of action for the resident should be:**
   A. Look up the data for the attending
   B. Log out of the network and allow the attending to login
   C. Look up the data then report the action to the program director
   D. D. Tell the medical student to look up the information

3. **A 60-year-old cirrhotic patient comes to the emergency room in severe septic shock and a perforated viscus and gross contamination. After massive fluid resuscitation and emergent source control, the patient's condition worsens. On maximal pressure support, his blood pressure continues to fall and you wish to call a family meeting. Which of the below are likely not stakeholders in this case to attend the meeting?**

   A. His wife
   B. His son
   C. His primary nurse
   D. His friend and neighbor

4. **In the case above, you believe cardiopulmonary resuscitation (CPR) would be futile. In this case, you should:**

   A. Give the family all treatment options and let them decide
   B. Tell them that CPR is not indicated, as it will only harm him
   C. Do not discuss CPR, as it is futile and you will not do CPR
   D. Do not discuss CPR, as you feel it will upset the family

5. **A 39-year-old motorcyclist is brought to the trauma center. He is obtunded, severely hypotensive, and has an open-book pelvic fracture, hemothorax, and multiple extremity fractures. He has lost a great deal of blood. Chest tube is inserted, a sheet is wrapped around his pelvis, and fractures are splinted. You receive information that someone told emergency medical services (EMS) he may be a Jehovah Witness. He will die without blood. What is not a fact in this case?**

   A. He is hemodynamically unstable
   B. He has life-threatening injuries
   C. He is a Jehovah Witness
   D. Practicing Jehovah Witnesses will not accept blood transfusions

6. **What is the best course of action for the patient?**

   A. Transfuse the patient
   B. Consult with elders in patient's community
   C. Consult with patient's spouse
   D. Do not give blood; he is a Jehovah Witness

7. **You are asked to consult on an 85-year-old male with moderate dementia for placement of a feeding tube in the OR. The patient is a DNR and does not have decisional capacity. The stakeholders do not include:**

   A. The medical student
   B. The surgeon
   C. The anesthesiologist
   D. The patient's son who is named in his advance directive as having health care decision power

8. **What is the best choice of action?**

   A. Honor the DNR order
   B. Refuse to do surgery w/o suspension of DNR order
   C. Negotiate a solution with the patient's son
   D. State that you are not obligated to honor the DNR order now that the patient is without capacity

9. **You find out during the preoperative work-up that one of your surgical clinic patients has HIV. He is married. You are concerned for his wife and other potential contacts. Who is not a stakeholder in this case?**
   A. The patient
   B. The wife
   C. You
   D. The state health authorities

10. **What is not an option in this case?**
    A. Encourage the patient to tell the wife and any other partners he can find
    B. Do nothing or you will be violating his confidentiality
    C. Inform the public health authorities if indicated per your local public health law
    D. If the patient does not do so, you inform his wife

ANSWERS

1. **Answer: C.** The resident does not know if the attending has patient's permission to see the results. Therefore, he could be violating the patient's privacy.

2. **Answer: B.** The best thing to do is offer your computer to the attending after logging out. Passing the buck to the medical student is not ethical and looking up the information is wrong, even if telling the program director.

3. **Answer: D.** Family and members of the health care team definitely should be present at the meeting. Unless the friend is designated power of attorney or there is some special reason, the friend does not need to be there.

4. **Answer: B.** The family should not be given options that the team feels are not helpful and are harmful. The issue must be discussed. CPR will not help a patient in this circumstance, and telling them so is your duty.

5. **Answer: C.** We do not know for sure the patient is a Jehovah Witness. It is hearsay.

6. **Answer: A.** The best course of action is to transfuse the patient and save his life with no other information to confirm or deny his religious status in this emergent situation.

7. **Answer: A.** The medical student does not have a stake in the decision but may want to be present to learn.

8. **Answer: C.** The best course of action is to negotiate a solution with the patient's son.

9. **Answer: D.** The patient, his wife, and you have a stake in the course of action chosen from the options. The state health authorities, though perhaps requiring reporting, do not have a direct stake in the discussion.

10. **Answer: B.** In this case, a breach of privacy and confidentiality is permitted to prevent serious, deadly harms to others.

INDEX

Page numbers followed by *f* and *t* indicate figures and tables, respectively.

A

AAAs grow. *See* Abdominal aortic aneurysms (AAAs) grow
Abdominal aortic aneurysms (AAAs) grow, 341
  rate of growth, 341
  retroperitoneal approach, 343
Abdominal colectomy, 275
Abdominal esophagus, 226
  arterial blood supply, 226
  venous drainage of, 227
Abdominal wall, 155–171
  anatomy, 155–157, 155*f*
  defects, 355
  desmoid tumor, 159
  diseases, 158–161
  doom borders, triangle of, 164
  layers of, 155
  malignancy, 159
  muscular layers of, 162*f*
  pain, triangle of, 164–167
  physiology, 157–158
  sarcoma, 159, 160
Abdominal x-ray (AXR), 253, 359
ABO system *vs.* HLA system, 1
Abscess complicating diverticulitis, 268
Acetylcholine, 177
ACGME core competencies of professionalism, 451
Achalasia, 48, 232*f*
  characteristics of, 231
  diagnosis of, 231
  pathogenesis of, 232
  symptoms for, 232
Acid-base disturbance, 145
ACTH-producing tumor, 146
ACTH stimulation test. *See* Adrenocorticotropic hormone (ACTH) stimulation test
Actin, 2
Actinomyces infection, 39
Acute mesenteric lymphadenitis, 160
Acute suppurative thyroiditis, treatment for, 133
Adenine, 2
Adenocarcinomas, 183
Adenoma, surgical treatment of, 257
Adenomatous gastric polyp, 183
Adenomatous polyposis coli (APC) mutation, 274
Adenomatous polyps, 182
Adhesion molecules, desmosomes/hemidesmosomes, 1
Adhesions, 255
Adjuvant therapy, 123, 149
Adrenal carcinoma, 89

Adrenal cortex, 145
  zona fasciculata, 145
  zona glomerulosa, 145
  zona reticularis, 145
Adrenal gland, 144–150
  adrenal insufficiency, 148
  adrenal tumors, 145–148
  adrenocortical carcinoma, pheochromocytoma, and MEN, 149–150
  anatomy and physiology, 144–145
Adrenal insufficiency, 148, 316
Adrenal mass, workup of, 145
Adrenal pheochromocytoma, 150
Adrenals, anatomy of, 144*f*
Adrenal tumor, 82
Adrenocortical suppression, 56
Adrenocorticotropic hormone (ACTH) stimulation test, 316
Adson test, 395
AF. *See* Atrial fibrillation (AF)
Aflatoxins, 85
AIDS, 262
  intestinal manisfestation, 40
  protozoal infection, 262
Air embolus, 310
Airway obstruction, 367
AJCC cancer staging, 119
AJCC Cancer Staging Manual, 183, 184
AJCC TNM staging system, 276, 277
  in colorectal, 275–277
AJCC TNM Staging System for Colorectal Cancer, 275
Albright syndrome, 392
Albumin, half-life of, 75, 191
Aldosterone
  renin ratio, 145
  suppression test, 145
  to-cortisol ratio, 146
Alemtuzumab, 26
Alkali ingestion, 237
Allen test, 385
Allograft nephropathy, 27
ALND, potential complications of, 115
Alternative hormonal/chemotherapy, 123
Alveolar hypoventilation, 59
Amebiasis, 195
Amebic abscess, treatment of, 195
American Cancer Society guidelines, 272
Amino acids, 73, 99
  transamination, 72
p-Aminobenzoic acid, 57

Aminoglycoside, resistance, 43
Aminoglycosides, mechanism of action, 41
Amphotericin B, mechanism of action, 39
Amsterdam criteria, 87
Amyand hernia, 166
Anal agenesis, 370
Anaphylactic shock, 194
Anaplastic thyroid carcinoma, 135
  prognosis for, 135
  treatment for, 135
Ancrod, 19
Anesthesia, 55–62
Anesthetics, local, 52
  mechanism of action, 57
Angiographic embolization, 299
Anion gap acidosis, 71
Annular pancreas, 374
Anocutaneous fistula, 370
Anomalies, VACTERL group of, 361
Anorectal agenesis, 370
Anterolateral thoracotomy, 348
Anteroposterior compression, 303
Anterosuperior mediastinum, 397, 399
Anthracycline containing chemotherapeutic
      regimens, 400
Antibiotics
  antibiotics/mechanism of action, 41–43
  antifungal, 39
  hepatitis/HIV/TB, 40–41
  mechanism of action, 41–43
  spontaneous bacterial peritonitis, 39–40
  wounds, 37–39
Anticoagulants, 13, 51
Anticoagulation, 18–19
  treatment, 19
Anti-D immune globulin, 434
Antiemetics, categories, 48
Antifungal, 39
Antihyperthyroid agents, 50
Antilymphocyte globulins, 24
Antimicrobial soak, 329
Antiplatelets, 51
Aortic dissection, classification of, 340
Aortic regurgitation, 310
APC gene, 274, 275
Apnea, life-threatening episodes of, 360
Apocrine sweat glands, 39
Apoptosis, 6
Apoptosis pathways, simplified view, 5*f*
Argatroban, 19
Arimidex/Femara, 123
Aromatase inhibitors, 123, 124
Arterial supply
  to cervix, 430
  to uterus, 429
Ascitic fluid protein, 40
Aspergillus species, 197
Astrocytomas, brain tumors, 423

Asystole/pulseless electrical activity, 313
Atonic bladder, 267
Atrial fibrillation (AF)
  management algorithm for, 314
  without hemodynamic instability, 314
Atrial natruretic factor, 319
Auditory ossicle bones, 103
Axial skin flap, 384
Axilla, boundaries of, 114
Axillary artery injury, 412
Axillary dissection, 115
Axillary lymph node groups, 114
AXR. *See* Abdominal x-ray (AXR)

B
Babygram, 357
Bactericidal antimicrobial agents, 41
Bactrim, mechanism of action, 42
Barium esophagram, 236
Barrett esophagus, 235, 239
Basal cell carcinoma, 379
  margins, 379
  morpheaform type, 379
  physical findings, 379
Basilar skull fracture, 283
Bassini repair, 167
Benign biliary disease, in hepatobiliary, 192–194
Benign chest wall tumors, 392
Benign esophageal disease, 225
Benign liver disease, in hepatobiliary, 194–197
Benign liver lesions, 195*f*
Benign liver tumor, 196
Benign neoplasm, 206
Benzodiazepine (BZ), 58
Bernard Soulier disease, treatment for, 18
Bevacizumab (Avastin), 277
Bilateral adrenalectomy, 143
Bile acids, 191, 249
Bile salts, 73, 192, 249
Biliary atresia, 373
Biliary tract disease, 158
BILIOUS vomiting
  malrotation, 357
  in newborn, 357
BIRADS. *See* Breast Imaging Reporting and
      Data System (BIRADS)
Black pigmented stones, 191
Bleeding disorder, 17
Bleeding time, 13
Bleeding, treatment of, 282
Blind loop syndrome, 261
  duodenal diverticula, complications of, 258
  manifestation, 260
Blood-borne organism, 40
Blood product contamination, 15
Blood, types, 16
Bloody diarrhea, 343
Bochdalek hernia, 166

Body fluid
  compartments, 63
    chemical composition, 64
  percentage, 63
Bone-to-bone contact, fracture, 304
Borchardt triad, 181
Bougienage, 236
Brachial plexus injuries, 395
Bradycardia, 313
Brain
  CO, percentage of, 310
  injury, 283
Branchial cleft cyst, 362
BRCA II mutation, 86
BRCA I mutation, 86
BRCA2 mutations, 121
Breast, 113–129
  anatomy/physiology, 113–115
  arterial supply to, 114
  cancer, 117–124
  diagnosis, 126
  embryologic structure, 113
  nodes in, 114
  screening/imaging, 115–117
  self-examination, 115
Breast biopsy
  indications for, 120
  sites of metastasis for, 120
Breast cancer, 86–87, 116*f*, 117–124
  common site, 119
  mammography for, 116
  percentage of, 115
  prognosis for, 121
  screening recommendations for, 115
  staging factor, 119
  type of, 124
  ultrasound, 117*f*
Breast-conserving therapy, contraindications for, 122
Breast Imaging Reporting and Data System
    (BIRADS), 116
Breast irradiation, complications of, 122
Breast lesion, 126
Breast reconstruction, postmastectomy, 384
Breath, with exertion, chest pain/shortness, 367
Breslow thickness, 380
Bromocriptine, 423
Bronchi, segmental anatomy of, 390*f*
Brown pigmented stones, 192
Brown-Séquard syndrome, 286
Brush border enzyme, 248
Budd-Chiari syndrome, causes of, 195
Bupivacaine, side effect, 57
Burkell classification, 398
Burns, 325
  classification, 325–326
  estimating extent, 327*f*
  fluid resuscitation, 328
  hydrofluoric acid, 330

  inhalation injury, 329–330
  injury, 326
  miscellaneous, 330–331
  pathophysiology, 326
  resuscitation formulas, 328*t*
  rules of nines, 327
  treatment of, 328–329, 329*f*
  wounds, evaluation of, 326–328
Butterfly fragment, 409
BZ. *See* Benzodiazepine (BZ)

C
Cadaveric kidney transplant, 27
Calcitonin, 140
Calcium gluconate, hydrofluoric acid burn
    treatment, 331
Calorie, requirement, 72
Cancer, 134–138
  cells, 73
  death, 87
  lung (*See* Lung cancer)
  thyroid (*See* Thyroid cancer)
  type of, 105
  viruses causes, 85
Cantrell pentology, 368
Caput medusae, 196
Carbapenems, 42
Carbohydrate digestion, 248
Carbon monoxide diffusing capacity, 391
Carboxypeptidase A, primary action of, 249
Carboxypeptidase B, primary action of, 249
Carcinogenesis, 85–86
Cardiac index (CI), 309
Cardiac output (CO), 309
Cardiac tamponade, 293
Cardiopulmonary bypass, 19
Cardiovascular failure, treatment of, 318*t*
Carotid sheath, 103
Carotid surgery, 103
Carpal tunnel syndrome, 385
Cartilaginous fractures, 290
Case-control studies, 443
Caspofungin, mechanism of action, 39
Castleman disease, 400
Catheter tip culture, 38
Caustic injury, 238
CBD diameter, 190
CBD stones, 193
Cecal bascule, 269
Cecal (cecocolic) volvulus, 269
  abdominal radiographs, 270
  treatment for, 270
Cefazolin, mechanism of action, 43
Cefotaxime, 40
Cell biology, 1–10
  cell cycle, 7–8
  cell structures, 2
  cell transport, 6

Cell biology (*Cont'd.*)
  cellular energy, 6–7
  cell wall, 1
  genetics, 2–4
  receptors and signals, 5–6
Cell-cell occluding junctions, 1
Cell, component, 2
Cell cycle, 7–8, 81–82, 81*f*
  control system, 8*f*
  part of, 7
Cell death. *See* Apoptosis
Cell membrane, lipid classes, 1
Cell structures, 2
Cell transport, type of, 6
Cellular energy, 6–7
Cell wall, capacitance in, 1
Central cord syndrome, 286
Central nervous system disease, 179
  anesthesia, 51–52
Central pontine myelinolysis, 67
Central/subareolar tumors, 120
Central venous catheter placement,
    complications, 310
Central venous pressure (CVP), 309
Cephalosporins, mechanism of action, 42
Cerebral perfusion pressure (CPP), 284
Cerebrospinal fluid (CSF), 107
  rhinorrhea, 38, 39
Cervical esophagus, 226
Cervical lymph nodes, regions of, 105
Cervical spine ligamentous injury, 283
Cetuximab (Erbitux), 277
CFUs. *See* Colony-forming units (CFUs)
Chance fracture, 410
Chemical carcinogenesis, 85
Chemokines, 24
Chemotherapeutic agents, 89, 207
  Classification of, 90*t*
Chemotherapeutic regimens, 122
Chemotherapeutics, 89–90
Chemotherapy, 277
Chest radiography, 392
Chest wall
  conditions, 391–394
  trauma, 291, 293
Childhood protein-energy malnutrition, 74
Chloramphenicol, mechanism of action, 42
Cholangiocarcinoma, 197
Cholecystokinin, 250, 251
Choledochal cyst, 193, 194
Cholelithiasis, diagnosis of, 192
Chondromas, 392, 393
Chondrosarcoma, 393
CHOP regimen, 90
Choriocarcinoma/testicular cancer, 82
Chromium deficiency, 75
Chromosomes, 82, 274
Chronic liver rejection, 29

Chronic lung rejection, 32
Chvostek sign, 69
Chylomicron, composition of, 249
Chylous ascites, 157
Chylous effusion, 239
Chymotrypsin, primary action, 248
CI. *See* Cardiac index (CI)
Circle of death, 164
Cisatracurium, 57
Cisplatin-based chemotherapy, 400
Claudication, 51
Clay shoveller fracture, 410
Clindamycin, mechanism of action, 43
Closed loop obstruction, 270
Clotting disorders, treatment, 16–18
Clotting time, 19
CO. *See* Cardiac output (CO)
Coagulation factors, 192
Coagulation pathway, 11–12
  extrinsic pathway, 12*f*
  intrinsic pathway, 11
  schematic, 11*f*
Cobalamin (B_{12}) deficiency, 75
Coldness, thoracic outlet syndrome, 395
Collagen
  accumulation, 96
  type of, 98
Colon cancer, 82, 87
  diagnosis of, 275
Colonic diverticulosis, 268
Colonic polyps, 274
Colonic pseudo-obstruction, 270, 271
Colon pharmacology, 49
Colony-forming units (CFUs), 37
Colorectal
  AJCC TNM staging system, 275–277
  anatomy and physiology, 265–268
  Crohn disease, 272–273
  diverticulitis, 268–269
  familial adenomatous polyposis
    (FAP), 274
  infectious and ischemic colitis, 273
  Lynch syndromes (hereditary nonpolyposis
    colon cancer), 273
  obstruction, 270–271
  polyps and colon cancer, 274–275
  ulcerative colitis, 271–272
  volvulus, 269–270
Compartment syndrome, acute, 414
Compound fractures, 409
Computed tomography (CT) imaging, 196
Concentric muscle bundles, 227
Concomitant neurologic/vascular injury, 304
Congenital bleeding disorder, 17
Congenital diverticulum, 258
Congenital hemolytic anemia, 217
Congenital hernia, 160
Constipation, definition of, 268

Continuous intravenous infusion, drug administration by, 47
Continuous positive airway pressure, 321
Continuous renal replacement therapy
    advantages of, 315
    disadvantages of, 316
Convergence point, 12
Cooper hernia, 166
Copper deficiency, 75
Cord lipoma, 163
Cori cycle, 6
Corrosive ingestion, 238
Corticotropin-releasing hormone (CRH) stimulation test, 148
Cortisol secretion, 148
Cosyntropin test, 50
Couinaud's liver segments, 189, 190f
CPP. See Cerebral perfusion pressure (CPP)
Cremaster muscle, 163
Crescent-shaped deformity, 286
CRH stimulation test. See Corticotropin-releasing hormone (CRH) stimulation test
Cricothyroid muscle, 132
Cricothyroidotomy, 282
Crigler–Najjar syndrome, 192
Critical care, 309–321
    acid/base physiology, 315
    arrhythmias, 313–314
    cardiac physiology, 311–312
    hemodynamic parameters, 309–310
    invasive monitoring, 310–311
    pulmonary physiology, 319–321
    renal physiology, 315–316
    sepsis, 319
    shock, 312–313
    vasoactive agents, 317–319
    ventilator management, 319–321
Crohn disease, 255, 256
    in colorectal, 272–273
    indications for surgery, 272
    massive bleeding from, 272
    sites of occurrence, 256
Cross-links fibrin, 12
Cryoprecipitate, 16
CSF. See Cerebrospinal fluid (CSF)
χ^2 test, 444
Cul-de-sac of douglas, 430
Cushing syndrome
    diagnosis of, 146, 147f
    signs/symptoms of, 144
CVP. See Central venous pressure (CVP)
Cyanide toxicity, treatment, 317

D
Daptomycin, mechanism of action, 42
DA receptors. See Dopamine (DA) receptors
Daunorubicin, 89
DCIS. See Ductal carcinoma in situ (DCIS)

DDT. See Dichlorodiphenyltrichloroethane (DDT)
Deep inferior epigastric artery perforator flap (DIEP), 384
    blood supply, 385
Demerol, metabolite, 58
De Quervain thyroiditis, 133
Desmoid tumor, 161
Desmopressin, 17
Dexamethasone, 316
    brain tumors, 423
    suppression test, 146, 148
Dextrose, 66
Diabetes, diagnosis of, 207
Diabetes, type 1, 30
Diagnostic peritoneal lavage (DPL), 295
Dialysis, 315
Dialysis–associated peritonitis, 157
Diaphoresis, 292
Diaphragm, 158
Diaphragmatic hernia, 355, 360, 361, 362
Diaphragmatic tears, 295
Diarrhea, definition of, 268
Diastasis recti, 159f
Dichlorodiphenyltrichloroethane (DDT), 149
DIC, treatment, 18
DIEP. See Deep inferior epigastric artery perforator flap (DIEP)
Dieulafoy lesion, 180, 181
Diffuse axonal injury, 423
Diffuse esophageal spasm, treatment for, 233
Dihydroxyphenylalanine (DOPA), 144
Distal cholangiocarcinoma, surgical management, 197
Distal pancreatic injury, treatment for, 298
Distal perfusion, 289
Distal rectosigmoid colon, 370
Diverticulitis
    in colorectal, 268–269
    Hinchey classification grading system for, 269
DNA, packaging, 4
DNR. See Do not resuscitate (DNR)
Dobutamine, 317
Donor-reactive antibodies, 33
Do not resuscitate (DNR), 451
DOPA. See Dihydroxyphenylalanine (DOPA)
Dopamine (DA) receptors, 317
Double bubble sign, 357
    abdominal radiograph, 357f
Double-stranded helical DNA, 2
Down syndrome, 355
Doxorubicin, 89
DPL. See Diagnostic peritoneal lavage (DPL)
Drugs, 132
    half-life, 48
    properties, 47
Dubin-Johnson syndrome, 191
Ductal carcinoma in situ (DCIS), 117
Duct of Santorini, 203
Duct of Wirsung, 203

Ductogram, 125f
Ducts of Luschka, 191
Dumbbell tumors, 398
Duodenal atresia, 357
Duodenal diverticulum, 258
Duodenojejunostomy, 262
Duodenum, 245
  injury scale, 296
  portions of, 248
  vascular supply of, 248
Dysplasia, 235

E
EA. *See* Esophageal atresia (EA)
Early-stage gastric MALT lymphoma, 186
Echinococcal cyst, 194
Ectopic gastric mucosa, 259
EDV. *See* End-diastolic volume (EDV)
EGD. *See* Esophagogastroduodenoscopy (EGD)
EGFR. *See* Epidermal growth factor
    receptor (EGFR)
Elastase, primary action of, 249
Elective laparoscopic cholecystectomy, 193
Electrocautery, 380
Electrolytes, 66–71
  composition, 65
  loss, 65
Eloesser flap, 397
Empty sella syndrome, 143
Empyema, 397
End-diastolic volume (EDV), 311
Endocrine, 131–153
  adrenal gland, 144–150
  cancer, 134–138
  drugs, 132
  hyperthyroidism/hypothyroidism and goiters,
      132–134
  parathyroid gland, 138–142
  pituitary gland, 142–143
  thyroid, 131–132
Endocrine pharmacology, 50
Endocrine tumors, surgical management, 210
Endoleak, four types of, 342f
Endometriosis, etiology of, 436
Endopelvic fascia, 267
Endoscopic retrograde cholangiopancreatography
    (ERCP)-induced pancreatitis, 192
Endotracheal tube (ETT)
  optimal distance, 55
Endovascular aneurysm repair (EVAR), 342
Entamoeba histolytica, 373
Enteric nervous system, 175
Enterocutaneous fistula, 259
  management of, 260
Enteroglucagon, 252
Eosinophilic granuloma, 393
Epidermal growth factor receptor (EGFR), 277
Epidural anesthesia

  advantage, 58
  side effects of, 58
Epidural catheter, 58
Epinephrine, 317
Epiphrenic diverticulum, 229, 229f
Epiphysis, 416
Epistaxis, 107
Epithelialization, 96, 97
Epstein-Barr virus, 86
ER. *See* Estrogen receptor (ER)
Erythromycin
    mechanism of action, 43
Esophageal atresia (EA), 361
Esophageal cancer, 239
Esophageal carcinoma, 232
Esophageal foreign body, 108
Esophageal injury, 237
Esophageal stricture, 239
Esophageal varices bleeding, 48
Esophageal web, 236
Esophagectomy, complications of, 239
Esophagogastroduodenoscopy (EGD), 180
Esophagus, 225–243
    acid/alkali injuries, 237–239
    anatomical narrowing, 227
    anatomy, 225–227
    arterial blood supply of, 225f
    benign disease, 231–237
    diverticulum, 228–231
        linear stapler, 231f
    layers of, 225
    malignant disease, 239
    peristaltic contractions, 228
    physiology, 227–228
    sympathetic innervation, 227
    tertiary contractions of, 228
    venous drainage of, 226f
Esophagus pharmacology, 48
Estrogen receptor (ER), 120
Estrogen replacement therapy, 86
Ethics
    decision making, SFNO approach, 449–450
    justifying decisions, 450
    principles, 449
    and professionalism, 450–451
ETT. *See* Endotracheal tube (ETT)
Eukaryotic gene expression, control, 3f
Euvolemic hyponatremia
    causes of, 66
    treatment of, 66
EVAR. *See* Endovascular aneurysm
        repair (EVAR)
Evidences levels, 444
Ewing sarcoma, 393
    malignant chest wall tumor, 393
Exploratory laparotomy/laparoscopy, 238, 239
External carotid artery, 104
Extracellular buffering system, 71

Extracellular fluid, 63
Extracorporeal circulation, 19
Extrafascial hysterectomy, 438

F
Facial nerve, 103
Factitious hyperinsulinemia, 209
Factors VII/X, deficiencies, 18
Factor V Leiden, 14
Familial adenomatous polyposis (FAP)
    in colorectal, 274
    syndrome, treatment of, 274
Familial juvenile polyposis, 274
Familial osteochondromatosis, 393
FAP. *See* Familial adenomatous polyposis (FAP)
Fasciocutaneous flap, 384
FAST. *See* Focused abdominal sonography for
    trauma (FAST)
Fatigue, thoracic outlet syndrome, 395
Fatty acids deficiency, 76
FDS. *See* Flexor digitorum superficialis (FDS)
Felty syndrome, 218
Female pelvis, avascular spaces of, 430*f*
Femoral canal, boundaries of, 163
Femoral hernias, 162, 163
Fetal circulation, 367
FFP, 17, 16
Fibrinogen, 12
Fibroblasts, filament in, 2
Fibromuscular dysplagia (FMD), 345
Fine-needle aspiration (FNA), 126
Finger fracture, 298
First-order kinetics, 47
Fisher exact test, 444
Flexor digitorum superficialis (FDS), 385
Fluids, 63–66
Flumazenil, 58
Fluoroquinolone, resistance, 43
FMD. *See* Fibromuscular dysplagia (FMD)
FNA. *See* Fine-needle aspiration (FNA)
FNH. *See* Focal nodular hyperplasia (FNH)
Focal nodular hyperplasia (FNH), 189, 196
Focused abdominal sonography for trauma
    (FAST), 295
Folate deficiency, 76
FOLFOX, 277
Follicle-associated epithelium, 250
Follicular cancer, malignancy in, 136
Follicular thyroid carcinoma, distant metastasis
    for, 136
Forced vital capacity (FVC), 319
Fractures, types of, 409–411
FRC. *See* Functional residual capacity (FRC)
Free flap failure, 384
FTSG, 383
Functional residual capacity (FRC), 320
Funnel chest, 391
FVC. *See* Forced vital capacity (FVC)

G
GABA receptor, 51
Gallbladder, 193
    parasympathetic innervation, 191
Gallstones, classification, 191
Galveston formula, 328
Ganglioneuroma, paravertebral region, 398
Gardner syndrome, 274
Gastric analysis, 177
Gastric cancer, 183
Gastric carcinoma, resections, 184–185
Gastric lymphoma, treatment for, 186
Gastric mucosa, 180
Gastric mucosal interneurons, 176
Gastric ulcer, Johnson classification for, 179*f*
Gastric ulcers, 178
Gastric volvulus, 181, 182
    diaphragmatic defect, 182
Gastrinomas, 209
Gastrin-releasing peptide, 251
Gastroesophageal (GE) junction, 174, 227
Gastroesophageal reflux disease (GERD), 360
    management of, 360
    preoperative evaluation, 360
Gastrointestinal pharmacology, 48–50
    colon, 49
    esophagus, 48
    intra-OP, 49
    pancreas, 49–50
    small bowel, 49
    stomach, 48–49
Gastrointestinal stromal tumor (GIST), 49, 91,
    173, 186, 257
    adjuvant therapy, 186
Gastrointestinal (GI) tract, 265
Gastroschisis, 355, 359
GE junction. *See* Gastroesophageal (GE) junction
Genetics, 2–4
Gentamicin, 43
GERD. *See* Gastroesophageal reflux disease (GERD)
GFR. *See* Glomerular filtration rate (GFR)
GI bleeding, 372
    secondary, 373
GIST. *See* Gastrointestinal stromal tumor (GIST)
GI tract, 182
    lymphoma in, 185
Glanzmann thrombocytopenia, 18
Glasgow coma scale (GCS) score, 281
Glioblastoma multiforme, 423
Glomerular filtration rate (GFR), 26
Glottic squamous cell carcinoma, 106
Glucagonoma, 208, 209
    diagnosis of, 208
    localization of, 208
Glucocorticoids
    anti-inflammatory effects, 26
Gluconeogenesis, 72
Glucose molecule, 6

Glycoprotein, 248
  antigen, 437
Gonadotropic hormone, 143
G6PD deficiency, 217
GpIb receptor, 12
Granular pneumocytes, 390
Graves disease
  etiology of, 132
  treatment for, 133
Greenstick fracture, 302
Grynfeltt triangle, 166
Guanine, 2
Gunshot wound, 413
Gustilo-Anderson classification, 412, 412*t*
Gut-associated lymphoid tissue, 250
Gynecology
  adnexal masses, differential diagnosis for, 435
  BRCA gene mutations, 437
  CA 125 tumor marker, 437
  cherney incision, 438
  conditions and complications, 435–438
  endometrial stroma and glands, 435
  endometriosis
    clinical features, 436
    etiology of, 436
  maylard incision, 438
  menopause, age, 436
  ovarian cancer, surgical staging/therapy, 437
  pfannenstiel, 438
  postmenopausal bleeding, differential, 436
  pregnancy (*See* Pregnant patient)
  ureteral injuries locations, operations, 438
  vertical midline incision, 438

H
Hairy cell leukemia, first-line therapy for, 218
Halo sign, 283
Hangman fracture, 410
Hashimoto thyroiditis, treatment for, 133
HCC. *See* Hepatocellular carcinoma (HCC)
Head, 103–111
  anatomy, 103–105
  infections, 108
  trauma, 107–108
  tumors, 105–107
Heart, CO percentage of, 310
Heart rate (HR), 312
Heart transplant, 31
  contraindications for, 31
  indications for, 31
  rejection, 31
Heimlich valve, 398
Heinz bodies, 218
Helicobacter pylori, 49
HELLP syndrome, 433
Hemarthrosis, treatment for, 17
Hematocrit, 18
Hematology, 11–21

  anticoagulation, 18–19
  clotting disorders and treatment, 16–18
  coagulation pathway, 11–12
  hypercoagulability disorders, 14
  laboratory tests and data, 13–14
  platelet function and dysfunction, 14–15
  red blood cell/blood products, 15–16
Hemispheric neurologic deficit, 289
Hemobilia, 299
  common cause, 194
  first-line therapy, 194
  test to rule, 194
Hemodynamic instability, atrial fibrillation with, 313
Hemolytic transfusion reaction, 16
Hemophilia A, preoperative treatment, 17
Hemophilia B, 17
Hemoptysis, treatment for, 310
Hemorrhagic shock, signs/symptoms, 312
Hemostasis, biology, 13
Henderson-Hasselbalch equation, 71
Heparin, 14, 18
Hepatectomy, 189
Hepatic adenomas, 196
Hepatic blood flow, 190
Hepatic gluconeogenesis, 7*f*
Hepatic hemangioma, 196
Hepatic portoenterostomy, 30
Hepatic resection, nomenclature/anatomy, 190*f*
Hepatic tumor, 197
Hepatic vein injury, 299
Hepatic veins, 190
Hepatitis B vaccination, 40
Hepatitis B virus (HBV) hepatitis, 196
Hepatitis/HIV/TB, 40–41
Hepatobiliary, 189–202
  anatomy, 189–191
  benign biliary disease, 192–194
  benign liver disease, 194–197
  malignant hepatobiliary disease, 197–198
  physiology, 191–192
Hepatocellular carcinoma (HCC)
  cause of, 197
  diagnosis of, 197
  treatment, 197
Hepatocellular disease, 12
Hepatoduodenal ligament, 189
HER-2. *See* Human epidermal growth factor
    receptor 2 (HER-2)
Herceptin (trastuzumab), mechanism of action, 87
Hereditary cancer, genes associated with, 83*t*–84*t*
Hereditary Nonpolyposis Colorectal Cancer
    (HNPCC), 273
  diagnosis of, 273
  screening recommendations for, 273
Hernias, 161–164, 237*f*, 259
  hernia repair, 167–168
  hydrocele, 368
  types of, 161

HER-2–positive breast cancer, 123
Hesselbach hernia, 166
Hesselbach triangle, 156, 156*f*, 162
Heterotopic kidney transplant, 26
Hiatal hernia, 237
Hidradenitis, treatment for, 381
Hinchey classification grading system, 269
Hindgut, 265
Hirschsprung disease, 370, 371, 372
    surgical correction of, 372
Hirudin, 19
Histamine, release, 58
HIV
    postexposure prophylaxis for, 40
    risk of transmission, 40
Hodgkin lymphoma, 400
Hoffman elimination, 47
Homan sign, 346
Homograft, 329
Hormonal therapy, 86
Hormone gastrin, 250
Hormone receptors, 86
Hormones, function of, 113
Howell-Jolly bodies, 218
Howship-Romberg sign, 166
H pylori
    duodenal ulcers, 178
    gastric ulcers, 178
HR. *See* Heart rate (HR)
Human epidermal growth factor receptor 2
        (HER-2), 121
    does overexpression, 87
    neu receptor, 86
Human neoplasia, 275
Humeral shaft fractures, 304
Hurthle cell carcinoma, 136
Hydatid cysts
    injection, 194
    percutaneous management, 194
    recurrence rate of, 195
    surgical options for, 194
Hydatid disease
    cause of, 194
    diagnosis of, 194
Hydrochloric acid, production, 177
Hydrofluoric acid burn, treatment of, 330
    calcium gluconate, 331
Hydroxylation, 98
Hyperaldosteronism, 145, 146
Hyperbilirubinemia, cause of, 191, 192
Hypercalcemia, treatment, 50
Hypercoagulability
    cause, 14
    disorders, 14
Hyperesthesia, cause of, 115
Hypergastrinemia, 176
Hyperglycemia, 30
Hyperkalemia

    causes of, 69
    EKG findings, 69
    signs and symptoms, 69
    treatment for, 69
Hypermagnesemia
    causes of, 70
    signs and symptoms, 71
Hypernatremia
    causes of, 67
    signs and symptoms, 67
Hyperparathyroidism, 139, 141
    chloride:phosphate ratio, 140
    type of, 140
Hyperphosphatemia
    causes of, 71
    signs and symptoms, 71
Hyperpigmentation, 274
Hyperplastic polyps, 182, 274
Hypersplenism, definition of, 217
Hypertensive LES
    findings with, 234
    treatment of, 234
Hyperthyroid conditions, 132
Hyperthyroidism, cause of, 132
Hyperthyroidism/hypothyroidism and goiters,
        132–134
Hypertrophic scar, treatment for, 381
Hyperventilation, 75
Hypervolemic hyponatremia, treatment of, 67
Hypocalcemia
    causes, 69
    EKG findings, 70
    mnemonic for, 70
    signs and symptoms, 69, 70
    treatment of, 70
Hypogastric, 429
Hypoglossal nerve, 103
Hypokalemia
    causes of, 67
    EKG findings, 67
    signs/symptoms, 67
    treatment for, 67
Hypomagnesemia
    causes of, 70
    signs and symptoms, 70
    treatment for, 70
Hyponatremia
    signs/symptoms, 66
    types, 66
Hypoparathyroidism, cause of, 142
Hypoparathyroid tetany, 50
Hypophosphatemia
    causes of, 71
    signs and symptoms of, 71
    treatment for, 71
Hypoproteinemic hypertrophic gastropathy, 186
Hypotension, treatment for, 58
Hypothyroidism, cause of, 133

Hypovolemic hyponatremia
 causes of, 66
 treatment of, 66
Hysterectomy, types, 438

I

Idiopathic thrombocytopenic purpura (ITP),
  215, 216
 first-line therapy, 216
 splenectomy for, 216
IgM, 216
Ileal carcinoids metastasize, 257
Ileocolic intussusception, 365
Ileum, 245
Ileus
 causes of, 255
 treatment for, 255
Iliac aneurysms, 343
Iliofemoral DVT, 347
Immunology
 graft and patient survival and complication
    rates, 27–28
 heart transplant, 31
 immunosuppressants, 24–26
 interferons and chemokines, 24
 interleukins, 23–24
 intestinal transplantation, 32
 liver disease, Child-Turcotte-Pugh score, 30
 liver transplantation, 29–30
 lung transplant, 32
 pancreas tranplant, 30–31
 potpourri, 32–33
 rejection after renal transplant, 27
 renal transplant, 26–27
Immunosuppressants, 24–26
Immunosuppressive drugs, 25t
Immunosuppressive regimen, 24
Imperforate anus, female, 370f
Incisional hernia, 165
Induction agent, 56
Ineffective esophageal motility, 234, 235
Infections
 and antibiotics, 37–46
  antibiotics/mechanism of action, 41–43
  antifungal, 39
  hepatitis/HIV/TB, 40–41
  spontaneous bacterial peritonitis, 39–40
  wounds, 37–39
 development, 37
 in head and neck, 108
 signs and symptoms, 38
Infectious and ischemic colitis, in colorectal, 273
Infectious diseases, types, 15
Inferior epigastric artery, 430
Inferior mesenteric artery, 267
Inferior vena cava, 429
Inflammation, 158
 signs and symptoms, 38

Inflammatory disease, 160
Infraumbilical lymphatic vessels, 158
Inguinal hernias, 161, 165
Inhalational agent, 55, 56
Inspiratory capacity, 320
Insulinomas, 209
 diagnosis of, 209
 surgical procedure of, 209
Interferon-α, β, 24
Interferon-γ, 24
Interferons, 24
Interleukins, 23–24
Intermittent hemodialysis
 advantages of, 315
 disadvantages of, 316
Internal carotid artery, 103
Intestinal anastomosis, techniques of, 358
Intestinal ischemia, form of, 273
Intestinal obstruction, cardinal symptoms, 253
Intestinal pacemaker cell, 257
Intestinal strangulation, signs of, 254
Intestinal transplantation, 32
Intra-abdominal abscess, 255
Intra-aortic balloon pump, ECG, 311
Intraductal papilloma, treatment for, 125
Intrahepatic cholangiocarcinoma, management
  of, 197
Intrahepatic presinusoidal hypertension,
  cause of, 195
Intramuscular injection, 19
Intra-OP pharmacology, 49
Intraosseous tibial plateau, 282
Intraparietal hernia, 167
Intravenous access, 282
Intrinsic kidney damage, 315
Intussusception, 365
 diagnosis, 364
  Meckel, incidental finding, 365
  nonoperative management, failure of, 364
  push/pull, 364
  ultrasound, 364
Ipsilateral amaurosis fugax, 424
Irreversible intestinal ischemia, 254
Ischemia, 273
Ischemic orchitis, 165
Ischemic pain, thoracic outlet syndrome, 395
Islet cell tumors, 209
I-131 therapy, indications for, 138
ITP. *See* Idiopathic thrombocytopenic purpura (ITP)
IVC filter, 19, 347

J

Japanese-style D2 resection, 185
Jefferson fracture, 410
Jejunoileal atresia, 355
Jejunoileal diverticula, 258
Jejunum, 245
Jeunoileal atresia, 357

K

Kasabach-Merritt syndrome, 196
Kasai procedure, 30, 373
    for biliary atresia, 373
    for biliary atresia die, 374
Keratin, 2
Keratinocytes, 96
Kidney
    CO percentage, 310
    failure, 348
    transplant, 28
        indications for, 26
        reason for, 26
Kidney-pancreas transplant, 31
Killian triangle, 230
Kleihauer-Betke (KB), 434
Knee dislocations, 411, 411*f*
Kohn pores, 390
Kussmaul sign, 293

L

Labile factors, 12
Laboratory tests, data and, 13–14
β-Lactams, mechanism of action, 42
Ladd procedure, for malrotation, 356*f*
Laparoscopic hernia, 164, 165
Laplace law, 271
Laryngeal injury, 290
Laryngeal nerve, 103
Laryngeal stenosis, cause of, 107
Larynx, sensory innervation, 104
Latissimus Dorsi, 384
LCIS. *See* Lobular carcinoma in situ (LCIS)
Left renal vein, 429
Left ventricular EDV (LVEDV), 311
Leiomyoma, 236*f*
    treatment for, 236
Lenticular/lens-shaped deformity, 286
Lentigo maligna, 381
LES. *See* Lower esophageal sphincter (LES)
Lethal gynecologic malignancy, 436
Levator ani complex, 430
LFTs. *See* Liver function tests (LFTs)
Lidocaine, 57
    overdose, 57
    toxicity, symptom, 57
    without epinephrine, 57
Lincosamides, mechanism of action, 43
Linezolid, mechanism of action, 43
Lipid propofol, 74
Lipogenesis, 75
Lipopolysaccharide complex, toxic
        portion, 1
Lisfranc injury, 409
Littre hernia, 166
Liver
    cancer, 82, 197
    disease, Child-Turcotte-Pugh score, 30

ligaments of, 189
lobes in, 189
Liver function tests (LFTs), 191, 381
Liver lesion, diagnostic workup, 198*f*
Liver transplantation, 29–30, 374
    vascular complication with, 29
Lobular carcinoma in situ (LCIS), 117
    treatment for, 118
Lobular hyperplasia, 118
Loop diuretics, 65
Lower esophageal sphincter (LES), 48
Lumpectomy, 122
Lung cancer, 401–403
    American Joint Committee on Cancer Staging
        System, 402
    cancer-related death, 401
    staging, regional lymph node stations location, 403*f*
    tumor stage, 401
Lungs
    maturity, 367
    parenchyma, 395
    segmental anatomy of, 390*f*
    transplant, 32
        anastomoses in, 32
        contraindications for, 32
        donor requirements for, 32
        indications for, 32
        postoperative complications, 32
    V/Q ratio, 310
LVEDV. *See* Left ventricular EDV (LVEDV)
Lymphatic malformation, 362
Lymphedema, 349
    incidence of, 115
    progression, 349
Lymphocyte-derived signals, 26
Lymphogranuloma venereum, 40
Lymphoma, surgical treatment of, 257
Lymphotoxin, 24
Lynch syndromes (hereditary nonpolyposis colon
        cancer)
    in colorectal, 273

M

Magnetic resonance cholangiopancreatography
        (MRCP), 192
Male gynecomastia
    causes of, 121
    treatment for, 121
Malignancy, 135
Malignant hepatobiliary disease, in hepatobiliary,
        197–198
Malignant hyperthermia
    treatment for, 56
    triggering agents, 56
Malignant pancreatic endocrine tumor, 210
Mallory-Weiss tear, 180
Mammography, 115
Mandibular injury, 287

Mangled extremity severity score (MESS), 413
  with high-energy, 413
  with pulselessness, 413
MAO. *See* Maximal acid output (MAO)
MAP. *See* Mean arterial pressure (MAP)
Marfan syndrome, 391
Mastitis, treatment for, 124
Mastodynia, treatment for, 125
Mathes muscle, 384
Maxillary fractures, LeFort classification, 290*f*
Maximal acid output (MAO), 177
Mean arterial pressure (MAP), 284, 309
Meckel diverticulitis, 259
Meckel diverticulum, 258, 372, 373
Meconium plug, 358
Median nerve injury, 412
Mediastinum, diseases of, 397–399
Medullary thyroid carcinoma (MTC)
  cytologic features, 135
  thyroidectomy for, 135
Melanocytes, 87
Melanomas, 82, 87
  diagnosis of, 88*f*
  skin lesion, 380
  subtypes, 89
  treatment algorithm, 88*f*
MELD score. *See* Model for end-stage liver disease
      (MELD) score
Membrane phosphoinositols, 5
MEN. *See* Multiple endocrine neoplasia (MEN)
Ménétrier disease, 186
Menopause, age, 436
Mesenteric hernia, treatment for, 160
Mesenteric ischemia
  acute, 344
  chronic, 344
Mesenteric panniculitis, treatment of, 160
Mesocolic (paraduodenal) hernia, location for, 160
MESS. *See* Mangled extremity severity score (MESS)
Metastatic disease, 392
  rib, 392
Metastatic melanoma, 380
Methimazole, mechanism of action, 132
Metronidazole, mechanism of action, 42
MI. *See* Myocardial infarction (MI)
Micelle, 249
Microadenoma *vs.* macroadenoma, 143
Microcytic anemia, 15
Microembolization, 343
Microtubules, 2
Midcarpal level, cross-section of, 386
Middle meningeal artery, 286
Midesophageal diverticula, 229
Midshaft humerus fracture, 412
Migrating motor complex, 250
Milrinone, 317
Minimal alveolar concentration (MAC), 52, 55
Misoprostol, uterine contractions, 434

Mitosis, 8, 82
Mivacurium, 57
MMC. *See* Myoelectric migrating complex (MMC)
Model for end-stage liver disease (MELD)
      score, 29
Mohs surgery, 380, 381
Mondor disease, 124
Monoamine oxidase inhibitors, 57
Monoclonal antibody, 24
Monro-Kellie doctrine, 284
Monteggia fracture, 409
Morbidity/mortality, 72
Morgagni hernia, 166
Morphine, 58
Motilin, 251
Motor examination, 285*t*
MRCP. *See* Magnetic resonance
      cholangiopancreatography (MRCP)
mRNA, ribosomes use, 4
MTC. *See* Medullary thyroid carcinoma (MTC)
Mucinous cystic neop, 208
Mucocutaneous candidiasis, treatment for, 39
Mucosal lacerations, 290
Mucous-secreting tumor, 157
Muffled heart tones, 293
Multinodular goiter, 134
Multiple endocrine neoplasia (MEN)
  manifestation of, 135
  syndromes, 203
Muscle, filament in, 2
Muscularis propria, 176
Myasthenia gravis, 398
Mycobacterium avium, prophylaxis for, 41
Mycobacterium tuberculosis, 262
Myocardial infarction (MI), 59
Myocutaneous flap, 384
Myoelectric migrating complex (MMC), 177, 178
Myosin, 2

N
Nahai muscle, 384
Narcan, atropine, vasopressin, epinephrine,
      lidocaine (NAVEL), 321
Nasal septal hematoma, 107
Nasogastric tube (NGT), 179, 359
Nasopharynx, tumor of, 106
Nasotracheal intubation, 281
NAVEL. *See* Narcan, atropine, vasopressin,
      epinephrine, lidocaine (NAVEL)
NEC. *See* Necrotizing enterocolitis (NEC)
Neck
  anatomy, 103–105
  cross-section, 108
  exploration, 288
  infections, 108
  lymph node compartments, 104*f*
  pediatric, 362
    midline neck mass draining pus, 362

trauma, 107–108
tumors, 105–107
Necrotizing enterocolitis (NEC), 358
Necrotizing pancreatitis, 50
Neoadjuvant therapy, 123
Neonatal intensive care unit, 359
Neonate, gastroschisis, 360
Neonates, respiratory distress, 366
Neovascularization, component in, 6
Nerve, artery, vein, extralymphatic space, lymphatics (NAVEL), 282
Nerve of Latarjet, 174
Neurilemoma, 398. *See* Schwannoma
Neuroblastoma, 85
Neurogenic tumors, 397
Neurologic injury, 282
Neurosurgery, 421
    arteriovenous malformation (AVM), 422
    brain tissue component, 421
    brain tumors, 423
    central cord syndrome, 424
    cerebral angiogram demonstrating, 422*f*
    cerebral blood flow, 421
    cerebrospinal fluid (CSF), 421
    cranium, types, 421
    drainage, 421
    Ehlers-Danlos/Marfan syndromes, 423
    head computed tomography (CT), 424
    hemorrhage, risk of, 423
    intracranial pressure (ICP), 421
    mean arterial pressure (MAP), 422
    Monro-Kelly doctrine, 421
    moyamoya, 423
Neurotensin, 252
NGT. *See* Nasogastric tube (NGT)
Niacin deficiency, 76
Nipride
    arterial/venous dilator, cardiovascular drug, 317
Nissen fundoplication, 233*f*–234*f*
Nitrofurantoin, mechanism of action, 42
Nitroglycerine
    arterial/venous dilator, cardiovascular drug, 317
Nitrous oxide, use, 56
Nodular sclerosing, 400
Nonblanchable erythema, 98
Noncomplicated radiation enteritis, acute treatment of, 261
Noncytotoxic drugs, 159
Nondepolarizing agents, 52
Nonmaleficence, 449
Nose and paranasal sinuses, 106
Nosocomial infection, causing death, 37
Nutcracker esophagus
    diagnosis of, 234*f*
    treatment of, 234*f*
Nutrition, 72–76, 365–374
    adequate fluid intake, 366
    caloric intake, 365

foregut, 366
hypothermia, 366
    higher risk for, 366
immune system, 366
infant, insensible losses, 366

O

Obstruction, 364
    in colorectal, 270–271
Obturator nerve, 431
Odontoid fracture, 287
Ogilvie syndrome, treatment for, 271
OKT3, 24
Omental cyst, 160
Omentum, malignancy of, 160
Omphalocele, 359
Open reduction plus internal fixation (ORIF), 417
Opisthorchis viverrini, 85
OPSI. *See* Overwhelming postsplenectomy sepsis (OPSI)
Optimal nutrition parameters, 95
Oral cavity cancer, 106
    incidence of, 106
    location for, 105
Oral contraceptive pill, 196
ORIF. *See* Open reduction plus internal fixation (ORIF)
Orthopedics, 409–417
    cross-section of mid-calf, 416*f*
    fractures, types of, 409–411
    injuries, mechanism/types of, 411–413
    lower extremity/compartment syndrome, 414–416
    mangled extremity severity score (MESS), 413–414
Osteochondroma, 393
Osteochondromatosis, 393
Osteosarcoma, 393
Ovarian cancer, 82
    risk of, 121
    surgical staging/therapy, 437
Overaggressive nasogastric tube, 65
Overwhelming postsplenectomy sepsis (OPSI), 218, 299
Oxygenated blood, 391
Oxygen delivery, 313
Oxygen-hemoglobin dissociation curve, 312
Oxytocin, uterine contractions, 434

P

Packed red blood cells (PRBC), 15, 16, 180
Paget disease, 124
Paget-Schroetter syndrome, 395
PAI. *See* Proximalization of the arterial inflow (PAI)
Pancreas, 203–213
    anatomy/physiology, 203–210
        benign pancreatic diseases, 204–206
        benign pancreatic tumors, 206–207
        malignant pancreatic tumors, 207–210
    arterial supply to, 203*f*
    blood supply to, 204

Pancreas divisum, 374
Pancreas graft, Bench preparation, 31
Pancreas pharmacology, 49–50
Pancreas transplant, 30–31
Pancreatic abscess, cause of, 206
Pancreatic cancer, 82, 207
  median survival time, 207
  signs of, 207
Pancreatic ducts, 206
  stricture, 205
Pancreatic endocrine tumor, 210
Pancreatic enzyme, 49
Pancreatic fistulas, 206
Pancreatic islet cell tumors, 210
Pancreatic islet transplantation, 31
Pancreatic necrosis, 206
  aspiration of, 206
  diagnosis of, 206
Pancreaticoduodenectomy, 208*f*
Pancreatic proteases, 248
Pancreatitis, acute
  antibiotics, 204
  diagnosis, 204
  etiologies of, 204
Pancreatitis, chronic, 205
  complications, 205
  surgical procedures, 205
Pancuronium, 57
Panel-reactive antibody, 33
Pantaloon hernia, 167
Papillary thyroid cancer, 136
Papillary thyroid carcinoma, 136
  histologic findings for, 136
  treatment for, 136
Pappenheimer bodies, 219
Parafollicular C cells, 131
Paralytic, administration, 56
Paralytic agent, 51
Parapharyngeal abscess, treatment for, 108
Pararectal space, boundaries of, 431
Parasympathetic fibers, 227
Parathyroid adenoma, risk for, 140
Parathyroid carcinoma, 142
Parathyroid gland, 138–142
  arterial blood supply to, 138
  embryology, anatomy, and physiology, 138–140
  hyperparathyroidism, 140–142
  to recurrent laryngeal nerve, 139*f*
Parathyroid hormone, half-life of, 139
Parathyroid tissue, autotransplantation of, 142
Paravesical space, boundaries of, 430
Paresthesia, thoracic outlet syndrome, 395
Parietal cells, 176
Parotid gland, 105
Parotid tumors, treatment for, 103
Partial portosystemic shunt, 197
Patent omphalomesenteric duct, treatment for, 158

PCWP. *See* Pulmonary capillary wedge pressure
  (PCWP)
Pectus carinatum, 392
Pectus excavatum, 367, 391, 392
Pediatric pneumonia, 368
Pediatrics, 355
  bilious vomiting, surgical emergency, 355
  meconium ileus, 355
Pediatric Trauma, 164. *See also* Trauma
Pedicle, 383
PEEP physiologic. *See* Positive end expiratory
  pressure (PEEP) physiologic
Pelvic floor, 267
Pelvis, muscles/vasculature, 429*f*
Penicillin, resistance, 43
Peptic ulcer disease, 48
  cause of, 178
Peptide YY, 252
Percutaneous nephrostomy, 301
Perforates, 385
Pericardial tamponade, 291
Perihilar cholangiocarcinoma, management of, 197
Peripheral nerve, regeneration of, 96
Peritoneal cavity, 266
Peritoneal dialysis catheter survival rate, 346
Peritoneum function, 157
Peritonitis, 269
Peritonsillar abscess, treatment, 108
Petit triangle, 166
Peudomyxoma peritonei, treatment for, 158
Pharmacologic pancreatitis, 50
Pharmacology, 47–54
  central nervous system/anesthesia, 51–52
  endocrine, 50
  gastrointestinal, 48–50
    colon, 49
    esophagus, 48
    intra-OP, 49
    pancreas, 49–50
    small bowel, 49
    stomach, 48–49
  mechanics, 47–48
  vascular, 51
Phenoxybenzamine, 50
Phenylephrine, 317
Phenylethanolamine-*N*-methyltransferase
  (PNMT), 144
Pheochromocytoma, ectopic sites, 149
Phosphate buffer system, 71
Phosphate deficiency, 76
Phrenic nerve, 103
Phyllodes tumors, 120
Physeal injuries, Salter-Harris classification of, 410*f*
Physis, 416
Phytobezoars, treatment for, 182
Pigeon breast, 392
Pituitary adenoma, 143

Pituitary gland, 142–143
  anatomy and physiology, 142–143
  pituitary pathophysiology, 143
  prolactinoma and pituitary lesions, 143
Plasma membrane
  nutrient composition, 1
  phospholipids in, 1
Plasmin, natural inhibitor, 12
Plastic surgery, 379
Platelet
  activation, thrombus function schematic of, 14*f*
  aggregation, 15
  count, 15
  dysfunction, 15
  factor, 96
  function and dysfunction, 14–15
  granule, type of, 96
  life span, 14
  plug, 14
  plug, formation, 15
Pleomorphic adenomas, 107
Pleural effusion, white blood cells (WBCs), 397
Plicae circulares, 246
Pneumatosis intestinalis, common site for, 260
Pneumocystis carinii, 41
Pneumocystis jiroveci (carinii), 26
Pneumocytes, 390
Pneumothoraces, bilateral simultaneous, 396
Pneumothorax, complications of, 396
PNMT. *See* Phenylethanolamine-*N*-methyltransferase
  (PNMT)
Poland syndrome, 392
Polycythemia, 18
Polyomavirus, 27
Polyps and colon cancer, in colorectal, 274–275
Popliteal aneurysms, 343
Portal hypertension (HTN), 181
Portosystemic shunts, categories, 196
Positive end expiratory pressure (PEEP)
    physiologic, 320
Positive predictive equation, 442
Postdural puncture, 58
Posterior sagittal anorectoplasty, 370
Postmenopausal bleeding, differential, 436
Postoperative hypocalcemia, 142
Postpartum hemorrhage, misoprostol, 434
Posttransplant lymphoproliferative disorder (PTLD), 27
Potpourri, 32–33
PPIs. *See* Proton pump inhibitors (PPIs)
PRBC. *See* Packed red blood cells (PRBC)
Prealbumin, half-life, 75
Preecalmpsia, 433
Pregnant patient. *See* Gynecology
  obstetrical conditions and complications, 433–435
  physiologic changes, 429
  physiology, 431–433
  pulmonary function, 432

Preoperative antibiotics, 165
Prevalence, definition, 442
Professionalism
  concepts, 451–452
  definition of, 451
  and ethical standards, 450
Progesterone receptor (PR), 120
Prolactinoma, treatment for, 143
Proline, hydroxylation, 99
Prophylactic antibiotics, 38
Prophylactic mastectomy, 122
Prophylactic platelet transfusions, 15
Propylthiouracil (PTU), mechanism of action, 132
Prostaglandin synthesis, 15
Prostate cancer, 82
  screening, 90
Protein-energy malnutrition, 74
Protein kinase C, 5
Prothrombin complex, 12
Prothrombin gene defect, 14
Proton pump inhibitors (PPIs), 48, 177
Proto-oncogene, 275
Proximal duodenum, 246
Proximalization of the arterial inflow (PAI), 345
Pseudocysts, 205, 206
Pseudohyponatremia, 66
P450 system
  inducers of, 47
  inhibitors of, 47
  role of, 47
PTEN mutations, 91
Pubic tubercle, 156
Pubococcygeal line, 370
Pulmonary artery catheters, 310, 311
  placement, 310
Pulmonary artery (PA) pressure, 309
Pulmonary artery sling, treatment of, 235
Pulmonary capillary wedge pressure (PCWP), 309
  respiratory cycle, 310
Pulmonary fibrosis, 89
Pulmonary physiology, 319
Pulmonary sequestration, 368
Pulse oximetry, 55
Purines, 82
Pyloric exclusion, 297*f*
Pyloric stenosis, 363
  electrolyte findings, 363
  paradoxical aciduria, 363
  pyloric channel, 363
Pyogenic liver abscess
  antibiotic course for, 194
  treatment of, 194
Pyridoxine (B$_6$) deficiency, 76
Pyrimidines, 82

Q
Quinolones, mechanism of action, 42

R
Radiation enteritis, treatment of, 261
Radical neck dissection, 106
Radiographic findings, 348
Radiotherapy, 394
Ranson criteria, 204, 205
Rapid sequence induction, 55
RAS. *See* Renal artery stenosis (RAS)
Rathke pouch, 143
Receptors and signals, 5–6
Reconstructive surgery, 379
    full-thickness and split-thickness grafts, 383*f*
    Z-plasty, 382, 382*f*
Rectobulbar urethral fistula, 370
Rectosigmoid junction, 266
Rectovesicular fascia, 266
Rectovestibular fistula, 370
Rectum, 265
    arterial supply to, 266*f*
Rectus abdominis, 384
Rectus sheath hematoma, 159
Red blood cell/blood products, 15–16, 191
Refeeding syndrome, 75
Renal allograft, 33
Renal artery revascularization, 345
Renal artery stenosis (RAS), 344
Renal failure, causes of, 33
Renal failure, postoperative, 315
Renal transplantation, 26, 27
Respiratory distress syndrome, 366
Retinol-binding protein, half-life, 75
Retrohepatic vena cava injury, 299
Retroperitoneal abscess, treatment for, 161
Retroperitoneal fibrosis, diagnosis of, 161
Retroperitoneal sarcoma
    prognostic factors for, 161
    treatment for, 161
Retroperitoneum, primary malignancy, 161
Retropharyngeal abscess, treatment for, 108
Retrospective cohort studies, 444
Retzius space, 430
Revision using distal inflow (RUDI), 345
Reynolds pentad, 193
Richter hernia, 167
Riedel fibrous struma, treatment for, 133
Right heart failure, acute, 292
Right upper quadrant (RUQ) palpation, 193
Rituximab, 26
RNA polymerase, 4
Rotter nodes, 114
RUDI. *See* Revision using distal inflow (RUDI)
Rule of twos, 259

S
SAAG. *See* Serum-ascites albumin gradient (SAAG)
Salivary glands
    benign tumor of, 107
    malignant tumor of, 107

Salivary tumors, 106
Salter Harris classification, 411
Sarcomas, 91
SBP. *See* Spontaneous bacterial peritonitis (SBP)
Scalene test. *See* Adson test
Scalenus anticus anteriorly, 394
Scaphoid fractures, 409, 410*f*
SCFA. *See* Short-chain fatty acids (SCFA)
Schatzki ring, 235, 236
    diagnosis of, 235
    indications for, 236
    treatment for, 235
Schistosoma haematobium, 85
Schwannoma
    morphologic patterns, 398
    vestibular, 423
Sciatic hernia, symptom of, 166
Sciatic nerve injury, 412, 431
SCIWORA. *See* Spinal cord injury without
        radiologic abnormality (SCIWORA)
SD. *See* Standard deviation (SD)
Secretin, 251
Selective venous catheterization, 146
Sensitivity, definition of, 441
Sensitivity equation, 441
Sentinel lymph node (SLN), 124
Sentinel lymph node biopsy (SNLB), 381
Sentinel node biopsy, 122
Septal hematoma, 287
Serologic tumor markers, 207
Serotonin, overproduction of, 90
Serous cystadenoma, treatment for, 206
Serum-ascites albumin gradient (SAAG), 157
Serum calcium, 69
Serum dehydroepiandrostenedione
        (DHEA-S), 148
SGAP. *See* Superficial inferior epigastric
        artery flap (SGAP)
Shock, categories of, 312
Short bowel syndrome, clinical hallmarks, 261
Short-chain fatty acids (SCFA), 266
Short gut syndrome, 261
Shouldice repair, 167
Sigmoid colon tumor, 275
Sigmoid volvulus
    recurrence rate for, 269
    treatment for, 269
Silver nitrate, adverse side effect, 382
Simple/total mastectomy, 121
Single pulmonary nodule, algorithm,
        401–403
Sinusoidal macrophages, 191
Skin cancer, 87–89
    form of, 87
    UV radiation, 379
Skin flaps, 383, 384
Skin grafts survive, 383
Skin infection, in burn patient, 382

Skin lacerations, 95
Skin pigmentation, 392
Sliding hernia, 163
SLN. *See* Sentinel lymph node (SLN)
Small bowel anastomosis, 96
Small bowel bleeding, cause of, 260
Small bowel carcinoids, 257
Small bowel fistulas, 260
Small bowel obstruction, 253*f*, 254*f*
   causes of, 252
   indications for, 254
   treatment for, 254
Small bowel pharmacology, 49
Small cell lung cancer, 423
Small intestine, 245–264
   anatomy, 245–248
   blood supply and luminal surface of, 246*f*
   embryology, 245
   layers of wall of, 247*f*
   lymphatic drainage of, 246*f*
   mucosa of, 247
   muscularis propria, 247
   physiology, 248–252
   small bowel, diverticular disease, 258–259
   small bowel fistula, 259–260
   small bowel neoplasms, 256–258
   small bowel obstruction/ileus, 252–256
Sodium abnormalities, evaluation of, 68*f*
So far no objections (SFNO) approach, 449
Soft tissue infections, 38
Solitary pulmonary nodules (SPNs), 401*f*
   algorithm for, 401*f*
   recommended management algorithm, 401*f*
Solitary thyroid nodule, management of, 134*f*
Somatostatin, 251
Somatostatinoma, diagnosis of, 209
Specificity equation, 442
Spectinomycin, mechanism of action, 43
Spermatic cord, 162
Spigelian hernias, 166
Spinal column injuries, 286
Spinal cord injury
   Brown-Sequard/hemitransection of, 424
   patterns, 424*f*
Spinal cord injury without radiologic abnormality
   (SCIWORA), 287
Spinal immobilization, 281
Spinal tumor characteristics, 425*t*–426*t*
Spiral fracture, anteroposterior x-ray of, 411*f*
Spleen, 215–223
   anatomy, 215–216
   arterial blood supply to, 215
   function of, 216
   nontraumatic diseases, 217–218
   physiology, 216–217
   postsplenectomy management, 218–219
   splenic artery and splenic vein, 215*f*
   splenic trauma, 219–221

Splenectomy
   expected response, indications for, 220*t*–221*t*
   indications for, 220
Splenic cyst, surgery for, 218
Splenic injury, nonoperative management, 219
Splenic Organ Injury Scaling System, 219*t*
Splenic tumor, 218
Splenic vein thrombosis, 181
SPNs. *See* Solitary pulmonary nodules (SPNs)
Spontaneous bacterial peritonitis (SBP), 39–40, 157
   antibiotic regime for, 40
Sports hernia, 167
Sprain, 416
Squamous cell carcinoma, 89, 379
   exposure, 379
   Mohs surgery, 380
   natural history of, 379
   risk factors, 379
Standard deviation (SD), 443
Statistical tests, types, 441
Sternocleidomastoid muscle, 362
Steroids
   inhibitory effects, 98
   supplementation, 316
Stomach, 173–188
   anatomy, 173–176
   arterial blood supply to, 173, 174*f*
   benign conditions, 178–182
   chief cells in, 176
   D cells in, 176
   endocrine cells in, 176
   G cells in, 176
   origin, 174
   pharmacology, 48–49
   physiology, 176–178
   proximal portion of, 176
   tumors, 182–186
   venous drainage of, 173
Strangulation, 255
Strap muscles, 104
Stress gastritis, 179, 180
Stress hypermetabolism, 72
Stricturoplasty, 256*f*
Stroke volume/EDV, 311
STSG, 383
Submandibular gland, 105
Submucosal hemorrhage, 273
Succinylcholine, 56, 57
Sulfonamides, mechanism of action, 43
Superficial inferior epigastric artery flap
   (SGAP), 384
Superior mesenteric artery (SMA), 204, 246
Supine chest radiograph, 294
Suppurative hidradenitis, 39
Suppurative parotitis, treatment for, 108
Supracondylar humerus fractures, 412
Supraumbilical lymphatic vessels, 158
Surgical airway, 281

Surgical oncology, 81–93
  breast cancer, 86–87
  carcinogenesis, 85–86
  cell cycle, 81–82
  chemotherapeutics, 89–90
  colon cancer, 87
  skin cancer, 87–89
  tumor markers, 82–85
Surgical procedure, for malrotation, 355
Surgical wound infections, 37
Suspensory ligaments, 114
SVR. *See* Systemic vascular resistance (SVR)
SVR index (SVRI), 309
Swallowing process., 227, 228*f*
Synchronous breast cancer, 118
Systemic antifungal therapy, 39
Systemic inflammatory response syndrome (SIRS), 319
Systemic vascular resistance (SVR), 309
Systolic blood pressure, 282

T

TAAs. *See* Thoracic aorta aneurysm (TAAs)
Tachycardia, with hypovolemic shock, 282
Tamoxifen, 86, 123
  blood clots, 123
Taxanes, mechanism of action, 89
TBSA. *See* Total body surface area (TBSA)
T-cell leukemia, 86
Tensile strength, 96
Terminal ileum, 248
Testicular cancer, 85
Tetracyclines, mechanism of action, 43
Thiamine (B_1) deficiency, 76
Thiazide diuretics, 70
Thoracic aorta aneurysm (TAAs), 340
Thoracic aorta injury, 294
Thoracic esophagus, 226
Thoracic EVAR (TEVAR), 340
Thoracic outlet syndrome (TOS), 394–395
  fatigue, weakness, coldness, ischemic pain, paresthesia, 395
  middle-aged women, 394
  neurologic, 394
Thoracic surgery, 389
  American Joint Committee on Cancer Staging System, 402*t*
  anatomy/physiology, 389–391
  chest trauma, 395–396
  chest wall conditions, 391–394
  lung cancer, 401–403
  mediastinum
    diseases of, 397–399
    divisions of, 398*f*
  pleural disease, 396–397
  single pulmonary nodule, algorithm, 401–403
  solitary pulmonary nodules (SPNs)
    recommended management algorithm, 401*f*
  test taking tip, 389

thoracic outlet syndrome (TOS), 394–395
thymoma staging, 399
Thrombin, 12
Thrombolytics, 19, 51
Thrombotic thrombocytopenic purpura (TTP)
  treatment, 217
Thymoma, 398
  staging, 399
Thyrocervical trunk, branches of, 104
Thyroid, 131–132
  arterial supply of, 132
  cancer, 136
  embryology, anatomy, and physiology, 131–132, 131*f*
  enlargement, 134
  venous drainage, 132
Thyroid cancer, papillary, 136
Thyroiditis. *See* Acute suppurative thyroiditis, treatment for
Thyroid nodule, evaluation of, 134
Thyroid storm, treatment for, 133
Thyroid tumors, TNM classification, 137*t*–138*t*
Tibial nerve, 304
Tietze syndrome, costochondritis, 394
Tis lesion, 275
Tissue factor pathway inhibitor, 12
Tissue plasminogen activator, 12
TLC. *See* Total lung capacity (TLC)
Toldt, white lines of, 265
Total body surface area (TBSA), 327
Total lung capacity (TLC), 319
Total parenteral nutrition (TPN), 321
  glucose administration for, 74
Toxic megacolon, operation for, 272
Toxoplasma gondii, 424
Trace element deficiencies
  manifestations, 63
Tracheoesophageal fistula (TEF), 360, 361
  surgical management of, 361
Tracheostomy, 108
Transcription, 4, 82
Transferrin, half-life, 75, 191
Transforming growth factor-β, 24
Transfusion
  hemolysis, treatment, 16
  reaction, symptoms, 16
  use, 16
Transjugular intrahepatic portosystemic shunt (TIPS), 196
Translation, 82
L, D-Transpeptidases, 42
Transplant, 23–36
  graft and patient survival and complication rates, 27–28
  heart transplant, 31
  immunosuppressants, 24–26
  interferons and chemokines, 24
  interleukins, 23–24
  intestinal transplantation, 32

liver disease, Child-Turcotte-Pugh score, 30

liver transplantation, 29–30

lung transplant, 32

pancreas tranplant, 30–31

potpourri, 32–33

rejection after renal transplant, 27

renal transplant, 26–27

Transplantation, contraindication to, 33

TransRectus abdominis myocutaneous flap (TRAM), 384

blood supply, 385

Transverse carpal ligament, 386

Transversus abdominis, 156

Trauma

abdomen, 295–300

chest, 290–294

evaluation of, 281

in head and neck, 107–108

mortality peak, 281

neck, anatomic zones of, 288*f*

neck exploration, clinical indications, 287

orthopedics, 302–304

pediatric, 362

airway, 362

IVF boluses, 362

nutrition, 365–374

physiology, 365–374

shock, 363

suspect child abuse, 363

urologic, 300–302

Trichobezoar, treatment for, 182

Trigeminal nerve, 103

Trisegmentectomy, 189

Trousseau sign, 69

Trypsin, primary action, 248

t tests, 444

Tuberculous peritonitis, treatment for, 157

Tubo-ovarian abscesses, management of, 429

Tubular necrosis, acute, 315

Tumor cells, 7

fuel source for, 86

Tumorigenesis, 87

Tumor lysis syndrome, 71

Tumor necrosis factor-α, β, 24

Tumor, node, metastasis (TNM) stage, 136

gastric cancer, 184*t*

Tumors

in head and neck, 105–107

markers, 82–85

in stomach, 182–186

Type 1 diabetes, 30

Typhoid enteritis, 262

Tyrosine kinase receptor, 5

U

UGI bleeding, 179

Ulcerative colitis

classes of drugs, 272

in colorectal, 271–272

diagnostic characteristics, 271

extraintestinal manifestations, 272

indications for surgery, 272

sine qua non, 271

Ulnar nerve, in hand, 385

Ultrasonography, 193

Umbilical granuloma, 158

Uncomplicated diverticulitis, treatment for, 268

Upper gastrointestinal (UGI) bleeding, 141, 173, 251, 262, 296, 355

cause of, 41

Uremia, 15

Uremic coagulopathy, 15

Urethral catheter, 26

Urethrocystography, 301

Urinary tract injury, 301

Urine osmolarity, 366

Uterine artery, anatomic relationship, 431

Uterus, 431

V

Vaginal arterial supply, 430

Vaginal lymphatics, 431

Vagina, sensory innervation, 431

Vagotomy, 175*f*

Vagus nerve, 175

Valveless venous plexus, 114

Vancomycin, mechanism of action, 42, 43

Vascular

aortic dissection, classification of, 340

cerebrovascular disease, 338–339

infrarenal aorta, 341–343

mesenteric arterial disease, 344

access, 345–346

renal arterial stenosis, 344–345

peripheral arterial occlusive disease, 335–338

peripheral venous disease, 346–347

lymphatics, 348–349

trauma, 347–348

pharmacology, 51

splanchnic, iliac, and peripheral artery aneurysms, 343–344

thoracic aorta, 339–341

Vascular plexus, 107

Vasoactive intestinal peptide, 252

Vasopressin, 317

Vein originates from, 430

Venous insufficiency, 346

Venous oxygen saturation, 309

factors influence, 309

Ventilator

IMV mode, 321

management, 319

Ventricular contraction, 311

Ventricular fibrillation/pulseless ventricular tachycardia, 313

Verner Morrison syndrome, 208. *See* VIPoma

Vesicocutaneous fistula, 159
Vesicoumbilical fascia, 164
Vestibular schwannoma, 423
Viable flap, 384
Video-assisted thoracoscopic surgery (VATS)
    biopsy, 397
Video-esophagram, 231
Vinblastine, 89
Vincristine, 89
VIPoma
    diarrhea of, 209
    localization of, 209
    treatment, 209
Virchow triad, 14
Vitamin A deficiency, 76
Vitamin B$_{12}$, 73, 250
Vitamin D
    deficiency, 76
    formation, 140
Vitamin E deficiency, 76
Vitamin K, 16
    deficiency, 76
    dependent factors, 12
Vitelline duct, 245
Volvulus, in colorectal, 269–270
Von Willebrand disease, 17
    inheritance, 17
    treatment, 17
Von Willebrand factor (vWF), 12
Voriconazole, mechanism of action, 39
vWF. *See* Von Willebrand factor (vWF)

W
Warfarin-induced skin necrosis, 19
Warthin tumor, 107
Waterhouse-Friderichsen syndrome, 143
Water, loss, 64
Weakness, thoracic outlet syndrome, 395
White blood cells (WBCs)
    in pleural effusion, 397
Whitesides' infusion technique, 414
Wilkie syndrome, diagnosis of, 262
Wilm tumor, 374
Wolff-Chaikoff effect, 132
Wound healing, 95–101, 381–382
    cellular, biochemical, and mechanical phases, 97*f*
    phases of, 95
    physiology of, 95
Wound infection, treatment for, 38
Wounds, 37–39

X
Xeloda, 277
Xenograft, 329

Y
Young males, 393

Z
Zenker diverticulum, 230, 230*f*
Zero-order kinetics. *See* Hoffman elimination
Zinc deficiency, 76
Z tests, 444